Adult
CCRN®
Prep

Sixth Edition

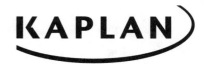

Adult CCRN® Prep

2 Practice Tests + Proven Strategies

Sixth Edition

© 2017 Kaplan, Inc.

Published by Kaplan Publishing, a division of Kaplan, Inc.
750 Third Avenue
New York, NY 10017

10 9 8 7 6 5 4 3 2 1

ISBN-13: 978-1-5062-2346-9

Kaplan Publishing books are available at special quantity discounts to use for sales promotions, employee premiums, or educational purposes. For more information or to purchase books, please call the Simon & Schuster special sales department at 866-506-1949.

Free Additional Practice

kaptest.com/CCRN6thEd

As owner of this guide, you are entitled to get more practice online. Log on to kaptest.com/CCRN6thEd to access an additional Adult CCRN practice test.

Access to this selection of online CCRN practice material is free of charge to purchasers of this book. You'll be asked for a specific password derived from the text in this book, so have your book handy when you log on.

Access to the online center is limited to the original owner of this book and is nontransferable. Kaplan is not responsible for providing access to customers who purchase or borrow used copies of this book.

For Any Test Changes or Late-Breaking Developments

kaptest.com/publishing

The material in this book is up-to-date at the time of publication. However, the AACN may have instituted changes in the test after this book was published. Be sure to read carefully the materials you receive when you register for the test. If there are any important late-breaking developments—or any changes or corrections to the Kaplan test preparation materials in this book—we will post that information online at kaptest.com/publishing.

Contents

PART III: ADULT CCRN SUBJECT REVIEW

PART IV: PRACTICE TEST

PART I

The CCRN: Information and Strategies

Introduction

ABOUT THE CCRN

If you have picked up this book, then you have probably decided that you are ready to take a step toward obtaining your CCRN certification. Congratulations! This is an exciting step, and this book will be instrumental in helping you succeed.

The CCRN certification exam is intended to gauge how well you can apply your medical knowledge, concepts, and principles to care for the complex needs of critically ill patients. By achieving certification, you will demonstrate to both patients and employers that you have the advanced knowledge and skills necessary to care for the acutely and/or critically ill, as well as demonstrate that you are competent in a specialized area of care.

CCRN certification is administered by the American Association of Critical-Care Nurses (AACN) Certification Corporation, although membership in AACN is not a requirement to take the exam. Currently, there are over 62,000 certified CCRNs. The certification was introduced in 1976, and it includes CCRN exams for adult, pediatric, and neonatal patients. Although the exam was introduced over 30 years ago, it is updated to keep pace with the changes in the health care world. It reflects the environment in which nurses care for acutely and critically ill patients—whether in an intensive care unit, trauma unit, or any other clinical arena.

WHAT IS CCRN CERTIFICATION?

The CCRN is a specialty certification, the goal of which is to validate the knowledge of the nurses who provide care to acutely and critically ill patients in areas such as intensive care units, cardiac care units, combined intensive care and cardiac care units, medical/surgical intensive care units, trauma units, and critical care transport and flight. In a sense, the certification provides hospitals, health care agencies, and health care consumers with a standard way of measuring qualifications.

Using CCRN Credentials

Once you pass the CCRN exam, you can—and should—list CCRN after your licensing title. Thus, Mary Jones, RN, would become Mary Jones, RN, CCRN, after passing the CCRN exam. Note that there are no periods in CCRN. You will receive a wallet card signifying that you are CCRN certified. Carry this with you in case you need to validate your credentials at any time.

REGISTERING FOR THE EXAM

To register for the CCRN certification exam, the AACN must deem that you are eligible to take the exam, which it does by reviewing an application. In this section, we'll outline the application and scheduling process for the CCRN exam.

CCRN Exam Eligibility Requirements

In order to be eligible to sit for the CCRN exam, you must meet certain requirements. To start, you must have unencumbered licensure as an RN or APRN in the United States. Not sure if your license is unencumbered? To be considered unencumbered, any RN or APRN licenses you hold cannot have any provisions or conditions that limit your practice in any way, and it cannot have been subjected to formal discipline by any Board of Nursing. If you meet the licensure requirement, you can look at the requirement for practice hours. The AACN states that CCRN candidates must meet one of the following **clinical practice requirement** options:

- **Option 1:** Practice as an RN or APRN for 1,750 hours in direct bedside care of acutely or critically ill patients (in the patient population of the exam for which you are applying: neonatal, pediatric or adult) during the previous two years. Of those hours, 875 must have taken place in the year immediately preceding your application.

- **Option 2:** Practice as an RN or APRN for at least five years with a minimum of 2,000 hours in direct bedside care of acutely and/or critically ill patients (in the patient population of the exam for which you are applying: neonatal, pediatric or adult) during the previous two years. Of those hours, 144 hours must have been accrued in the most recent year preceding application.

On occasion, a question arises for those individuals who work in a management or educator position as to whether this experience would qualify for eligibility. The response is that their experience qualifies them if they are actively involved in caring for patients at the bedside, such as by demonstrating nursing care interventions or supervising new registered nurses. In addition, only hours that take place in a U.S.- or Canada-based (or comparable) facility will count.

The Application Process

While the application process is not overly complicated, there are a few key steps that you will need to take to ensure that you are properly registered for the exam.

First, request an application (available from the AACN Certification Corporation at *aacn. org*) or print out the online version. To access the online CCRN registration, enter the following URL into your web browser:

https://www.aacn.org/certification/preparation-tools-and-handbooks/
exam-scheduling-and-cancellation

You will need to set up an online registration in order to use the website. This process is straightforward and requires basic information, such as your name and address. You will choose a member name and a password to use for when you return to the site. Once you have registered to use the AACN website, you can apply for the exam. Note that the online registration can only be used to apply to take the computer-based CCRN exam. If you know that you need to take the paper-and-pencil exam, you will need to apply the old-fashioned way—using a paper form available from AACN.

You will need to submit your application, along with a one-page honor statement listing your verifier information and RN or APRN license information and your application fee, to the AACN Certification Corporation. AACN accepts applications via fax at (949) 362-2020 or via postal mail at

AACN Certification Corporation
101 Columbia
Aliso Viejo, CA 92656-4109

Peace of Mind

You can buy yourself some peace of mind by sending your application via certified mail or by requesting a return receipt. These options will inform you when your application has been received by the AACN Certification Corporation. You can purchase these mailing upgrades at your local post office for a nominal fee.

AACN takes approximately two to three weeks to process applications. (Online applications are processed more quickly than paper applications.) Once the application has been processed, the AACN will notify Applied Measurement Professionals, Inc. (AMP), the company that administers the exam for AACN, of all the eligible exam candidates. If you are deemed eligible to take the exam, AMP will send you a postcard and an email informing you that your application has been approved. If, for some reason, AACN finds that you are not eligible to take the exam or if it has questions about any part of your application, you will be contacted in writing. You should respond to any requests from AACN quickly and thoroughly.

CCRN Certification Application Honor Statement

The Honor Statement is a form that you fill out, certifying that you have met the minimum requirements for taking the CCRN exam. You do not need to write the statement yourself; you will use the preprinted form from the AACN Certification Corporation, which is available in its text booklet and online. You will fill in your name, AACN number (if applicable), and contact information for a professional associate who can verify that you have actually met all of the eligibility requirements. It doesn't matter whether your verifier is an RN colleague or a clinical supervisor (RN or physician); the person you choose must be able to verify accurately and truthfully that you are eligible to take the exam.

If you are aware that you are not fully eligible for the exam, you should not apply for it. All applications are subject to a random audit of eligibility. If you are selected, you will be notified in writing and have 60 days to respond. Your verification contact will be asked to confirm your eligibility in writing, and you will be asked to submit a copy of your RN or APRN license.

Application Fees

The application fees are the same, whether you take the neonatal, pediatric, or adult CCRN exam. The CCRN computer-based exam fee is $230 for AACN members and $335 for nonmembers. The retest fee and the current CCRN renewal fee are both $170 for members and $275 for nonmembers.

For the paper-and-pencil exam, however, the fees may be higher. The fees depend on the number of people taking the exam simultaneously at one location. If you need to take the paper-and-pencil exam, you should inquire about pricing when applying.

Scheduling Your Exam

Once you have received notification that you are eligible to take the CCRN exam, you need to schedule a time to do so. As with most things, however, it is wise to stay flexible and plan ahead. Before scheduling your exam date, visit the AMP website to see what exam locations are near you. There are over 190 testing centers in the United States where you can take the computer-based exam. To find exam locations and schedule your exam online, type the following URL into your web browser:

www.goamp.com

Make a note of one or two specific locations so that you'll have this information handy when you schedule your test date. Be advised that although you can sometimes schedule your exam almost immediately, in other cases dates may not be available for several weeks. It all depends on the availability of slots at the location you choose, as well as how popular that exam location and time period are with other examinees.

Exams are given by appointment only, which must be made *at least* two days before your chosen testing date. It is important to note that your exam eligibility only lasts for 90 days, so you should schedule your exam immediately after receiving your postcard and email. Both the postcard and the email will clearly note the expiration date of your eligibility period. Since the exam is offered twice a day, five days a week throughout the year, you should not have a problem scheduling your exam within your eligibility period.

That said, if you are unable to schedule your exam during the 90-day eligibility period, you should call AACN to request a new 90-day period. You are allowed to do this only once, and you must pay a $100 change fee for the new eligibility period.

In addition to listing the exam locations, the AMP website has a user-friendly interface for scheduling and even rescheduling your exam. If you prefer to schedule your exam by phone rather than online, call 888-519-9901. Before calling or going online, make sure you have your confirmation postcard handy. You will need your AACN customer number (which will be printed on your postcard) in order to schedule your exam.

If the testing center closest to you is more than a three-hour drive one way, you can apply to take a paper-and-pencil exam. To do so, you need to apply for authorization *at least three months* in advance of the test date by calling 800-899-2226. This is true for people who live outside of the United States as well.

GENERAL CCRN EXAM CONTENT

You will have three hours to complete 150 multiple choice questions, 125 of which will be scored. The remaining 25 unscored questions are used by the AACN to plan for future exams.

CCRN at a Glance

Examination Length: 3 hours
Number of Questions: 150 total (125 scored, 25 unscored)
Question Types: Multiple-choice

Which CCRN Exam Should I Take?

The exam that you take should correlate with your experience. You should take the adult exam if you have experience in direct bedside care of acutely or critically ill adult patients. Do not register for an exam for which you do not have adequate experience.

The CCRN Adult Exam consists of two sections: Clinical Judgment, which is 80 percent of the exam questions, and Professional Caring and Ethical Practice, which is the remaining 20 percent of the exam questions. The questions in the Clinical Judgment section are specific to the adult population. The questions in the Professional Caring and Ethical Practice section, however, can be about patients of any age.

CCRN Adult Exam

The following is a brief overview of the content of the CCRN Adult Exam, along with the percentage of questions that are in each category. These percentages correspond to the 2017 test plan changes.

Clinical Judgment (80% of the exam)

Cardiovascular	18%
Pulmonary	17%
Endocrine/Hematology/ Gastrointestinal/Renal/ Integumentary	20%
Multisystem	14%
Musculoskeletal/Neurology/ Psychosocial	13%

Professional Caring and Ethical Practice (20% of the exam)

Advocacy/Moral Agency
Caring Practices
Collaboration
Systems Thinking
Response to Diversity
Clinical Inquiry
Facilitation of Learning

YOUR CCRN SCORE

At the end of the day, what you really want to know is whether or not you passed the exam. Luckily, if you take the computer-based exam, you will receive your score report immediately upon completion. Those who take the paper-and-pencil exam will have to wait three to four weeks for their results to be sent in the mail.

Duplicate score reports are available for both the computer-based and the paper-and-pencil exams. You may request a duplicate report from AMP within 12 months of sitting for your exam. Your request should be made in writing and should include the following:

- Your name
- AACN customer ID number
  (preceded by the letter *C*, as listed on your initial eligibility confirmation postcard)
- Your address
- Your telephone number
- The date and type of exam that you took
- Check or money order for $25, made payable to AMP

Be sure to sign your request and mail it to

Applied Measurement Professionals, Inc.
18000 W. 105th Street
Olathe, KS 66061

You should receive your duplicate report in approximately two weeks.

Passing Score

If you pass the CCRN exam, you will receive a wallet card and wall certificate stating that you are certified within six to eight weeks. Your certification is good for three years, starting the first day of the month in which you passed the exam. So, if you take the exam in April 2016 and you pass, your certification will last from April 1, 2016, through March 31, 2019.

What to Do If You Fail

The first thing to do if you fail the exam is keep your chin up! Don't be discouraged; you can take the CCRN exam up to four times in a 12-month period. So, if you don't pass on your first try, spend a little more time preparing and then register to take the exam again.

If you do fail the exam, you won't be allowed to appeal your score. You can apply for a retest and receive discounted retest fees.

RENEWING YOUR CCRN CREDENTIAL

Your CCRN certification is good for three years. When the time comes to renew your certification, you have two options to choose from. Briefly, you will be able to choose either

1. *CCRN renewal by Synergy CERPs* (Continuing Education Recognition Point), which involves meeting eligibility requirements for CCRN recertification and completing the Synergy CERP Program; or

2. *CCRN renewal by exam,* which involves meeting the eligibility requirements for CCRN recertification and successfully completing the CCRN certification exam before your scheduled renewal date.

You can also choose these nonrenewal options:

1. *Inactive CCRN status,* which is available to those nurses who do not meet the CCRN recertification eligibility requirements and who wish to keep their CCRN certification status.

2. *Alumnus CCRN status,* which is available to nurses who no longer provide bedside care to critically ill patients.

3. *Retired CCRN status,* which is available to current CCRN nurses who are retiring or retired from nursing.

You should plan to review the renewal criteria from AACN throughout your three-year certification period to keep abreast of any changes to the requirements.

HOW THIS BOOK CAN HELP YOU

This book is designed to make your dream of CCRN certification a reality. In chapter 2, we'll cover the ins and outs of the exam's computer interface so you can enter the testing environment feeling comfortable with computer-based testing. Chapter 3 will provide you with specific exam strategies and advice for test day. Chapters 4 through 13 are content-based; each of these chapters covers a particular category of the exam, from the cardiovascular system to multiorgan, providing you with in-depth content and sample questions to study for the exam.

The CCRN Computer Interface

In recent years, most medical licensure and other professional certification organizations have switched from paper test booklets to computer-based testing (CBT). From the testing organization's viewpoint, CBT offers many advantages. First, it takes place year-round in hundreds of sites throughout the United States and the world. Every test site offers standard testing conditions in terms of the computer equipment used and the rules governing the behavior and monitoring of examinees. There is also increased security as compared with paper tests because completed exams do not need to be physically shipped back to testing agencies for scoring. Instead, examinee data are sent electronically to the testing agency, thus reducing the chance that grid sheets and exam booklets could be lost during shipping. Additionally, examinees often receive their scores immediately, as compared with the six- to eight-week waiting period for paper tests. In the case of the CCRN, as stated in chapter 1, the scores are available immediately after taking the computer-based CCRN exam.

The future holds even more opportunities that make CBT attractive. Paper test booklets must be assembled and printed many months before testing dates; therefore, typographic corrections or other changes are difficult to make or must await a new test-creation cycle. With electronically based testing, test developers have quicker and more numerous options for making changes, such as adding fresh photographic material, replacing poor items, or simply correcting typographic mistakes.

Because most medical licensing organizations now require not only initial certification by examination but also periodic recertification testing to maintain professional certification on a regular basis, there is good reason to become comfortable with these types of tests and with effective ways to review for and deal with multiple-choice questions. After all, if you can't avoid it, you may as well take steps to become good at it!

The CCRN exam is given in a CBT environment, except in special situations when candidates request and are authorized to take a paper-and-pencil version of the exam. The paper-and-pencil version is an option for those candidates who live more than three hours (one way) from a testing center. Unless you meet this criterion, you should be prepared to take the computer-based exam.

This chapter will explain what you can expect from the testing environment and what to look out for on the day of the exam.

THE CCRN TESTING ENVIRONMENT

As we mentioned earlier, the CCRN certification exam is administered by AMP. The exam locations are set up to be conducive to test taking, but there are a few things that are worth noting to make your exam experience as stress-free as possible.

Know Where You're Going

When you register for the exam, you will select an exam location. You will want to keep the address of the exam location and the directions to it handy. If you misplace either piece of information, you can look up the address and find directions on the AMP website at *www. goamp.com.* This information is very important because you need to know exactly where you are going on the day of the exam. Ideally, you should be familiar with the area so you will know how long it will take you to get to the exam location. If you are not familiar with the area, you should attempt to cover the route to the location prior to the day of the exam, whether by car or mass transit, so you will know what to look out for, where to park, what the travel time will be, and the possible alternate routes to get to the testing location (in case there is a traffic emergency, roadblock, or detour). It is critical that you know how long the trip will take you because you do not want to be late reporting to the exam. In fact, if you arrive more than 15 minutes late, you will not be allowed to take the exam.

Arriving at the Exam

At the exam location, you will be asked to *show two forms of identification,* one of which must be a photo ID. The forms that you choose must be current and show your signature, and the name on the identification must be the same as the one that you registered with. So, for example, if you recently were married and changed your name, and then you registered for the exam with your new name, both forms of identification would need to show your new name. If you had not yet gotten around to changing your name on your driver's license, however, you would not be able to show that card as a form of identification. Make sure that you have your IDs in order well in advance of test day.

ID Savvy

You must bring two forms of identification with you to the CCRN exam. One of the IDs has to be a photo ID. The AACN accepts the following as photo IDs:

- Driver's license
- State identification card
- Passport
- Military identification card

For your non-photo ID, you can show a credit card or any other card that has your current name and signature.

Inside the Testing Area

We suggest that you dress in layers on test day so that you can adjust accordingly if the center feels either too warm or too cool for you. Except for the identification needed when you check in, all other personal items should be left in your car or at home. You will be allowed to carry only your identification with you into the examination room.

Food and beverages are not allowed in the testing rooms. You can choose to leave exam location to get a drink, take medication, or use the restroom, but the amount of time allowed for the exam is not stopped when you are away from your computer. Because your computer is still running, inadvertent data entry from your keyboard can also occur, so it is recommended that you try not to take a break unless you absolutely must.

You are not allowed to bring any scratch paper, or any other materials, into the testing room. Instead, you will be provided with scratch paper for making notes. This paper must be turned into the proctor after you complete the exam in order to receive your score report.

Once you are brought to the testing cubicle designated for your use, center staff will start your testing software. In the unlikely event that there is a hardware or software problem during your exam, center staff should be notified immediately so that they can correct the problem and so that you will not lose valuable test response data or testing time.

Although center policies are designed to provide all examinees with a comfortable test area equipped with functioning equipment and a reasonably quiet environment, don't expect a soundproof cubicle. Other examinees are taking exams or may be taking breaks, so you should expect some background noise.

Don't Be Dismissed!

After all of your preparation for the exam, you don't want to run the risk of being dismissed from the exam and having your exam score rendered null and void. According to the AACN, exam candidates can be dismissed from the exam for any of the following:

- Entering the exam without authorized admission
- Taking the exam for someone else
- Recording test questions or making notes
- Bringing notes, unauthorized electronic devices (PDAs, hand-held computers, cell phones, pagers, etc.), or other resources into the exam location
- Creating any sort of disturbance, including being abusive or uncooperative
- Leaving the exam location without notifying the proctor
- Giving or receiving help

Cancellations

Should an emergency or illness prevent you from keeping your exam appointment, you will be allowed to reapply to take the exam in the future. If you reapply for the CCRN exam within one year of your original application, you reactivate your application by simply paying the initial exam fee. However, if you reapply more than one year after your original application, you will need to resubmit a full application and pay the initial exam fee again.

What about cancellations of the exam itself? If inclement weather or an emergency on the day of the exam warrants cancellation of the exam, it will be rescheduled. AMP offers a 24-hour weather hotline available by calling 800-380-5416. If you think that there is a chance the exam may be cancelled, call the hotline to check. It is only in rare circumstances that the exam actually has to be cancelled, but if it happens to you, you will be notified of the rescheduled date or how to reapply for the exam.

THE BASICS OF THE COMPUTER-BASED CCRN EXAM FORMAT

Once you have checked in at the exam location, you will have to log in at the computer terminal assigned to you for the exam. You will be directed to enter your AACN customer identification number, preceded by the letter *C*. This is the number that was printed on your eligibility confirmation postcard. If you failed to bring the postcard with you and you do not remember your AACN number, the exam proctor should be able to give it to you. However, you should plan to bring the postcard with you to the exam location on test day.

After you enter your AACN number, your photograph will be taken by the computer. This photo will stay on-screen during your exam and will be included on your score report. This helps ensure that you are not taking the test for someone else or that someone else is not taking the exam for you.

Test Items

The CCRN exam is comprised of 150 multiple-choice questions. Test items may contain a variety of information sources. Some items include colored photographs, diagrams, or other reference material that may be useful in answering the item. Only one item will be shown at a time. The question number will appear in the lower right-hand corner of the screen. The entire test item, including the question and four answer choices labeled A, B, C, and D, should appear on the screen. To answer a question, use the mouse to click on the answer or use the keyboard to input the letter (A, B, C or D) of your answer. After doing so, you will see your answer in the lower left-hand corner of the screen.

Changing your answer is simple. To do so, click on a different answer or enter a different letter as many times as you want. Before second-guessing yourself (or third- or fourth-guessing!), review our thoughts about it in chapter 3 on page 24.

When you have answered a question, you can move on to the next item by clicking on the forward arrow (>) in the lower right-hand corner of the screen or by clicking on the "NEXT" key. This will move you ahead one item. If you change your mind and need to go back to a previous item, click on the backward arrow (<) in the lower right-hand corner of the screen. As with moving forward, this will move you backward by one item. Repeat either action if you need to move forward or backward by more than one item.

Timed Exam

As you know, the CCRN exam is a timed exam. The computer that you are using will monitor the time and will automatically end the exam if you run out of time. Therefore, you will need to work quickly and efficiently.

If you have not taken a computer-based exam before or you are not comfortable with computers, you may be worried that your lack of familiarity with the computer-based testing process will put you at a disadvantage. Don't worry. At the start of the exam, you will be given a practice test so you can gain comfort with the computer-based testing process before you start the actual exam. Further, by practicing at home prior to arriving at the exam, you can increase your familiarity with the computer-based testing format and help decrease your anxiety even more. The time that you spend on the practice test does not count as part of the timed exam. So, relax and practice using the computer interface until you feel comfortable with it. All of the instructions that you need for the exam will be available on-screen once you finish the practice test and begin the actual exam.

At any point during the exam, you can display a digital clock showing the time remaining by clicking the "TIME" button in the lower right-hand corner of the screen or selecting the "TIME" key. This will allow you to watch your pace so you can keep on track. If you decide that you no longer want to have the clock displayed, you can turn it off by clicking the "TIME" button or key again at any time.

DURING THE EXAM

After making sure you have adequate experience, studying hard for months, and gearing yourself up to take the CCRN certification exam, the last thing you want to do is jeopardize your score by making a silly error at the testing site. Here is a quick look at some of the things you are allowed and, perhaps more important, not allowed to do during the exam:

During the exam you CAN . . .	During the exam you CANNOT . . .
Dress in layers. Dressing in layers is a good idea so you can make adjustments if the room is hot or cold.	**Take purses, briefcases, or jackets into the testing room.** You are not allowed to bring any personal items into the test area. Leave all such items either at home or in your car.
Use a calculator. This comes with some stipulations. Your calculator must be nonprogrammable, silent, hand-held, and either solar or battery operated, and it must not have printing capabilities or an alphabetic keypad.	**Take books, papers, or any reference books or materials into the testing room.** The CCRN is definitely not an "open book" test. Leave all study aids and other books and materials at home.
Comment on any item on the exam. Click on the exclamation point to the left of the TIME button to open a dialogue box to leave your comments.	**Ask questions about content.** You may not ask the proctor any questions about the exam content during the exam.
Make notes. The proctor will give you scratch paper to use for notes during the exam. This is the only paper that you may use, and it must be returned to the proctor at the end of the exam in order to receive your score.	**Take notes or other material home with you.** You cannot take any material related to the exam, including the scratch paper provided to you for making notes, out of the testing site.

During the exam you CAN . . .	During the exam you CANNOT . . .
Take a break. If you need to take a break, you must request authorization to do so. However, it is important that you understand that breaks count toward your total exam time. If you take a break, you will not be allowed any extra time on the exam.	**Leave the exam location without permission.** If you take a break or leave the testing site for any reason without authorization, your score will automatically be rendered null and void.
End the exam early. If you are a quick test taker and you finish before the allotted time, you may opt to end the exam early. To do so, click on the COVER button on the computer screen.	

AFTER THE EXAM

When you have completed the exam, you will undoubtedly be anxious to receive your score report. You will need to be patient and take one additional step before seeing your score; you will need to complete an evaluation of your testing experience. The evaluation is brief and should not take you too much time.

When you are done with the evaluation, the proctor will give you your official score report, showing the percent of correct answers for each major category.

FINAL THOUGHTS

Now that you know what to expect from the exam location, the computer-based testing environment, and the CCRN certification exam itself—we're ready to review some exam strategies. In chapter 3, we'll show you some tips and techniques to ensure that you pass the CCRN.

CCRN Exam Strategies

3

To get to where you are in your career, you have prepared for and passed many examinations over the years. You probably have an established method for test preparation that has worked well in the past, so you may feel little need to create a specific plan for the CCRN. However, it is important to realize that while you may be able to rely on your previous test-taking skills, you should adapt them to the CCRN.

SPECIFIC STRATEGIES FOR THE CCRN

The CCRN assesses your knowledge of the skills and abilities necessary to practice in acute and critical care settings. The questions will require more from you than simple recall. The questions are designed to elicit *critical thinking* and to assess your ability to apply knowledge in a wide variety of contexts and patient-care situations.

To be able to walk into the exam location on test day with confidence that you will do well, you need a plan. This chapter will help you to develop a study plan and manage where you most need to invest your review time so that your efforts result in a score that truly reflects the knowledge, skills, and abilities that you have worked so hard to acquire.

Develop a Study Plan

An effective study plan involves the following key factors:

- Determining how much time you need for each area
- Establishing a good study process
- Maximizing recall
- Monitoring your performance
- Determining when you are ready to take the exam

Familiarize Yourself with Exam Content and Weight Your Review

A key strategy for the CCRN certification exam is to become familiar with the exam content. In this book, each system is covered in a chapter, allowing you to progress from the cardiovascular system to pulmonary to endocrine and so on. Studying everything equally wastes limited review time by investing the same amount in every subject. As we showed in chapter 1, not every subject appears on the exam in equal proportion. You should weight your review time more heavily toward the subject areas that are emphasized on the exam and toward areas in which you are weaker. By thinking carefully about what needs more time and what needs less, you will derive the maximum benefit from your review.

In the past, nurses were required to have accomplished a specific set of technical skills before they were allowed to take the CCRN exam. This is no longer the case. However, having experience with certain skills and technologies will most likely improve your score on the exam. The AACN has a list of experiences that it suggests that CCRN certification exam candidates have. The lists for adult, pediatric, and neonatal are available on the AACN website at *www.certcorp.org*. Navigate to the CCRN Eligibility Requirements to review the list of suggested experiences. If you do not have experience in these areas, it may be to your benefit to seek them out prior to taking the exam.

Establish an Effective Study Process

One of the most common myths about studying and test performance is the belief that merely going through the material results in being able to apply the learned material successfully to test items. If this were true, then doing well would require only that you reviewed good notes or a good review book. This myth assumes that reviewing equals the ability to apply, which is not the case.

Nearly everyone has had some experience with individuals who seem to be able to do well on examinations even when they study less than many others. Are they simply geniuses, or do they possess photographic memories? Usually neither. Most of these individuals have discovered that the key to doing well on exams lies in the study process itself.

A good study process involves using your time strategically, systematically working to address your weak areas, and understanding major concepts and key definitions. The other component of a good study process is using practice questions (like those included in this book) to test how well you can apply what you are studying. In this way, you will not be simply studying in isolation from the application. You will engage the material, which will help you learn and remember it so that you can be one of those test takers who achieves a top score on the CCRN exam!

Actively Engage with the Material

So, you understand that you need to engage with the material that you are studying. But what does that mean? This means you *should not* simply run your eyes along the words you are reading and, in effect, merely follow what is being said. Simply reading your review material will do you little good. You have to *do* something with what you are reading. Here are some methods:

- Transform the material by extracting key aspects into a briefer, personally meaningful version.

- Use arrows and boxes to diagram a process.

- Stop after reviewing a topic and summarize out loud.

- Answer practice questions that relate to what you just read and clarify any misunderstandings or forgotten elements by searching your notes or the review book.

- Make quiz cards with a topic or item on one side and key features on the other. Looking at the item side of the card, try to recite the features.

- If you are currently working in a clinical setting caring for critically ill patients, use the material to approach your patient care (e.g., if you are caring for a patient in septic shock or severe sepsis, review the orders, labs, and plan of care either proactively to ensure they address a multisystem approach or retrospectively based on the patient outcome for appropriateness of care).

Any other study methods that call for you to make judgments about the material, express it in your own words, show linkages between things, or mimic the demands of actual test items are all effective techniques to use. You may find that one method works better for you than others. Or you may find that you need variety so you'll try all the methods listed. Do whatever makes you comfortable.

Beware of Passivity

Passive study methods are deceptive because you tend to assume that you know the material well when, in reality, you only followed along and recognized the material as familiar. If what you do when you study results in frequent nodding off or mind wandering, then you need to change your methods. Perk it up so you can ensure you are really learning, and retaining, the material. Oftentimes this has to do with what time of day you study. Some people are more effective if they study in the evening or night, and others are more effective if they study in the morning or afternoon. You need to decide this for yourself if you have not already figured it out.

Methods of Remembering

Everyone must deal with forgetting. Because there is so much information to review, whatever you study first is going to fade away to some degree by the time you finish studying everything else. To combat this problem, you must create a *greatly condensed* summary of notes that you can use later on to refresh your memory during the final days before the exam. Tackling practice questions on a regular basis that cover all previously reviewed material is another method of keeping material fresh in your memory. If you don't address the problem of forgetting information, your performance will reflect how recently you studied each area, with earlier topics yielding a lower performance than the topics you studied closer to the day of the exam.

Know When You're Ready

The final aspect of a solid study plan is determining if you are ready for the exam. The most reliable way to do this is to take a full-length practice test like the one at the end of this book. How well you do on the practice test will be a pretty good indicator of how well you might score on the actual examination.

Don't wait until a day or two before the exam to take your practice test. You will want to make sure that you have enough time to analyze your errors and clarify any misunderstandings or forgotten elements.

Answer All the Questions

Your CCRN exam score is based on the number of questions answered correctly. Therefore, you will want to answer all of the questions on the exam, but that doesn't mean you have to answer a question the first time you see it. You can leave items unanswered as you progress through the exam and return to them later. This approach will allow you to skip difficult questions and move on to the questions to which you know the answers. Then, if you have time at the end of the exam, you can return to the difficult questions that you left unanswered.

By clicking on the blank square to the right of the TIME button, you can bookmark an item so you'll know to return to it at the end of the exam. If you do have time to review your unanswered items, click on the hand icon or select the NEXT key. Doing so will show you your first unanswered item. Continue to click on the NEXT key or the hand icon to progress through all of your unanswered items. You will need to practice this before you get to the test so you are familiar with the software!

At the end of the exam, you will receive a report of the number of items that you have answered. If there is still time remaining, you can go back and answer any unanswered questions. Even if you do not know the answer to a question, if you have time to answer it, you should. Remember, your score is based on the number of *correct* answers you select. There is *no penalty for guessing*, so take a chance and answer every question that you can. You never know—you may even guess correctly!

GENERAL TEST-TAKING STRATEGIES

Test-taking is a performing art. To perform well, you must practice the skills, get feedback, and try again until the whole thing becomes internalized and finely tuned and every aspect of the piece has been rehearsed in advance. The following general test-taking strategies are designed to help you do just that!

Identify and Correct Your Error Patterns

As you progress with your practice questions and studying, you should routinely analyze your errors and look for patterns among the items that you missed. Some possible error patterns might include the following.

Test Anxiety

If many of your errors occurred on items early in the exam, this may be an indicator of test anxiety, which is often most strongly felt during the early stages of taking an exam. Alternatively, it may simply reflect the fact that difficult content happened to be asked early in the test. However, most often the answer is test anxiety.

Pace Yourself and Avoid Mental Fatigue

If many of your errors occurred on the final pages of the exam, and you answered the items in numerical order instead of jumping around, then mental fatigue may be a problem for you. Are you getting enough sleep at night? Are you finding that you run short of time near the end of the exam, causing you to rush through answering the final items? Did you feel that the most difficult material was covered mainly in the final portion of the exam? Try finding a better pace to ensure that you have enough time to answer all of the questions without having to rush. If fatigue is an issue for you, practice more to raise your testing endurance, or plan to get more sleep in the weeks leading up to the exam.

Misreading

Reading mistakes are more common during exams than most people think. After all, people feel nervous, rushed, or simply tired toward the end and may easily misread a word or key phrase—or even answer the question they *expected* to be asked rather than the one *actually* asked. How can you tell if an error was made because of a reading mistake? Read the item and note the correct answer, as well as the answer you selected. If your choice makes no sense, given what was asked, then it is highly likely that you misread the question at the time.

Beware of misreading. Only a few letters in a prefix or suffix can change the entire meaning of a question (e.g., *hyper* versus *hypo*). Negatively phrased items (e.g., "What is the least likely diagnosis?") can trip people up, too. Read the questions carefully to avoid this common mistake.

Frustration

Were there any items on the exam that at the time made you upset or frustrated? Test takers often describe such questions as picky, tricky, or unfair. The reason you should identify these anger-triggering items is that test takers frequently make silly mistakes on items following the ones that made them upset. So the test takers pay the price for the tricky, unfair, or frustrating item because their strong emotions interfered with their concentration on subsequent items.

Second-Guessing Yourself

Most test takers second-guess themselves at some point. Unfortunately, most second-guessing does not lead to more correct answers. Instead, when people change answers, they often change a wrong answer to another wrong answer and sometimes a correct answer to a wrong answer. Here is a way for you to identify what happens when you second-guess yourself.

When you take a practice test, make a mark (such as a triangle in the margin) so that you will be able to spot all items where you changed your initial answer. Now tally the three possibilities:

- Wrong to wrong
- Wrong to right
- Right to wrong

Don't be surprised if you discover that most changed answers end as the first option. These reflect knowledge gaps, not a problem with whether you do or do not change answers. Next, if the sum of those that fit the second possibility is greater than those that fit the third possibility, then you are using good judgment and don't have a problem with answer changing. If the sum of those that fit the third possibility is greater than those that fit the second possibility, however, then you have an answer-changing problem. The solution? Simple: Adopt a rule, based on the data you've collected and analyzed, that you will change answers more critically.

Knowledge Gaps

Are many of the errors you make referring to a common topic or similar kind of material? For example, you might notice that test after test, you tend to answer questions on the renal system incorrectly. This pattern clearly signals its own solution—you must spend more time studying the renal system if you want to improve. Adjust your study strategy accordingly and put more time into practicing the problematic areas identified in your error analysis.

Other Obstacles

The potential patterns identified in error analyses can't all be described here. Not every test error will fall into a pattern. But the process of scanning your performance for patterns is extremely worthwhile if you have adopted active, sound study strategies and you try to anticipate what might be asked, yet your test performance is still not improving.

Master the Multiple-Choice Format

The CCRN certification exam consists solely of multiple-choice questions, so you will want to get experience with that format in your study plan. Let's look at the approach to questions used by many test takers and focus on why it works.

The Basic Steps

1. Read the question stem carefully to locate important clues.

2. Make sure you fully understand what is being asked.

3. Before looking at any answer choices, put the clues together with what you are being asked and allow your mind to form some kind of answer.

4. Look at the choices offered, and if one of them fits your anticipated answer, mark it.

5. If no choice is a good fit, use general knowledge, larger concepts, and logic to eliminate as many choices as you can.

6. Select an answer from the remaining choices.

Interestingly, not all of these steps will necessarily be used in every question. However, in most standardized exams, many questions will ask you to assess specifics that you won't be able to recall. It is in dealing with these that good test takers have a real advantage over those who aren't as adept. So, just what methods are used to get more correct answers?

The Methods

Unconfident test takers are prone to an "either/or" mindset when they encounter questions. If, after reading the question, they aren't sure of an answer based on what they recall, they quickly give up and guess. Good test takers don't admit defeat that quickly. Instead, they use information presented in the question itself or more of their general knowledge to chip away at the question. By persevering and exploiting whatever they can to eliminate choices, they more frequently end up with correct answers. Here are some methods for you to follow to get more correct answers on the CCRN exam:

- *Recognize a question in disguise.*
  It is crucial that you fully understand what is being asked in every question. Take your time to read and re-read the questions, if you need to. Ask yourself, "What is really being asked?" Once you are confident that you know what the question is, then you can move on to find the answer.

- *Eliminate distracters.*
  Distracters are designed to do just what their name implies—to distract you from the correct answer. For most questions, you can eliminate at least one or two of the distracters by applying your basic knowledge of the subject area.

- *Visualize the correct situation.*

  As you read through a question, visualize the information that is being presented. Imagine what a patient looks like in the situation being described; visualize any injuries or symptoms. Then, follow up by visualizing the proper response to the question that is being asked. If you can see the situation in your mind, you will often be able to see the answer, too.

- *Be wary of suspicion.*

  People who have struggled on multiple-choice exams often carry around strong negative emotions about having to take these kinds of tests. Sometimes they feel that the items are designed to trick them into choosing wrong answers. In fact, it is often those feelings that cause them to choose the wrong answer. A suspicious test taker will read a clue in the question stem and immediately reason that it was put there to lure them into making a mistake. So, instead of using the clue to select the right answer, the suspicious test taker will choose another answer, the wrong one.

- *Don't let sharp turns confuse you.*

  While we don't want you to be too suspicious, we do want you to look out for what is often referred to as a "bait-and-switch" question. In such questions, the focus in the point of view changes, usually sharply and sometimes slyly. These types of changes require you to read the question very closely to ensure that you really do understand what is being asked. In these types of questions, one or more of the answers will relate to the focus *prior* to the sharp turn. If you don't notice that a change has occurred, you may choose the wrong answer. So, read carefully and follow all the twists and turns of the question.

ADVICE FOR TEST DAY

As the CCRN exam day approaches, many test takers become increasingly anxious. This is a natural reaction, but it is wise to recognize the symptoms of pre-exam anxiety and to take steps to manage it. You don't want your nervous feelings to lead to counterproductive behaviors that can decrease your exam performance.

Mental Turmoil

One of the most common symptoms of test anxiety is a tendency to lose focus and concentration. Rather than thinking about the material they are studying, people find their minds racing with thoughts about the material they still haven't mastered, questioning whether they should stop studying this topic and review another topic instead, or worrying about what they will do if they fail the examination. Their regimen of studying, taking breaks, and practice testing also tends to become harder to adhere to, so many people abandon their study plans and begin to flit from one thing to another. Others may decide to do only practice questions from dawn to dusk, believing that the more items they see in the final days, the more likely it is that they will encounter similar items on the actual exam. Still others engage in polling their colleagues, feeling that whatever their friends are doing in these final days must be the right thing for them to do as well. All of these behaviors are symptomatic of test anxiety and often result in feeling less and less in control at the worst of times. *Remember that your goal is to adhere firmly to your study plan and to allow the structure it provides to help you rein in the pre-exam jitters.*

Nutrition

Eating habits affect everyone's ability to deal with life's challenges, whether they involve sports, taking a test, avoiding fatigue and moodiness, or becoming more vulnerable to illness. Diabetics must monitor their food intake closely to prevent dangerous fluctuations in their blood glucose levels, but all of us are affected by the ups and downs of our blood sugar levels and excessive intake of junk foods. Caffeine, alcohol, too much sugar, and not enough variety in your diet can all disrupt your metabolism and leave you feeling short on energy or, in some cases, overstimulated.

Taking a long exam like the CCRN burns many calories, so it's a good idea to think ahead about fueling up properly before the exam. Since you will not be allowed to bring any food or drinks into the testing site, make sure that you eat enough before you arrive. Avoid heavy foods or eating a large meal before the exam, both of which can leave you suffering from postprandial droop, resulting in grogginess or abdominal discomfort. Finally, be sure to drink enough fluids; dehydration is another potential cause of fatigue, headache, and general listlessness.

Insomnia

People's personalities vary greatly, with some reacting to increased stress by seeking out favorite activities that help them mentally regroup and feel physically tired, allowing them to fall asleep and regain their equanimity. Other people turn to drugs or alcohol, self-medicating to bring on sleep. Nearly everyone occasionally finds sleep elusive when they are worried about something they must deal with soon, such as a certification exam. Although most adults can function on six hours of sleep, some individuals require eight or nine to feel fully rested and alert. Tune into your own sleep requirements and make sure that in the weeks and days leading up to the CCRN exam, you are allowing yourself ample rest.

Prescribed medications can alter sleep requirements, making it difficult to fall asleep or to wake without grogginess. Perhaps the best advice that can be given to test takers who fear they will not be able to fall or stay asleep the night before the exam is to avoid foods or beverages containing caffeine later than mid-afternoon the day before the exam.

The day before the exam, take some extra steps to ensure that you wake well rested. First, avoid strenuous exercise too close to bedtime. While exercise may help tire you out, therefore helping you sleep, if it is done too close to retiring, vigorous exercise can actually overstimulate you, making it even harder for you to fall asleep. The most important thing to avoid doing late on the day before your exam is studying. Whatever material you madly race through that evening is not going to settle into your long-term memory. Instead, bits and pieces of it will still be spinning around in your working memory the following morning, and this can directly interfere with recall of the far larger body of information that you spent the last few months and weeks working with. In addition, cramming the night before the exam may overstimulate your mind so that you have trouble relaxing and falling asleep.

Your best bet for a good night's sleep the night before the CCRN exam? Have a relaxing evening that doesn't veer too far from your normal routine but that doesn't include any last-minute cramming.

Five Tips for Concentration, Pacing, and Test Anxiety

Tip One: Reflect on Your Strengths

Several weeks before the exam, use an index card to list several of your greatest personal strengths and attributes, such as "I'm an intelligent person who reacts well under pressure," or "I am an excellent nurse, and I have the experience and knowledge required for CCRN certification." Keep this card handy so that whenever negative thoughts intrude while you are studying, you can pull the card out, read each statement, and reflect on their truth. Luxuriate in the calm, positive feelings you associate with each of the statements. Fairly soon, you won't even need the card because you will know all the statements by heart and will be able to review them mentally as an antidote to negative thoughts and self-doubt.

Tip Two: Become Aware of Mind-Wandering

Keep a master tally sheet nearby each time you sit down to study. Make a check or a hash mark each time you find yourself engaging in negative thinking, daydreaming, or otherwise mentally escaping from the study situation. For many people, the very act of counting the frequency of mind-wandering actually reduces the frequency of those behaviors. This is a mild form of behavior modification that you can apply to your own study behavior. Although simple, it works well for many people.

Tip Three: Relive Your "Hero" Moments

As you prepare for the exam, spend some quiet time thinking back over your life experiences to find one event in which you were the "hero" of the situation. Perhaps you walked in on a serious fight between two friends and were able to bring about a peaceful resolution. Perhaps you'll recall the first time you successfully intubated a patient with respiratory failure or the time you successfully led a fund-raiser for your favorite charity. Whatever life event you select, it must be a situation in which your abilities and actions solved a problem or redeemed a bad situation.

Spend 10 minutes each day in a quiet place reliving this event, trying to bring back the memory in as much detail as possible. What time of year or day was it? What were you wearing? What was the setting like? As you practice this, it will take less and less time for you to retrieve the memory in graphic detail. The purpose of this exercise is to allow you to mentally revisit the event quickly because stored with this remembered event are all of the associated psychological feelings of being in control, being a successful problem solver, feeling confident, and in general, winning over adversity. When you retrieve this memory as part of a time-out taken during the exam when anxious feelings arise, positive emotions serve to counteract the negative emotions associated with the test-taking process.

Tip Four: Go at Your Optimal Pace

To find your optimal pace, be sure to work through several practice tests during your preparation. This book is filled with sample questions; use them not only to test yourself but also to learn how long it takes you to answer the questions as well. With practice, you will sense the right pace and will be able to walk into the exam location on test day confident that you can handle it because you have already done so in practice mode.

During the actual exam, use the same pacing plan that you used in practice over the final week or two of studying. Worrying about running out of time contributes to anxiety and often leads to time-wasting behaviors, such as checking the clock every few minutes. This nervous habit continually interrupts your thought process and often results in the need to re-read once you return to the question.

Tip Five: Take Time Out

If you feel anxiety during the exam that is interfering with your ability to concentrate on the questions, take a brief mental time out. Shut your eyes, lean back, and slowly rotate your neck and roll your shoulders to relax them. Take several slow, cleansing, deep breaths and exhale each breath slowly. Recall your "hero" moment if you think it will help reinvigorate you. This time out helps break the cycle of anxiety and will usually help you return to the task at hand with a greater sense of calm and improved concentration.

Signs of Anxiety That May Require Professional Help

For some anxiety symptoms, such as muscle twitching, chronic insomnia, nausea, hyperventilation episodes, or chest tightness, self-help tactics may not be enough. If you experience several of these symptoms and they are severe, seek professional help from a psychiatrist or a cognitive psychologist who is experienced in helping people overcome situational anxiety.

Therapies may include anti-anxiety medications, self-hypnosis instruction, behavioral retraining, or a variety of other interventions. But don't delay making an appointment—each of these treatment modalities requires time before it becomes effective. In seeking a professional, don't see just anyone. The professional you choose should have experience in treating this type of problem.

Managing Time during the Examination

Don't skip around frantically searching for easier items to answer. Doing this can result in missing items and will leave you feeling out of control in the test situation—something you definitely want to avoid. Also, because you won't easily be able to estimate how many items you have left to answer at any given point, skipping around makes following any pacing plan very difficult.

Decision Rules

Use decision rules to make the most of your testing time. Everyone needs at least two deciding rules. *Rule One* is used when you have thought about the question and are able to narrow the possible answers to two options. At this point, self-honesty is paramount. If you have already used recall and any strategies appropriate to such a question, it's time to choose and move on. Rule One gives you a way to decide, preventing you from reading and re-reading the item, hoping that something else will occur to you that will help you decide between the final two choices. To apply Rule One, mark the *upper* of the final two choices and move on to the next question. Then, the very next time that you are faced with the same final two choices dilemma, you should mark the *lower* of the final two choices. This is actually a time-management rule, designed to prevent you from endlessly obsessing between the final two choices.

Rule Two pertains to questions about material that you've never come across before. Fortunately, you are unlikely to encounter very many of these "clueless" items (especially since you are using this book!). Most test takers report that on standardized examinations, they encounter only a handful of items that they truly have no idea how to answer. If you encounter a question dealing with totally unknown content, then have a favorite among A through D in mind, mark the answer that corresponds to your favored letter, and move on. There is little to be gained from reading and re-reading the question multiple times in hopes that lightning will strike your synapses and make the correct answer apparent. Cut your losses (time loss in this case), so that you can address subsequent items that you have a far stronger chance of answering correctly without rushing through them.

FINAL THOUGHTS

In this chapter, we covered the importance of developing a solid study plan and following a good study process as well. We outlined several test-taking skills that you can employ to enhance your chances of acing the CCRN certification exam. We also looked at how to improve your concentration, find your optimal pacing, and reduce your anxiety on test day. All of these issues are important for you to consider as you prepare for the CCRN exam. Now that you are aware of them and understand what and how you need to study, we'll move on to the exam content, starting with the cardiovascular system.

Remember: Engage with the material and answer the practice questions, and you will do well. Good luck!

PART II

Diagnostic Test

Adult CCRN Diagnostic Test

4

Before beginning your review, take this 25-question diagnostic test to assess your current strengths and weaknesses in the Adult CCRN content areas. Choose a quiet area free of distractions and silence all your devices. The results will show what your weakest areas are—and where to focus the most time and effort in your exam preparation.

Directions: Each question or incomplete statement below is followed by 4 suggested answers or completions. In each case, **highlight** the statement that best answers the question or completes the statement. Allot 30 minutes to take the diagnostic test.

1. A patient's ECG heart rhythm is shown below after an initial shock of 120 joules was delivered. What should the nurse do next?

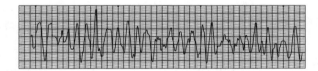

A. Get the patient intubated ASAP by the anesthesiologist.

B. Check the blood pressure and heart sounds.

C. Prepare to transfer the patient to the intensive care unit.

D. Perform cardiac compressions for 2 minutes.

2. What is the **most** definitive treatment for the ECG rhythm shown below in a patient without a pulse?

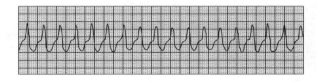

A. cardiac compression

B. cardioversion

C. intubation

D. defibrillation

3. The nurse noted the ECG rhythm strip shown below in a patient. Which of these medications should the nurse withhold (not give) for this patient?

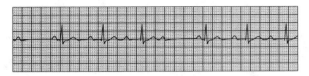

A. lisinopril

B. metoprolol

C. ondansetron

D. methylprednisolone

4. What is the correct interpretation of the ECG rhythm strip shown below?

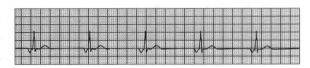

A. accelerated junctional

B. junctional tachycardia

C. junctional escape rhythm

D. junctional rhythm

5. Based on the ECG rhythm strip shown below, which health education topic is **most** appropriate for the nurse to provide to the patient?

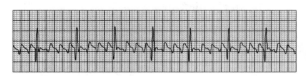

A. stroke

B. sudden cardiac death

C. cardiomyopathy

D. hypertension

6. Which of these laboratory results in a patient diagnosed with disseminated intravascular coagulation (DIC) will require immediate attention?

A. International Normalized Ratio (INR) of 2.0

B. platelets of 8,000

C. activated partial thromboplastin time (aPTT) of 60 seconds

D. fibrinogen 300 mg/dL

7. The nurse teaches a patient recovering from diabetic ketoacidosis (DKA). Which information should the nurse tell the patient about preventing recurrence of DKA?

A. The patient can have better health outcomes by adopting a vegetarian diet and exercising twice daily.

B. The patient should check glucose levels every 2 hours while at home.

C. Effective communication between the patient and provider is important during intercurrent illness.

D. A salt-free diet is vital during periods of nausea.

8. While recovering from an episode of diabetic ketoacidosis (DKA), the patient calls the nurse and reports feeling anxious, nervous, and sweaty. Which action should the nurse do **first**?

A. Obtain a glucose reading using a fingerstick.

B. Administer 1 mg of glucagon subcutaneously.

C. Let the patient eat a candy bar immediately.

D. Ask the patient to drink 8 ounces of orange juice.

9. The nurse cares for a patient with rhabdomyolysis who has a serum potassium of 7.0 mEq/L. Which medication would the nurse anticipate administering?

    A. calcium gluconate

    B. magnesium sulfate

    C. sodium chloride

    D. NPH insulin

10. The nurse reviews the laboratory values of a patient diagnosed with rhabdomyolysis. Which of these lab values would the nurse be **most** concerned about?

    A. BUN of 50 mg/dL

    B. creatinine of 2.0 mg/dL

    C. potassium of 6.9 mEq/L

    D. calcium of 7.5 mg/dL

11. The nurse cares for a patient diagnosed with rhabdomyolysis who just received a 1 liter bolus of normal saline. The central venous pressure (CVP) after the bolus was 7 mm Hg, and then subsequently dropped to 1 mm Hg after 1 hour. What is the correct interpretation of this finding?

    A. It is a sign of improvement in hydration status.

    B. The patient is progressing into severe sepsis.

    C. It is time to do a bladder scan to monitor output.

    D. The patient requires more intravenous (IV) fluid.

12. A patient on mechanical ventilation has the following ventilator settings: assist control (AC) of 20, FiO_2 of 40 percent, tidal volume (TV) of 400 mL, and positive end-expiratory pressure (PEEP) of 5. The ABG results are: pH of 7.50, PaO_2 of 95 mm Hg, $PaCO_2$ of 29 mm Hg, and HCO_3 of 23 mmol/L. Which ventilator setting change would the nurse anticipate?

    A. Increase the FiO_2.

    B. Increase the TV.

    C. Decrease the AC rate.

    D. Extubate the patient ASAP.

13. A patient is placed on assist control (AC) mechanical ventilation with a rate of 14, positive end-expiratory pressure (PEEP) of 15 cm H_2O, tidal volume (TV) of 450 mL, and FiO_2 of 60 percent. Which information indicates that a change in the ventilator settings may be required?

    A. The ECG shows sinus bradycardia at 56/minute.

    B. The blood pressure is 88/40 mm Hg.

    C. The respiratory rate is 14/minute.

    D. The patient is calm and arousable to touch.

14. The nurse cares for a patient with small bowel obstruction. Which statement accurately describes the abdominal pain associated with mechanical obstruction of the bowels?

    A. steady dull pain

    B. colicky pain

    C. pain worsened by food intake

    D. pain during the middle of the night

15. A patient admitted for possible bowel obstruction has 3/10 abdominal pain. The vital signs are: temperature 101 °F (38.3 °C), pulse 130/minute, respirations 34/minute, and blood pressure (BP) 98/64 mm Hg. Blood cultures were drawn. Which provider order should the nurse implement **first**?

    A. Infuse 500 mL of saline over 1 hour.

    B. Administer morphine 6 mg IV push.

    C. Give intravenous ceftriaxone 1 gram.

    D. Give acetaminophen 650 mg rectally for fever.

16. The nurse cares for a patient with bleeding esophageal varices who is receiving a vasopressin IV infusion. Which of these actions is **most** appropriate for the nurse to take to monitor for adverse reactions of vasopressin?

    A. Monitor the patient for chest pain.

    B. Check the patient's potassium.

    C. Send blood for type and screening.

    D. Weigh the patient every day.

17. To manage high blood pressure in a patient with stroke, the nurse anticipates a provider order to give which medication?

    A. ACE inhibitors

    B. labetalol

    C. diltiazem

    D. metoprolol

18. The nurse receives a patient from the operating room who had an intraventricular catheter (external ventricular drain) inserted. Which action is the **priority** of the nurse in measuring the intracranial pressure (ICP)?

    A. Position the head of the bed at a 45-degree angle.

    B. Position the transducer at shoulder level.

    C. Position the transducer at the level of the tragus.

    D. Position the transducer with the phlebostatic axis.

19. The triage nurse just evaluated a patient for suspected stroke. At which benchmark period should the patient have a noncontrast CT scan of the head ordered by the provider?

    A. 90 minutes of arrival

    B. 60 minutes of arrival

    C. 10 minutes of arrival

    D. 5 minutes of arrival

20. The nurse cares for a patient who has acute kidney injury secondary to an adverse reaction to intravenous contrast media. Which of these lab results reflects the type of renal failure in this patient?

    A. blood urea nitrogen of 20 and creatinine of 0.9

    B. blood urea nitrogen of 47 and creatinine of 3.8

    C. blood urea nitrogen of 60 and creatinine of 1.5

    D. blood urea nitrogen of 90 and creatinine of 2.5

21. Which outcome is most appropriate to establish for a patient on therapeutic hypothermia who is being considered for rewarming?

    A. Turn and reposition the patient every 2 hours.

    B. Gradual warming goal is 0.5 °C per hour.

    C. Restore body temperature to 37 °C in 2 hours.

    D. Assess sedation level using RASS every hour.

22. Which is the cause of anemia of chronic inflammation (also known as anemia of chronic illness) commonly seen in older adults and critically ill patients?

    A. poor intake of iron, calcium, and vitamin C in anorexic older adults

    B. chronic iron deficiency secondary to occult gastrointestinal bleeding

    C. increased levels of inflammatory cytokines due to comorbid illness

    D. uncontrolled diabetes mellitus (DM) and the resulting kidney disease

23. Which of these pathophysiologic changes meet the diagnostic criteria for acute respiratory distress syndrome (ARDS)?

    A. PaO_2/FiO_2 ratio of less than 300 mm Hg

    B. pulmonary wedge pressure of 20 mm Hg

    C. fraction of inspired O_2 requirement of more than 50 percent

    D. mechanical ventilation for more than 1 week

24. The nurse cares for a patient immediately after an open-heart surgery. The patient has the following hemodynamic parameters: central venous pressure (CVP) 1, pulmonary artery systolic pressure (PAS)/pulmonary artery diastolic pressure (PAD) 19/6, pulmonary artery occlusion pressure (PAOP) 3, arterial BP 78/41, and cardiac index 1.63. Urinary output is 10 mL/hour. Which intervention should the nurse anticipate?

    A. Check the patient for signs of infection from the surgery.

    B. Administer fluid challenge and titrate the vasopressors.

    C. Flush the Foley catheter to make sure output is accurate.

    D. Give the patient a bolus of pain medication as ordered.

25. The nurse cares for a patient in the intensive care unit (ICU) who is terminally ill. The family expressed concerns regarding the invasive procedures that the patient is going through. The nurse listened attentively and informed the family that she would share their concerns in the next ICU "huddle." Which of these characteristics does the nurse's action represent?

    A. collaboration

    B. advocacy

    C. system thinking

    D. clinical inquiry

Diagnostic Test
Answers and Explanations

ANSWER KEY

1.	D	14.	B
2.	D	15.	C
3.	B	16.	A
4.	D	17.	B
5.	A	18.	C
6.	B	19.	C
7.	C	20.	B
8.	A	21.	B
9.	A	22.	C
10.	C	23.	A
11.	D	24.	B
12.	C	25.	B
13.	B		

1. D

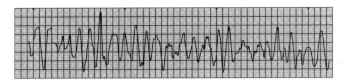

The ACLS algorithm indicates that after the initial shock/defibrillation, the rescuers should perform cardiac compressions for 2 minutes or 5 cycles. Intubation (A) is not the next action, but the airway should be kept patent. BP check and listening to heart sounds (B) is not warranted during ACLS. Once stabilized, the patient may be transferred to a critical care setting (C).

2. D

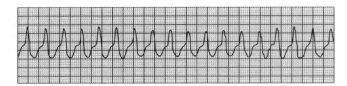

The definitive treatment for pulseless ventricular tachycardia (V-tach) is defibrillation. Cardiac compression (A) is done for 2 minutes, in between shocks, but only defibrillation can convert V-tach to a viable rhythm. Cardioversion (B) is done for rapid atrial fibrillation, atrial flutter, and supraventricular tachycardia. Intubation (C) is done to keep the airway patent and deliver O_2, but intubation alone will not convert V-tach to a viable rhythm.

3. B

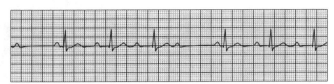

The ECG rhythm shown is second-degree AV block, Mobitz type I. Metoprolol should not be given as it may further slow down the pulse rate (PR) or worsen the heart block. Lisinopril (A) does not prolong the PR interval and has no chronotropic effects. Ondansetron (C) prolongs the cardiac output (QT) interval, not the PR interval. Methylprednisolone (D) has no heart rhythm adverse effects.

4. D

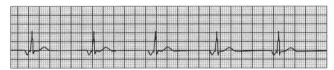

Inverted P waves signify a junctional rhythm when the pulse rate (PR) is 40–60 beats per minute (bpm). If the PR is 60–100 bpm, it is called accelerated junctional (A). When the PR is greater than 100 bpm, it is called junctional tachycardia (B). Junctional escape rhythm (C) or escape beats occur when the AV junction takes over after a significant pause in electrical activity. A junctional escape rhythm is a sequence of 3 or more junctional escapes occurring by default at a rate of 40–60 bpm.

5. A

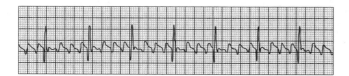

The ECG shown is atrial flutter. Along with atrial fibrillation, they put the patient at risk for strokes. Sudden cardiac death (B) is a risk for those who have a history of V-tach or ventricular fibrillation (V-fib) and cardiomyopathy (C). Hypertension (D) is a risk factor for developing atrial flutter, not the other way around.

6. B

A platelet level of 8,000 is critically low (normal range: 150,000–450,000/mL) and warrants immediate attention due to the risk of intracerebral bleeding. An INR of 2.0 (A) is high (normal range: 0.6–1.7) and cause for concern, but it is not critical. An aPTT of 60 seconds (C) is high (normal range: 25–35 seconds), but it is not critical. Fibrinogen of 300 mg/dL (D) is normal (normal range: 200–400 mg/dL).

7. C

Close collaboration between the patient and the primary care provider will allow for prompt intervention of clinical situations that might put the patient at risk for DKA. There is no evidence to support that adopting a vegetarian diet (A) prevents DKA. Continuous glucose monitoring (B) may be useful; however, checking it every 2 hours is excessive. A salt-free diet (D) is not compatible with life.

8. A

To rule out if the symptoms are related to hypoglycemia, the nurse should check the glucose fingerstick first. Glucagon injection (B) is given only after the patient is confirmed to be hypoglycemic. Before the nurse gives the patient something to eat or drink (C and D), assessment should be done.

9. A

Intravenous (IV) calcium gluconate will prevent ventricular dysrhythmia by stabilizing the action potential of the myocardial cells. Magnesium sulfate (B) is given for confirmed hypomagnesemia and for torsade de pointes. Sodium chloride (C), by itself, is not clinically indicated in hyperkalemia. Critically high levels of potassium are treated with dextrose 50 percent, IV regular insulin (not NPH insulin, D), and IV calcium gluconate.

10. C

Potassium of 6.9 mEq/L is critically high and can lead to life-threatening dysrhythmia such as heart blocks and ventricular tachycardia. A BUN of 50 mg/dL (A) is high, but it does not require emergency measures. Creatinine 2.0 mg/dL (B) is high, but it does not require emergency measures. Calcium of 7.5 mg/dL (D) is low, but it does not require emergency measures.

11. D

The drop in CVP signals the need for more fluid boluses, as the patient is most likely hypovolemic or has ongoing fluid losses. A drop in CVP indicates the patient is "dry" and needs more IV fluids; it is not a sign of improved hydration status (A). Severe sepsis (B) is diagnosed when there is organ dysfunction in a patient with sepsis, not by the level of the CVP. Output is monitored by measuring hourly urine drainage, not by scanning the bladder (C).

12. C

The patient is in respiratory alkalosis. To reduce hyperventilation, the assist control (AC) rate can be reduced to minimize excess respiratory CO_2 losses. The patient is not hypoxic (PaO_2 of 95), so there is no need to increase the FiO_2 (A). A TV of 400 mL is adequate for the average-size adult, so there is no indication to increase the TV (B). Before extubation (D), it is best to place the patient on an intermittent mechanical ventilation (IMV) setting first.

13. B

Hypotension is an adverse effect of high positive end-expiratory pressure (PEEP). Either the PEEP can be reduced or the patient will require an IV fluid bolus to maintain a viable BP. Bradycardia of 56/minute (A) is not a critical finding and not directly related to mechanical ventilation. The respiratory rate (RR) of 14/minute (C) means all the patient's breath is coming from the ventilator. No change in rate is required. A calm and arousable patient (D) is a desired outcome, not a complication from mechanical ventilation.

14. B

Colicky pain characterizes mechanical bowel obstruction. Steady dull pain (A) is typically seen in ileus. Pain worsened by food intake (C) is associated with gastric ulcers. Abdominal pain experienced during the middle of the night (D) or a few hours after meals is associated with duodenal ulcers.

15. C

The nurse should give the antibiotic first due to risk of sepsis from the bowel obstruction. Antibiotics should be administered within 60 minutes from the time sepsis is recognized. The patient's BP is not critically low. Normal saline bolus (A) is not the highest priority. Pain of 3/10 (B) is not severe, and morphine 6 mg is most likely too much considering the BP is only 98/60. The patient will need acetaminophen for fever (D), but the first thing the nurse should give is the antibiotic.

16. A

Vasopressin may cause coronary vasoconstriction; therefore, the nurse should monitor the patient for chest pain. Potassium (B) is not directly affected by vasopressin infusion. Type and screening (C) are helpful in possible transfusion, not for monitoring for the adverse effect of vasopressin. There is no indication in the scenario to weigh the patient daily (D).

17. B

IV labetalol is the first-line medication of choice in managing hypertension in stroke patients because it is titratable. ACE inhibitors (A) are not used to manage malignant hypertension seen in some stroke patients. A calcium channel blocker such as diltiazem (C) is not the first-line medication to give in malignant hypertension. Metoprolol (D) cannot be given in continuous infusion, but labetalol can be given as a drip.

18. C

Accurate ICP reading is best obtained when the transducer is leveled with the tragus. Typically, the head-of-bed is placed at a 30-degree angle to measure the ICP, not a 45-degree angle (A). If the transducer is lower than the tragus (B), the ICP will be falsely high. Phlebostatic leveling (D) is applicable for hemodynamic monitoring (e.g., CVP, arterial line), not for ICP monitoring.

19. C

A noncontrast CT should be ordered within 10 minutes of arrival or upon recognition that the patient is having a stroke. At 90 minutes to 3 hours post-tPA (A), the stroke pathway should already be in place. The stroke algorithm suggests that at 60 minutes (B), the CT scan should have been read already and tPA given if there are no contraindications. At 5 minutes of arrival (D), a rapid neurological assessment should be done for suspected stroke patients.

20. B

A blood urea nitrogen (BUN) of 47 and creatinine of 3.8 has a ratio of 12.3:1, indicating an intrarenal failure pattern. Contrast media is nephrotoxic and can cause an intrarenal failure pattern in the BUN:creatinine ratio. In *intrarenal* failure, the ratio is less than 20:1. In *prerenal* failure, the ratio is greater than 20:1. A BUN of 20 and creatinine of 0.9 (A) are normal. A BUN of 60 and creatinine of 1.5 (C) have a ratio of 40:1, indicating a prerenal pattern. A BUN of 90 and creatinine of 2.5 (D) have a ratio of 36:1; it is also a prerenal pattern of kidney failure.

21. B

Gradual rewarming is important in therapeutic hypothermia, keeping a 0.5 °C per hour increase. Turning and repositioning (A) are not appropriate goals during the rewarming. Rapid rewarming (C) can lead to electrolyte abnormalities, cerebral edema, and seizures, and it defeats the benefits of therapeutic hypothermia. Sedation level assessment using the Richmond Agitation-Sedation Scale (RASS) is essential; however, it is not the priority care outcome during rewarming (D).

22. C

Increased levels of inflammatory cytokines in chronic illness lead to reduced hematopoiesis. Malnutrition (A) is not the main reason for anemia of chronic illness; multi-morbidity and inflammation are. Occult GI bleeding (B) is a confounding problem in anemia of chronic disease, not the main cause. DM and kidney failure (D) confound anemia of chronic disease; they are not the main causes.

23. A

Diagnostic markers for ARDS include a PaO_2/FiO_2 ratio of less than 300 mm Hg. Pulmonary wedge pressure (B), also called pulmonary occlusion pressure (PAOP), is not part of the ARDS diagnostic criteria. The amount of FiO_2 given (C) is not part of the ARDS diagnostic criteria. The patient does not need to be on the ventilator for 1 week (D) to be diagnosed with ARDS.

24. B

The patient has volume deficits as evidenced by a critically low arterial BP of 78/41 and low hemodynamic pressure readings. Normal hemodynamic pressures are: CVP 2–8 mm Hg, PAS/PAD 20–30/5–20, PAOP 5–12 mm Hg, and cardiac index 2.2–4 L/min/m^2. Signs of surgical site infection (A) are usually not apparent immediately after surgery. There is no indication to suspect that the Foley is clogged in the scenario described (C). Pain is not a concern in the scenario described (D).

25. B

The nurse's action represents advocacy/moral agency characteristics based on the AACN's Synergy Model for Patient Care. Advocacy/moral agency means acting on another's behalf, representing the concerns of the patient/family and nursing staff, and serving as a moral agent in identifying and helping to resolve ethical and clinical concerns. Collaboration (A) focuses on working with others in a way that promotes each person's contributions toward achieving goals. System thinking (C) allows the nurse to manage system resources that exist for the patient/family and staff, within or across healthcare systems and non-healthcare systems. Clinical inquiry (D) is the ongoing process of questioning and evaluating practice and providing informed practice.

PART III

Adult CCRN Subject Review

The Cardiovascular System

Knowledge and the ability to apply information regarding the cardiovascular system is extremely important for the CCRN. Approximately 20 percent of the total number of scored questions on the CCRN examination involve the cardiovascular system. You will need to master a basic understanding of cardiovascular anatomy and physiology, electrocardiography (ECG) interpretation, and advanced cardiac life support (ACLS), as well as more complex physiology and disease management, to do well on the CCRN.

Understanding major concepts such as preload and afterload, diagnostic and clinical complications associated with myocardial infarction in particular anatomical areas of the heart, pharmacological effects and shock states based on hemodynamic parameters, and differences between right and left heart failure are also important. It is also imperative to know that when terms such as *pulsus alternans*, *pulsus paradoxus*, *narrowed pulse pressure*, and *Lewis lead* appear on the exam, they relate to specific cardiovascular conditions. Knowing the particular conditions that these terms apply to is paramount in mastering cardiology for the CCRN; for example, pulsus paradoxus is an indication of pericardial effusion.

ANATOMY OF THE CARDIOVASCULAR SYSTEM

The position of the heart is slightly left of the midline, above the diaphragm, and within the anterior thoracic cavity behind the sternum. With this positioning, the right atrium and ventricle are primarily inferior and anterior, while the left atrium and ventricle are posterior and anterolateral. This will be important when the location of myocardial ischemia or damage is identified. To locate the point of maximal impulse (PMI), the health care provider places his fingers over the apex of the heart, which is located at the left fifth intercostal space in the midclavicular line. This provides information as to the possible dilation of the left ventricle. As the left ventricle dilates, the PMI will be located more laterally and inferiorly. When describing the size of a normal adult heart, the clenched fist can be used as a guide for approximate size. Weight varies based on whether there are conditions that enlarge the heart, such as heart failure or cardiomyopathy. In general, a male heart weighs slightly more than the female heart. There are four layers of the heart with different functions and attributes:

Pericardium

The pericardium is composed of two layers and forms a pericardial sac. The two layers of the pericardium are the fibrous and serous pericardium. The serous pericardium is further broken down into two layers: the parietal (outer) and visceral (inner, sometimes referred to as the epicardium) pericardium. Since the parietal layer is fused to the fibrous pericardium, you can think of the heart as essentially having two membrane layers: the parietal/fibrous pericardium and the visceral pericardium. The area between these two layers forms the pericardial sac, which holds approximately 10–15 mL of viscous fluid. Not only do the layers of the pericardium provide protection, but the fluid between the parietal and visceral layers allows the chambers of the heart to fill with blood and contract smoothly, and it prevents the heart from overexpanding. However, when there is a pericardial effusion, fluid or blood accumulates between these two membranes and impedes cardiac function by not allowing the chambers of the heart to fill normally. As a result, cardiac tamponade occurs (a critical emergency). Typically, once this condition is diagnosed, a directed needle pericardiocentesis will be done to aspirate the fluid temporarily and allow normal contraction of the heart. A more permanent pericardial window might be required to prevent recurrence.

Myocardium

This is the muscle layer of the heart. The contractile muscle fibers are located in this layer and arranged in multiple, interlacing levels. These are effective in pushing the blood flow through the chambers and into the lungs for reoxygenation and to the critical organs and extremities for oxygenation. This is the layer that is damaged in acute myocardial infarction. A blockage in coronary blood flow is the most common cause of this damage.

Endocardium

The innermost lining layers of the heart are called the endocardium. This lining forms a continuous layer with the vessels and intracardiac structures such as the papillary muscles and heart valves.

The anatomical structures within the heart include heart chambers, cardiac valves, nervous conduction system, and coronary vessels. There are two upper chambers of the heart that are considered low pressure chambers. The right atrium receives deoxygenated venous blood from the superior/inferior vena cava and coronary sinus, while the left atrium receives oxygenated blood from the pulmonary veins. The right atrium and ventricle are separated by the tricuspid valve, while the left atrium and ventricle are separated by the mitral valve. These valves initially open during ventricular diastole (relaxation) and close during ventricular systole (contraction). Approximately 80–85 percent of the blood is received passively from the atria. The contraction of the atria is responsible for "pushing" the remaining 15 percent of the blood from the atria into the ventricles; this is often referred to as the "atrial kick." The loss of this "kick" due to heart irregularities such as atrial fibrillation or flutter may cause a significant drop in cardiac output, which causes the patient to become symptomatic. The valves that separate the outflow tracts of the right and left ventricles are the pulmonic and aortic valves, respectively. These are referred to as semilunar valves. Chordae tendineae and papillary muscles join the valves to the wall of the ventricles.

The muscular wall of the left ventricle is three times thicker than that of the right ventricle. The right ventricle forms the greatest majority of the anterior surface of the heart. There are three types of cardiac muscle: atrial muscle, ventricular muscle, and excitatory and conductive muscle fibers. The atrial and ventricular muscle contracts similarly to skeletal muscle, except that the duration of the contraction is longer. The excitatory and conductive muscle exhibits autonomic electrical discharge, which controls the rhythmical beating of the heart.

Coronary Vasculature

The coronary arterial system originates from the base of the aorta immediately above the aortic valve. There are four major vessels: right coronary artery (RCA), left coronary artery (LCA), left anterior descending artery (LAD), and the left circumflex artery (LCX). There are also collateral arteries that support circulation and may enlarge when there is damage to the other major vessels. During myocardial ischemia or infarction, it is possible to tell where the symptoms are originating from by changes on the ECG related to the location of the symptoms. For example, anterior changes on the ECG in "V" leads or a right bundle branch block may indicate blockage in the LAD. The RCA feeds the posterior wall of the myocardium, the AV node, and the SA node in approximately 55 percent of adults. The LCA branches into the LAD and the circumflex arteries. The LAD supplies the anterior septum, anterior wall of the left ventricle, right bundle branch, and the anterosuperior left bundle branch.

The coronary veins serve to return the deoxygenated blood from the heart to the right atrium. The major vessels in this system include the great cardiac vein, small and middle cardiac veins, and the thebesian veins. These veins join to form the coronary sinus.

The important fact to remember about the coronary blood flow system is that there is a reserve that, when necessary, *can increase* the circulation to the heart by as much as six times normal. Myocardial oxygen demand may *increase* during hyperdynamic states such as strenuous exercise and conditions such as sepsis. Coronary blood flow may *decrease* during states such as decreased tissue perfusion (hypotension), decreased left ventricular diastolic pressure, increased myocardial mass (heart failure), or mechanical obstruction (valvular disease).

FIGURE 5.1 *Arterial Supply to the Heart*

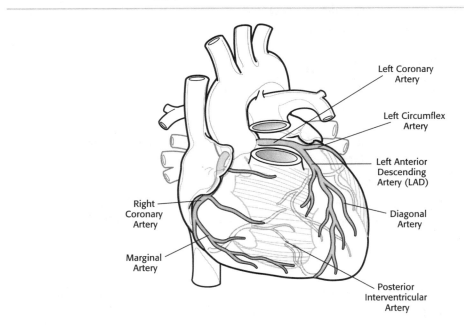

PHYSIOLOGY OF THE CARDIOVASCULAR SYSTEM

Conduction System

The cardiac cycle is initiated in the healthy heart by the **sinoatrial** (SA) **node**, which is located in the mouth of the vena cava on the posterior aspect of the right atrium. The SA node is considered the heart's natural pacemaker due to its characteristics of high automaticity and/or intrinsic heart rate. Typically, this heart rate is 60 to 100 beats per minute (BPM). The SA node contains two very specialized types of cells: **specialized pacemaker cells** and **border zone cells.**

Once the SA node cells are depolarized, the impulse generated is conducted down through the border of the atrium to four specialized pathways: Bachmann's bundle toward the left atrium and three internodal pathways directed to the atrioventricular (AV) node. The AV node is located posteriorly on the interatrial septum. Between the atria and ventricle are nonconducting tissues, and, therefore, the impulse travels to ventricle via the AV node. The AV node also contains pacemaker cells, but their intrinsic rate is lower than the SA node. The AV node is technically reset by the functioning SA node to prevent it from initiating its own impulse. However, in the event the SA node is nonfunctional or dysfunctional, the AV node will stimulate the impulse to the ventricles at a rate between 40 to 60 BPM. There is a slight delay in the conduction as the impulse travels through the AV node. The effect of this delay is to allow time for optimum ventricular filling and, in turn, ventricular ejection during contraction.

FIGURE 5.2 *Cardiac Conduction System*

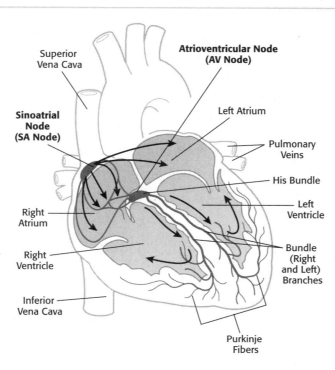

The normal AV node contains only one pathway to the ventricle for conduction. If there is an additional abnormal pathway, it is considered to be an accessory pathway. These circular pathways can allow the impulse to reenter the atrial circuit and cause rapid dysrhythmias, which would then override SA node function. An atypical situation may develop where the pathway travels between the atria and ventricles, but outside the AV node. This dysrhythmia is called Wolfe-Parkinson-White (WPW) syndrome and can cause premature impulses in the atria or ventricle, causing tachydysrhythmias. An ECG of a person with WPW will demonstrate the presence of delta waves just immediately preceding the QRS complex.

The final conduction pathway is through the bundle of His, bundle branches, and Purkinje fibers. This pathway runs through the subendocardium down the right side of the intraventricular septum. The two bundle branches follow toward the right apex and the left ventricular wall. These branches narrow into a thin anterior branch and a thick posterior branch. A serious conduction defect, called a hemiblock, can occur when the left bundle is blocked. With any blockage in the bundles, a widening of the QRS complex will occur on the 12 lead ECG, indicating a lengthening of conduction. Eventually the right and left bundles divide into the Purkinje fibers, which attach to the subendocardial surface of both ventricles. The Purkinje fibers, which provide for rapid depolarization of the ventricles, have the fastest conduction velocity of all heart tissues.

Nervous Regulation

Within the regulatory nervous system there are two systems that can directly impact cardiovascular functions. These are the **sympathetic nervous system** (SNS) and the **parasympathetic nervous system** (PNS). Typically, the PNS has the effect of *decreasing* most of the cardiovascular functions such as automaticity, contractility, rate, and velocity of contraction. The SNS has the opposite effect and will *increase* all of these functions.

Parasympathetic fibers are located at the level of the SA and AV node and, more specifically, the right and left vagus nerves. Sudden bradycardia can occur with stimulation of the vagus nerve. Sympathetic fibers parallel the coronary circulation before the fibers innervate the myocardium. It appears that the right chain of these fibers tends to affect rate while the left chain impacts contractility.

Within the nervous system there are also intrinsic regulatory reflexes, which provide feedback to the brain and work to maintain blood flow and perfusion. The first of these are called **baroreceptors**. As the name indicates, they are sensitive to pressure and are located in the aortic arch and carotid sinuses. These receptors sense changes in volume, as a measurement of pressure, and will respond through stimulation of the autonomic nervous system. If a sudden drop in blood volume should occur, such as in gastrointestinal bleeding, the baroreceptors would stimulate an increased heart rate through the vasomotor center in the medulla. The second of these reflexes is the **chemoreceptors**, located in the aortic arch; these are provided a rich blood supply and innervated by the PNS. They have the ability to detect oxygen tension and respond to a decreased oxygen tension by the stimulation of respiration. The Bainbridge reflex causes reflex tachycardia in response to increased right atrial pressure. This reflex is designed to protect right heart function.

Although not specifically a reflex, another control mechanism of the heart involves the atrial release of a hormone called atrial natriuretic factor, also called alpha natriuretic peptide. The response is due to an increase in atrial pressure. The effects are that sodium and water are excreted by the kidneys and vasodilation occurs. The dual effect of reducing extracellular fluid volume and improving the capacity of the venous system results in a restoration to the blood volume. Alpha natriuretic factor antagonizes the effects of antidiuretic hormone (ADH) and aldosterone, resulting in natriuresis and diuresis.

Concepts of Cardiac Output

The definition of cardiac output is fairly simple; however, the actual potential of cardiac output has many factors. **Cardiac output** (CO) is the volume of blood that is ejected by the heart over 1 minute and is reported in liters/minute. Considering this definition, the two major components of the equation are *heart rate* and *stroke volume*. A calculation can be made for cardiac index (CI), which is the CO divided by the patient's body surface in square meters (m^2). The normal range for CO is 4–8 L/min, and the average CI is 2.5 to 4.0 L/min/m^2. Additionally, there is a component of efficiency involved. Simply increasing CO does not necessarily mean increased functional capacity of the heart. Eventually, the resultant increase could lead to decompensation of the heart, resulting in clinical heart failure.

Preload

Preload was not recognized as a fundamental concept until the early 1900s. The researcher who wrote about his findings with relation to preload was Ernest Starling. Starling's law is still recognized today as one of the primary concepts in cardiac function. The basis for this law is that the heart will respond to an increased volume and compensate for a period of time to improve CO until a certain point, at which time the contractility actually diminishes and the heart function decreases. These changes occur on a molecular level with the actin and myosin cross-bridges in the myofilament. Therefore, preload is a combination of blood volume entering the left ventricle and the contractility of that ventricle. It is also known as left ventricular end diastolic pressure (LVEDP), and it can be measured with the use of a pulmonary artery catheter and pulmonary capillary wedge pressures (also called pulmonary artery occlusive pressure). Factors that affect preload are venous return, total blood volume, "atrial kick" (mentioned earlier), and compliance of the ventricles.

Afterload

Afterload of the heart is the pressure or stress that the ventricular wall faces when ejecting its blood volume. Afterload may be considered the resistance in the circulation as well. Factors that impact afterload include increased systemic vascular resistance (SVR) or vasoconstriction, increased blood volume, aortic impedance such as with aortic valve sclerosis/stenosis, and septal hypertrophy. Along with increased afterload and work of the heart comes increased myocardial oxygen demand; therefore, the goals for reducing afterload should include decreasing SVR with the use of vasodilators, reducing blood volume, or repairing valvular dysfunction with valve replacement.

The concepts of preload and afterload are important aspects of CO, and in most abnormal heart and circulation functions, one or both are severely altered from normal.

Contractility

Contractility is essentially the ability of the heart to contract and the subsequent force of contraction. The body will compensate for decreased contractility by increasing heart rate to a certain point, as discussed earlier with Starling's law. This is done via stimulation of the SNS. In critical care patient management, pharmacologic agents that function similarly to the SNS stimulus may also be used to increase cardiac contractility. Pharmacologic agents that increase cardiac contractility are referred to as inotropic agents.

The above definitions and concepts are important for the critical care RN to understand, particularly in the administration and titration of medications based on the response to the CO and other hemodynamic measurements, such as mean central venous pressure (CVP).

For example, if the patient you are caring for has been diagnosed with septic shock, your first line of treatment is administration of large volumes of crystalloid solutions (normal saline), which will improve the intravascular fluid volume deficit. This deficit is caused by severe vasodilation and venous pooling. At the point where 30 mL/kg of fluid has been infused and the patient remains hypotensive or the mean arterial pressure is < 65 mm/Hg, a norepinephrine infusion is indicated. Norepinephrine is a potent alpha-adrenergic stimulant that increases systemic vascular resistance through vasoconstriction, while not increasing heart rate significantly as dopamine (beta-adrenergic agonist) does. Without the knowledge of the concepts of preload, afterload, and cardiac output, the critical care RN will not be able to make informed decisions on the administration and titrations of inotropic and vasoactive drugs (or pharmacologic agents).

CARDIOVASCULAR CONDITIONS

Hypertensive Crisis/Emergency

Hypertensive crisis, otherwise known as hypertensive emergency, is a sudden event involving a critically elevated blood pressure and requires immediate medical attention. Hypertensive emergency is diagnosed when there is a critically elevated blood pressure associated with end-organ damage. Hypertensive crisis was once known as malignant hypertension (higher than 250/150 mm Hg causes hypertensive encephalopathy). The presenting clinical manifestations include altered level-of-consciousness or disorientation, seizure, vomiting, severe headache, epistaxis, visual disturbances, and diastolic blood pressure exceeding 120 mm Hg. Hypertensive encephalopathy as well as irreversible end-organ damage to the brain, kidneys, and heart or death can result if not corrected.

The primary cause of hypertensive crisis is most often due to untreated or uncontrolled hypertension. Secondary causes include renal dysfunction or endocrine disorders. Risk factors associated with hypertensive crisis include diabetes, smoking, obesity, oral contraceptive agent use, hypertension during pregnancy, and hyperlipidemia. Hypertension enhances sympathetic stimulation causing systemic vasoconstriction, which decreases blood flow to vital organs. Complications of hypertensive crisis include cerebrovascular accident (CVA), increased intracranial pressure (IICP), intracerebral or subarachnoid hemorrhage (SAH), myocardial infarction (MI), decreased mesenteric blood flow, and renal failure. The goals of treatment are to (a) determine the cause, either primary or secondary; (b) immediately detect and prevent clinical sequelae; (c) reduce the blood pressure no more than 25 percent in the first one to two hours of presentation; and (d) provide patient teaching to decrease risk factors and promote compliance with prescribed medical regimen.

A common treatment for hypertensive crisis is the administration of a potent vasodilator such as *nitroprusside (Nipride)* or *fenoldopam mesylate (Corlopam)*. Nipride works in seconds and its drug action lasts 1 to 5 minutes. It should be titrated to lowest dose.

The bag and tubing must be protected from light. Other agents that can be used in the treatment of hypertensive crisis include nitroglycerin (produces more venodilation than arteriolar dilation), nicardipine, labetalol, esmolol, and enalaprilat. Hydralazine is reserved for use in pregnant patients. Phentolamine is the drug of choice for a pheochromocytoma crisis. However, nitroprusside can cause fetal renal impairment and should not be used in pregnancy for this reason. Nipride also causes cyanide toxicity (confusion, seizure activity, visual disturbances, and tinnitus) and requires thiosulfate as an additive to prevent cyanide toxicity. Fenoldopam isn't always preferred due to its longer half-life (5 to 10 minutes) and hypokalemic effects. Other effects of fenoldopam are headaches and reflex tachycardia. Hypotension caused by fenoldopam can be treated with IV fluids and Trendelenburg position. *Nicardipine hydrochloride (Cardene)*, a calcium channel blocker/antihypertensive, is gaining popularity as a choice infusion for the treatment of hypertensive crisis due to gentler effects and lack of toxicity. Other useful agents include *nitroglycerin (Tridil), ACE inhibitors (lisinopril, captopril, enalapril, enalaprilat), beta-blockers (labetalol, esmolol, and metoprolol), calcium channel blockers (nicardipine and amlodipine), and diuretics (furosemide and bumetanide).*

Chronic Stable Angina Pectoris

Chronic stable angina pectoris is chest discomfort that does not increase in severity or frequency over time. This type of angina is predictable and typically follows some type of exertion (physical activity, stress, anxiety, extreme emotions or a meal). This type of chest pain is easily relieved with *nitrates (nitroglycerin)* and rest. During the episode of chest pain, the patient's ECG may reflect the following changes: T wave inversion or ST segment depression in ECG leads correlating with decreased coronary blood flow and oxygen delivery (myocardial ischemia).

Myocardial ischemia causes the symptom known as angina or chest discomfort. Most victims of chronic stable angina pectoris describe this discomfort as a pressure, indigestion, heaviness, or achy feeling across the chest lasting anywhere from 5 to 20 minutes. Others describe the discomfort by location: chest, jaw, arms, substernal, back, or epigastric region. Accompanying symptoms include nausea, diaphoresis, shortness-of-breath, and dizziness. Angina occurs as a result of the myocardium lacking blood supply due to coronary artery disease (CAD), namely, atherosclerosis. It may also occur as a result of an embolus and/or vasospasms of the coronary arteries. Atherosclerosis results in the loss of elasticity of the vessel and progresses as we age. The result of this type of angina is that myocardial oxygen demand exceeds supply. Coronary artery disease (CAD) is the most prominent risk factor associated with chronic stable angina pectoris. Most importantly, serum cardiac biomarkers (CK and CK-MB isoenzymes, myoglobin, and T/I troponins) are not elevated with episodes of stable angina.

The goal of treatment for this type of angina is to increase myocardial oxygen supply (nitrates) and decrease demand (nitrates, calcium channel blockers, and beta-blockers). This can also be accomplished by lifestyle modification teaching, such as smoking cessation, diabetes education, weight control, stress or anxiety reduction, promotion of a nonsedentary lifestyle, proper diet, and blood pressure, and cholesterol control. Illicit drug use is often associated with this condition; therefore, a thorough patient history is necessary. Prinzmetal's angina (coronary vasospasm) is primarily seen with illicit drug use. Oftentimes, *antiplatelets like aspirin 81 mg daily and/or clopidogrel 75 mg daily* may be prescribed. Aspirin is the first-line antiplatelet agent except in patients who have recently had a myocardial infarction or undergone stent placement, in which case clopidogrel is recommended. Adequate nitroglycerin instruction is needed for patients with chronic stable angina pectoris. Angiography and percutaneous coronary interventions (PCIs), such as percutaneous transluminal coronary angioplasty (PTCA), laser angioplasty, cutting balloon angioplasty, bare-metal stent placement, drug-eluting stent placement, brachytherapy, and directional and rotational atherectomy, can be the treatment for this condition as well as coronary artery bypass grafting (CABG).

Acute Coronary Syndromes

Acute coronary syndrome (ACS) is described by the American Heart Association as an "umbrella term which describes any group of clinical symptoms compatible with acute myocardial ischemia." Examples of the conditions that fall under this generic descriptor include unstable angina pectoris (UA), ST segment elevated myocardial infarction (STEMI), and non-ST segment elevated myocardial infarction (NSTEMI). UA and NSTEMI are grouped together under the term non-ST elevation acute coronary syndromes (NSTE-ACS). Acute coronary syndromes may result from coronary artery disease (CAD), thrombosis, atherosclerotic plaque, vasoconstriction, and occlusion. The goal of treatment of ACS is to identify rapidly the cause of the chest pain or associated symptoms, exclude nonischemic chest pain, stratify patients with coronary ischemia, and provide immediate treatment, including interventional procedures such as percutaneous transluminal coronary angioplasty (PTCA) or CABG if necessary to prevent further damage.

Unstable Angina Pectoris

UA is often referred to as "crescendo or preinfarction angina," since this type of chest discomfort becomes more difficult to relieve and lasts longer. Often this pain is a symptom of multicoronary artery disease. Unstable angina does not cause elevations in cardiac biomarkers (CK, CK-MB isoenzymes, myoglobin, and T/I troponins), nor does it cause myocardial cell death (necrosis). Patients do, however, present with similar symptoms as acute myocardial infarction. Current recommendations for treatment by the American College of Cardiology include initial diagnostic testing to rule out infarction, biomarkers, ECG, stress test, and radionuclide angiogram. Medical treatment also includes initial diagnostic testing, physical examination, ECG, biomarkers of myocardial necrosis, and imaging. The course of UA is unpredictable; therefore, the need for initial invasive or conservative measures must be determined quickly. Medical treatment also includes administration of oxygen, antiplatelet agents (aspirin or clopidogrel), anticoagulants, anti-ischemic and analgesic medications (nitrates, morphine), beta-blockers, and lipid-lowering statins, and discontinuation of nonsteroidal anti-inflammatory drugs (NSAIDs). Early cardiac catheterization is recommended to evaluate presence of coronary blockage and the need for stenting. At the time of discharge, the patient should be started on protective medications such as angiotensin-converting enzyme inhibitors (ACEIs) or angiotensin receptor blockers (ARBs). The chain of blood pressure–regulating hormones is referred to as the renin-angiotensin-aldosterone (RAA) hormonal system, which regulates the blood pressure in the body. ACEI and ARB drugs have the most substantial effects on the RAA system.

Non-ST Segment Elevation Myocardial Infarction (NSTEMI)

The major difference between UA and NSTEMI or STEMI is the myocardial cell death or necrosis associated with the latter two (hence the term *myocardial infarction*). In NSTEMI, troponin T and I levels are more than 0.1 ng/mL. These elevations are present for 4 to 12 hours after the onset of symptoms and are generally trended over 24 to 36 hours to determine the peak. If the patient has evidence of renal insufficiency, these levels may be difficult to interpret, as they are elevated from the excretion of troponin from the kidneys into the bloodstream. ST segment changes sometimes occur with chest pain and ST segment depression, or inverted T waves may be present.

NSTEMI presents a twofold challenge. First, elevation in troponins may not be detected for up to 12 hours after presentation, so at initial presentation it can be difficult to distinguish between UA and NSTEMI. Second, ECG may or may not show evidence of acute myocardial injury or ischemia. The sensitivity of the biomarker test used to evaluate patients with ACS determines whether a given patient is diagnosed with UA or NSTEMI. In practice, UA and NSTEMI present on a pathophysiologic continuum and are often indistinguishable.

The acronym MONA is often used as a guideline for treating patients who present with acute chest pain. It helps the nurse recall easily the treatment regimen, which includes morphine, oxygen, nitroglycerin, and aspirin. During states where the myocardium may be experiencing reduced blood flow and myocardial oxygen is limited, supplemental oxygen will help improve the availability of oxygen to the bloodstream. Morphine serves both to reduce pain and as a mild vasodilator that helps reduce venous return or preload. Nitrates relax smooth muscle and cause venodilation, thus also decreasing the venous return to the heart and, in turn, reducing myocardial oxygen demand and consumption. In cases of myocardial artery spasm, nitrates may help reduce the spasm and assist in improving blood flow and oxygenation to the tissue of the myocardium. Aspirin prevents platelet aggregation and should be given in the prehospital environment.

The mortality associated with NSTEMI is, in fact, greater than that with STEMI due to the more standardized approach to the STEMI and the goal of door to balloon within 90 minutes. Since the presentation of NSTEMI is more difficult to assess, clinical protocols are not as structured. The approach to NSTEMI is similar to the new recommendations for unstable angina and include clopidogrel, aspirin, and a glycoprotein IIb/IIIa antagonist (recommended for ST depressions greater or equal to 0.5 mm, elevated troponins, and diabetes). Appropriate diagnostics should be done including, as mentioned above, cardiac markers, ECG, stress testing, radionuclide angiogram, and early catheterization.

ST Elevation Myocardial Infarction

In STEMI, ECG changes correlate with the location of the blockage and potential necrosis. Table 5.1 demonstrates the association between the location of the infarction and ECG leads. Patients diagnosed with acute inferior myocardial infarction should also be routinely screened with a right-sided ECG due to the possibility of a right ventricular infarction. As mentioned above, the goal of treating the STEMI is to identify quickly myocardial ischemia or infarction and intervene rapidly with interventional procedures to open the occluded vessel(s). National standards for STEMI include door-to-balloon angioplasty within 90 minutes. The following criteria conclude the diagnosis of STEMI or NSTEMI acute myocardial infarction: (a) a change on the ECG indicating myocardial ischemia or injury (ST elevation, ST depression, presence of Q wave), (b) elevated cardiac biomarkers, and (c) symptoms of acute coronary syndrome lasting longer than 20 minutes or chest discomfort that occurs at rest. The pain associated with ACS is typically described by patients as chest "pressure," and they may feel as if someone is "sitting on their chest."

Differentiation of a transmural (endocardium to epicardium) from a nontransmural (subendocardial) myocardial infarction is dependent upon the extent of the necrosis. In the past, the medical terms *transmural* and *subendocardial* were used to be synonymous with *Q wave* and *non-Q wave*, respectively, based upon the presence or absence of Q waves. Currently Q-wave detection is pathologic and mainly associated with larger infarctions. If Q waves become apparent, then they appear within hours of myocardial infarction. Abnormal Q waves greater than 0.04 sec. in duration and 25 percent at the height of the R wave develop within the first 24 hours.

A low percentage of people with chest discomfort who seek medical attention may present with normal ECG rhythms initially. Therefore, a normal ECG does not rule out acute myocardial infarction.

The use of beta-blockers (e.g., atenolol, metoprolol) is standard in the treatment of acute MI patients. Beta-blockers reduce heart rate and contractility, thus reducing myocardial oxygen demand and afterload. These drugs are contraindicated in the patient with AV blocks or hypotension. Non-cardioselective beta-blockers should not be used in patients with a history of COPD or asthma. In addition, patients with a reduced ejection fraction should also be treated with ACEI/ARBs at the time of discharge.

Acute mitral regurgitation (AMR) caused by papillary muscle rupture (PMR) is a rare but life-threatening mechanical complication of myocardial infarction. Patients typically present with an inferior infarction resulting from right coronary artery occlusion; most patients are older, with limited ejection fraction. Most ruptures occur within five to seven days after MI, but a delayed rupture several weeks or months after MI is also possible. The patient may present with a systolic murmur and dyspnea; echocardiography is useful to diagnose papillary muscle rupture. Despite high risks, immediate surgical intervention is the optimal and most rational treatment for acute PMR; however, mitral valve repair may lead to better postoperative left ventricular function.

TABLE 5.1

Area of Infarction	Indicative Changes (ST segment elevation)	Reciprocal Changes (ST segment depression)	Coronary Artery Involved
Inferior wall	II, III, aVF	I, aVL, V5, and V6	RCA or Circumflex
Septal wall	V1 and V2	II, III, aVF	LAD
Anterior wall	V2–V4	II, III, aVF	LAD
Lateral wall	I, aVL, V5, and V6	II, III, aVF	Circumflex or Obtuse Marginal
Right ventricle	V3–4R	I, aVL	RCA

Heart Failure

Heart failure is one of the most predominant conditions in the Medicare population. In fact, it is the most frequent diagnosis-related group (DRG) for acute care hospital admission in this population. Heart failure is a general term that describes an impaired cardiac function where either one or both of the ventricles are unable to maintain an adequate cardiac output to meet the metabolic demands for the body. Classification of heart failure is done with the use of the New York Heart Association (NYHA) Functional Classifications: Classes I–IV.

AHA/ACC Stages of Heart Failure

The American Heart Association (AHA)/American College of Cardiology (ACC) staging system for heart failure focuses on the progression and worsening of the condition over time. The AHA/ACC staging system moves forward from one stage to the next based on the progression of the disease. It helps doctors identify people who are at high risk for heart failure but don't have the condition yet (Stage A), those with heart damage but no symptoms of heart failure (Stage B), and those with heart damage and symptoms of heart failure (Stages C and D).

AHA/ACC HEART FAILURE STAGES	
Stage	**Description**
A	People at high risk for developing heart failure but who do not have heart failure or damage to the heart
B	People with damage to the heart but who have never had symptoms of heart failure; for example, those who have had a heart attack
C	People with heart failure symptoms caused by damage to the heart, including shortness of breath, tiredness, inability to exercise
D	People who have advanced heart failure and severe symptoms difficult to manage with standard treatment

New York Heart Association (NYHA) Classification System

The NYHA classification system is used to classify symptoms of heart disease, including heart failure. Symptoms are graded based on how much they limit your **functional capacity** (your ability to perform basic physical tasks). Unlike the AHA/ACC staging system, the NYHA classification can often shift from one level to another; for example, if you respond well to treatment and your symptoms improve, your NYHA class can go down. If you don't respond well and your symptoms continue to worsen, your NYHA class can go up.

NYHA HEART FAILURE CLASSIFICATION	
Class	**Description**
1 (Mild)	No limitation of physical activity, ordinary physical activity doesn't cause tiredness, heart palpitations, or shortness of breath
2 (Mild)	Slight limitation of physical activity, comfortable at rest, but ordinary physical activity results in tiredness, heart palpitations, or shortness of breath
3 (Moderate)	Marked or noticeable limitations of physical activity, comfortable at rest, but less than ordinary physical activity causes tiredness, heart palpitations, or shortness of breath
4 (Severe)	Severe limitation of physical activity, unable to carry out any physical activity without discomfort, symptoms also present at rest; if any physical activity is undertaken, discomfort increases

The highest classification (Class 4) describes a patient who remains symptomatic even at rest. Heart failure can be due to either a systolic dysfunction, such as cardiomyopathy or vavular disease, or diastolic dysfunction, such as acute myocardial infarction or drug abuse (cocaine).

When educating patients about heart failure and how this impacts their future quality of life, it is best to discuss the preservation of ejection fraction. This education should focus on diet, exercise tolerance, compliance with medication, daily weight monitoring, and when to discuss changes in their weight or breathing with their primary care physician. Noncompliance with medications can play a large role in heart failure hospital admissions; hence, it is important to discuss clearly the medication and diet regimen with each patient diagnosed with heart failure.

The pathophysiology of heart failure is complex and cyclical, which often leads to involvement of other organs, particularly when there is chronic fluid overload. The primary indicator of heart failure is ejection fraction. Normal ejection fraction (EF) is 50% to 70%. This is assessed with the use of a transthoracic echocardiogram (TTE), commonly referred to as "echo." The TTE will describe systolic and ventricular function, valvular dysfunction, and chamber sizes, and it may be able to estimate pulmonary artery pressure. Table 5.2 lists the clinical manifestations of left- and right-sided heart failure.

TABLE 5.2

LEFT-SIDED HEART FAILURE		RIGHT-SIDED HEART FAILURE
Systolic	**Diastolic**	
Fatigue, weakness, lethargy	Exercise intolerance	Easily fatigued
Orthopnea	Orthopnea	Dependent/pitting leg edema
Tachycardia on exertion	Tachycardia on exertion	Anorexia, GI distress
Basilar rales, rhonchi, crackles, and wheezes	Basilar rales, rhonchi, and wheezes	Weight gain
Elevated PAOP	Elevated PAOP	Oliguria
Murmur of mitral insufficiency	Holosystolic murmur if evidence of tricuspid or mitral regurgitation	Venous distension
Skin cool, moist, cyanosis		Extra heart sounds—S3
Hypoxia, respiratory acidosis	Hypoxia, respiratory acidosis	Elevated CVP, right atrial and right ventricular pressures

Left-Sided Heart Failure—Systolic

Left-sided heart failure is demonstrated by a series of events that ultimately leads to a failure of the left ventricle (poor contraction). Examples of etiologies of this type of heart failure include **idiopathic dilated cardiomyopathy** and **myocardial infarction**. This type of heart failure begins with a reduction in left ventricular contractility, resulting in an impairment of the cardiac output. The ejection fraction (EF) then falls to below normal (normal range = 50–75 percent). The ventricle compensates by dilating, and the heart rate increases as it attempts to maintain an adequate cardiac output. As discussed earlier, based on Starling's law, initially the contractility of the heart will increase, thereby increasing the stroke volume and cardiac output. However, if the dilation persists, the contractility will begin to decrease, further depressing the cardiac output. These responses may be satisfactory to increase the cardiac output, despite a poor EF. As stroke volume and heart rate increase, myocardial oxygen demands may increase. In addition, left atrial and pulmonary venous pressures increase as a result of myocardial dilatation and/or decreased left ventricular compliance. Pulmonary congestion and edema occur as these pressures rise and fluids leak into the pulmonary interstitial space. Subsequently the patient may demonstrate signs and symptoms of right-sided failure as a result of fluid overload and increased pulmonary pressures.

Left-Sided Heart Failure—Diastolic

In this type of heart failure, the ventricle is considered stiff or noncompliant (impaired filling). Etiologies of this type of heart failure include mitral stenosis, constrictive pericarditis, hypertrophic cardiomyopathy, or restrictive cardiomyopathy. The condition results in inadequate filling pressures and rising diastolic pressures. With increasing diastolic pressures also come increased left atrial, pulmonary venous, and pulmonary capillary pressures. In these cases, the systolic function may remain normal or be hyperdynamic.

Right-Sided Heart Failure

The etiology of right-sided heart failure can be varied but commonly is caused by fluid overload such as in renal failure, cardiomyopathy, or valvular disease. It can also result from pulmonary hypertension. In these conditions, the patient's right ventricle is unable to pump blood adequately into the pulmonary bed, which causes a drop in cardiac output. As a result, the right ventricle enlarges, in turn resulting in peripheral edema and elevated jugular venous pressure and corresponding distention. Occasionally in left ventricular myocardial infarction, the patient may show evidence of a right ventricular infarction, which could also result in right-sided heart failure. Another indication of right-sided heart failure is the presence of the hepatojugular reflex. Place the patient at a 30–45 degree angle, compress the right abdomen, and observe for distension of the neck veins. Positive distention of the jugular veins is indicative of heart failure.

Typically when a patient is admitted with heart failure, the first line of treatment is pharmacological. Initial treatment focuses on reducing the preload and afterload with diuretics and vasodilators for symptomatic relief and then inhibiting the renin-angiotensin-aldosterone system and sympathetic nervous system with ACEIs/ARBs, beta-blockers, and aldosterone antagonists. Once the causative condition is determined, the appropriate medications can be administered.

Pharmacologic Management

- *Diuretics* can be ordered either intravenously or orally based on the severity of the fluid overload. For severe cases, initial IV administration of a loop diuretic is preferred because the presence of bowel edema inhibits absorption of the oral form. Thiazide diuretics may be preferred in patients with mild fluid retention because of the persistent antihypertensive effects of these drugs. Transition to oral diuretics is made when the patient reaches near-normal blood volume. (The oral dose equivalent is usually equal to the IV dose.) Careful monitoring of electrolytes, particularly sodium, potassium, and magnesium, is necessary to ensure balance. Low-dose morphine (3–5 mg IV) produces a mild vasodilation and decreases venous return to the heart, anxiety, and pain.

- *Vasodilators* such as nitroprusside, nitroglycerin, or nesiritide may be considered in addition to diuretics in patients with acute heart failure or for symptom relief. *Nitroprusside* may be used to reduce afterload, especially if the patient is hypertensive. This effect occurs due to arterial dilatation and reduction of systemic and pulmonary vascular resistance. Rate of this infusion is 0.1 mcg/kg/min with a maximum dose of 8–10 mcg/kg/min. Like dopamine, this drug causes tissue sloughing and necrosis with extravasation. *Nesiritide* can be effective in patients with acutely decompensated heart failure who experience shortness of breath at rest. This drug is a recombinant form of the natural human peptide, hBNP. Nesiritide relaxes smooth muscle and causes both venous and arterial dilation (both of which cause a reduction in systemic vascular resistance), and it may be effective for patients where other therapies have not reduced the symptoms of heart failure. One of the significant side effects of nesiritide is hypotension, so it is critical that this patient be monitored closely. An IV bolus may be required to treat the hypotension, which may last for a period of time due to the half-life of the drug.

- Inotropic agents increase myocardial contractility. Phosphodiesterase inhibitors such as milrinone can improve contractility without increasing pulse. It will also relax vascular smooth muscle and cause vasodilatation. Dobutamine (Dobutrex) can increase contractility and stroke volume and reduce systemic vascular resistance (SVR). The patient should be monitored for hypotension, tachyarrhythmia, and ventricular ectopic beats.

- Vasopressors such as dopamine (Intropin) or phenylephrine (Neo-Synephrine) may be also used in heart failure to improve blood pressure. Phenylephrine effectively improves BP without causing tachycardia. For patients receiving dopamine, it is important to note that extravasation can cause tissue necrosis and sloughing. In the event of extravasation, stop the infusion immediately and prepare to give phentolamine.

ACC/AHA guidelines advise against the use of regularly scheduled intermittent intravenous infusions of positive inotropic drugs. Instead, the guidelines recommend use of positive inotropic agents (other than digoxin) only as palliative agents in patients with end stage disease who cannot be stabilized with standard medical treatment. NSAIDs, calcium channel blockers, and most antiarrhythmic agents (other than amiodarone and beta blockers) can exacerbate heart failure and should be avoided in most patients.

With all of the above intravenous medications, it is imperative for the critical care RN to closely monitor blood pressure and ECG to observe for hypotension and arrhythmias such as conduction defects. Neurological status should be monitored for decreased cerebral perfusion as well. Laboratory tests to evaluate electrolyte levels should be scheduled and replacement therapies ordered to ensure adequate blood levels, particularly when the patient is receiving diuretics or other medications which deplete electrolyte stores.

Cardiogenic Pulmonary Edema

As the name implies, cardiogenic pulmonary edema is the result of some type of cardiac dysfunction that occurs in late-stage heart failure. Typically, this occurs suddenly after an event that causes temporary overload of the work of the heart. It then becomes a vicious circle as the patient is unable to compensate for the changes. The cycle begins as a temporary increase in the load on the heart, often due to decreased pumping capacity of the heart (e.g., myocardial infarction, heavy exercise, or severe infection). The result is backing up of blood into the pulmonary bed. The increased blood in the lungs causes pulmonary capillary pressure to increase. Leaking of fluid begins to occur in the tissues and alveoli. Blood flowing through the capillary bed then cannot be oxygenated, and as a result, the body tries to conserve oxygen by causing peripheral vasodilatation. To compensate, the body tries to increase venous circulation from the periphery. There is more evidence of damming of the blood within the lungs. Further leaking occurs, and the cycle becomes circular. Symptoms the patient may experience include acute shortness of breath; frothy, pink-tinged sputum; and hypotension. The patient often requires immediate intubation and control of airway.

Late End Stage Heart Failure

In late stage heart failure, all reserves are exhausted, and the patient becomes end stage. Alternatively, or if the patient is determined to be a good candidate for transplantation, more interventional procedures such as insertion of a left ventricular assist device, right ventricular assist device, or biventricular assist device can be done to allow more time until an organ becomes available.

Left Ventricular Assist Device (LVAD)

The use of LVADs to bridge the period between end stage heart failure and transplant has decreased, and the goal of LVAD has changed to become a standard treatment for heart failure patients and permanent definitive therapy. Despite these advances, the mortality rate for heart failure patients remains high at 70 percent. Not all heart failure patients are candidates for ventricular assist devices. Younger patients with fewer morbidities are the best candidates for LVADs.

The criteria for insertion of LVAD include a lack of response to conventional medical therapies, as discussed above. Additionally, if the purpose of this device is a bridge to transplantation, the patient must meet the transplant criteria as well. It is also important that the patient not suffer from deterioration of renal and hepatic function, as these functions will be critical in the recovery during the postoperative period and for quality of life in the long run. If the patient has suffered respiratory failure requiring ventilation prior to transplant, the mortality risk significantly increases.

The device is typically inserted via a sternotomy while patient is on cardiopulmonary bypass. The inflow cannula is inserted into the left ventricle and tunneled to the external pump, while blood is returned via an outflow tract that has been inserted subcostally into the ascending aorta. The patient must be anticoagulated to prevent clot formation either in the blood exterior to the body or in the vasculature where the devices lie. The cannulas are connected to an external pump, via a pneumatic hose, to a blood sac, which pumps via alternating pressure and vacuum. The cannulas are covered with a synthetic material that encourages endothelial cell ingrowth, thus sealing the tract of the cannula to the mediastinum. This process can take up to 10 days.

Electrical backup is also required for the device, even though it primarily runs on a pneumatic system. The pump can be run on either a manual fixed rate that does not respond to the patient's own intrinsic heart rate or the preferred trigger, which is that when the device blood sac reaches full fill, the device then pumps the blood back to the patient. The second method reduces the chances of thrombus formation.

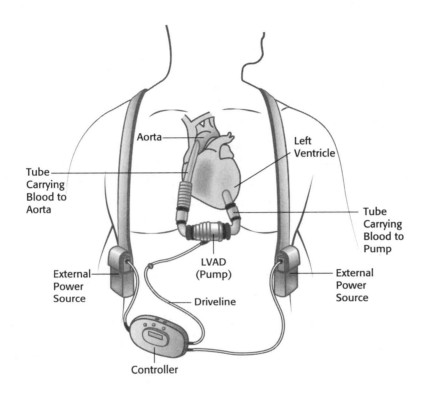

There are also totally implantable devices, which are electrically driven pulsatile LVADs made of titanium. The patient wears an external battery pack that is connected to the system controller. This is positioned either in the left upper abdominal quadrant or intra-abdominally. The insertion of this device requires entry into two compartments (thoracic via a sternotomy and abdominal via a laparotomy), which increases the opportunity for infection. Similar positioning of the cannulas occurs during insertion of the device. In these devices, air is displaced through a pump, and the air reenters through the same housing as a space is created by the ejection of the blood from the pump. The device also has the capability to be hand pumped in emergencies or be reconnected to a pneumatic device for patients who have to be rehospitalized.

Complications of the LVAD postoperatively include multiorgan failure, which is often due to preoperative conditions such as low perfusion states, right ventricular failure (especially if there is evidence of respiratory failure requiring mechanical ventilation preoperatively), bleeding due to anticoagulation or prolonged cardiopulmonary pump time, infection, neurologic events, arrhythmia, thromboembolism, and device malfunction. These are best managed with standard approaches to the patient's care in medical centers that are known for their expertise in use of these devices.

Right Ventricular Assist Device (RVAD)

Unfortunately one of the complications of LVADs is right-sided heart failure. This is often due to the fact that the failing heart, particularly the right side, does not have the capability to provide enough blood flow through the pulmonary circuit to fill the device. Occasionally, the patient can be managed with inotropes, nitrous oxide, or prostaglandins to increase the cardiac output and RV function. The effect of nitrous oxide is lowering of the pulmonary vascular resistance and mean pulmonary artery pressure, thus increasing LVAD flow. The RVADs currently in use require external drive systems. The RVAD receives blood from the right atrium, diverting it from the right ventricle, and delivers it to the pulmonary artery for distribution by the pulmonary vasculature. The device is connected to the right atrium and the pulmonary artery via vascular grafts from one of the passageways of the RVAD and exits via either a sternotomy or parasternal incision. Similar complications may develop with the use of RVADs as with LVADs and include thrombosis, bleeding, infection, secondary organ failure, and air emboli.

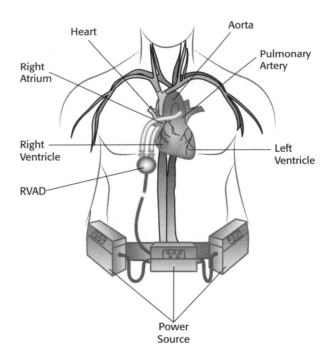

Biventricular Assist Device (BiVAD)

In conditions when there is failure of both ventricles, such as extensive cardiomyopathy or cardiogenic shock, biventricular assist devices can be used to bridge the period prior to transplantation or extend the period of cardiovascular support to promote recovery of the patient's own heart. Occasionally, these devices are used when the patient cannot be successfully removed from the cardiopulmonary bypass devices intraoperatively. Based on the location of the cannula placement at the time of insertion, either one or both ventricles can be bypassed. The system consists of two single-use blood pumps, cannulae (which are used to secure openings into the ventricles), aorta and pulmonary artery, and a pneumatic drive console.

Nursing Considerations with VADs

It is imperative that critical care nurses caring for the patient with VADs are familiar with the technical aspects of the device that their organization uses to provide ventricular assist. There are specialists who typically work in the cardiovascular operating arena called *cardiac perfusionists* who are specially trained with these types of devices and will serve as a resource. Additionally, device vendors typically have clinical nurse specialists who will assist with training on the devices.

Hemodynamic monitoring is continuous, and the frequency is based on the patient's clinical condition but should include vital signs, cardiac output measurements, hemodynamic measurements including pulmonary artery (PA) pressures, pulmonary artery occlusion pressures (PAOP) except in RVAD use, central venous pressure (CVP), and arterial pressures, intake and output, circulatory checks, and monitoring of arrhythmias.

The patient must be able to support a reasonable cardiac output for consideration for weaning to occur, as well as a mean arterial pressure > 60 mm Hg. Similar to ventilator weaning, the ventricular assist device flow rate is decreased gradually to ascertain if the patient's own ventricles will be able to sustain the cardiac output.

Peripheral Vascular Disease (PAD)

Similar to coronary artery disease, peripheral vascular disease develops most commonly due to atherosclerotic vessel disease. As a result of the narrowing or occlusion of the vessels, decreased perfusion to the extremities will occur, and damage to tissues most likely will result.

Arterial versus Venous Occlusion

Peripheral vascular disease (PVD) is divided into two categories: arterial and venous. Venous peripheral disease is chronic, evolves over time, and can be managed on an outpatient basis once diagnosis is made and the patient is adequately anticoagulated. On the other hand, arterial peripheral vascular disease may require acute intervention for a thrombotic occlusion to preserve the limb. PVD may occur in any peripheral vessel but most often occurs in the lower extremities.

Acute Arterial Occlusion

Vessels that are most commonly affected from arterial peripheral vascular disease are the superficial femoral artery, popliteal artery, distal aorta, and iliac arteries. In arterial peripheral vascular disease, blood flow is occluded either by a thrombus or narrowing of the vessel and ischemic muscle pain ensues. These symptoms appear after 75 percent of the vessel is occluded. The pain from ischemia can be extreme. If the vessel is not totally occluded, the patient may experience claudication, which is an intermittent aching pain when walking. Claudication can be relieved by rest and may remain unchanged for many years. Arterial peripheral vascular disease can be clinically assessed using Doppler ultrasound to calculate ankle-brachial indices (ABI). Low ABI are diagnostic of arterial PVD.

TABLE 5.3 *Comparison between Arterial and Venous Leg Ulcers*

	Arterial Ulcers	**Venous Ulcers**
Site	Any part of the leg, usually between the toes or at the end of the toes	Ankle (gaiter area), around the medial malleolus
Size	Usually small	Usually large
Edges	Deep, with "cliff" edge	Shallow with diffuse edges
Edema	Localized	Generalized
Staining	None	Brownish pigmentation
Ankle Brachial Index (ABI)	<0.8	>0.8
Pain	Present, especially at night	Some, especially when standing
Pulses	Reduced or absent	Normal
Wound Surface	Dry/necrotic	Exuding/granulating

Acute arterial occlusion is evidenced by sudden onset of severe pain, loss of pulse to the extremity, cold skin, pallor of the skin, and impaired motor and sensory function. These symptoms are also known as the five "P's": pain, pallor, pulselessness, paresthesia, and paresis. This condition is a surgical emergency and requires immediate intervention to remove the obstruction or to stent the artery. Without rapid intervention, the patient will likely suffer the loss of the limb due to excessive tissue damage and gangrene, which can lead to sepsis.

Severe blockage due to plaque in the femoral artery is treated with femoral popliteal bypass surgery. This open vessel surgery attaches a piece of another blood vessel above and below the blocked portion of the artery, rerouting the blood flow around the blockage through the new vessel. Percutaneous transluminal angioplasty (PTA) is a minimally invasive procedure used to open the blocked or narrowed femoral artery and to restore blood flow to the distal leg without open vascular surgery. A catheter with a tiny balloon at its tip is inserted into the femoral artery; once in place, the balloon is inflated and the fatty tissue in the artery is compressed, making a larger opening. Following surgery, peripheral pulses (or Doppler ultrasound signals) should be checked frequently. Routine medications include an antiplatelet agent, a beta-blocker, and a statin.

Venous Occlusion

One of the most common forms of venous occlusion is the **deep vein thrombosis** (DVT). The etiology of DVT is often immobility when blood flow is diminished to the vessel for hours and venous stasis occurs. Clots form and can occlude lower extremity vessels even as far up as the iliac vein and the inferior vena cava. These clots can also become systemic and cause pulmonary embolism, which may be life threatening. The acute treatment for venous occlusion is anticoagulation with *enoxaparin* or *heparin*. Heparin is primarily indicated for renal patients or patients who may require surgical intervention and, thus, rapid reversal of the anticoagulation. Prevention is the most appropriate treatment, including early mobilization and prophylaxis with low molecular weight heparin; this is why all bedfast critically ill patients should be on this medication unless contraindicated. Hospitals have also begun to institute the use of sequential compression devices (SCDs) to inflate and compress the veins of the lower extremities intermittently, simulating muscular contraction during ambulation. For patients where anticoagulant therapy is contraindicated, the physician may insert an inferior vena cava (IVC) filter to prevent the movement of thrombi from the lower extremities to the lungs.

Arterial Aneurysm

An aneurysm is described as a weakening of a vessel wall resulting in a bulging and wall stress at the site. Within the body there are several sites where aneurysms can develop as a result of atherosclerosis. These include the following vessels: thoracic and abdominal aorta, femoral and popliteal arteries, and the circle of Willis (berry aneurysm). Several potential complications can occur as a result of arterial aneurysms, including rupture, dissection, and stenosis. Location of the aneurysm and expediency in the treatment will determine the outcome for the patient if one of these complications occurs. Dissections and ruptures especially require immediate surgical intervention to prevent rapid blood loss. The mortality rate remains high for these situations, up to 80 percent. We will focus our discussion in this section on the complications associated with aortic dissections.

Aortic Rupture

When the wall of the vessel weakens beyond a certain point, the vessel ruptures and immediate arterial blood loss occurs. Rupture more likely occurs if the vessels are dilated beyond 5–6 cm. Immediate treatment would include fluid and blood replacement and surgical intervention. With aortic rupture, a significant amount of blood loss results in hypoperfusion to key end organs, including the brain and kidneys. If the patient survives the initial event, end organ failure is likely to occur as a result of lengthy hypoperfusion.

Aortic Dissection

The primary difference between aortic rupture and aortic dissection is that in aortic dissection, a tear likely occurs in the intima of the vessel, which then moves up and down the vessel causing a larger tearing and leaking of blood into the column of the intima. The patient will describe the pain from this dissection as "tearing or ripping" whose onset is sudden and abrupt. This pain may also be described as radiating to the back between the blades of the scapula. In addition to noting the distinctive pain pattern, the critical care nurse may note a significant difference in the interarm blood pressures. It is imperative to communicate your findings emergently to the physician, as immediate surgical intervention is required. Perfusion to key organs may still occur. However, if the bleeding extends into the valves and pericardium, ischemia may occur, and end organ damage will result. The most significant risk factor for aortic dissection is hypertension. Cocaine use has also been identified as a risk factor, as it produces a sudden elevation in blood pressure. The patient can be initially managed with antihypertensives and pain control. However, immediate surgical intervention is required. Even with surgical intervention, the mortality for aortic dissection remains at approximately 80 percent.

Carotid Artery Stenosis

Similar to the above-referenced peripheral vascular conditions, the carotid arteries may also develop atherosclerosis and plaque. Symptoms that may develop as a result of carotid artery stenosis are primarily neurological since these vessels provide blood flow to the brain. With significant blockage, the patient may experience transient ischemic attacks (TIAs) or stroke. Permanent brain damage can occur as a result of lengthy hypoperfusion to the brain. Often, if the occlusion or stenosis is gradual in onset, collateral circulation will develop and provide adequate circulation. Stenotic areas of more than 75 percent in the vessels are more prone to the development of thrombosis due to the sluggish blood flow and adhesion of platelets and fibrin. Diagnosis is made by carotid Doppler studies.

Carotid Stent

If the carotid artery blockage is due to stenosis, the physician may elect to implant a stent to provide a more permanent means to keep the artery open. This is a minimally invasive procedure done under local anesthetic. An incision is made in the femoral artery, and a guide wire is threaded to the site of blockage. A balloon is used to dilate the artery, and a stent is inserted to keep the vessel open.

Endarterectomy

Another surgical procedure to clear the blockage in the carotid artery is called an endarterectomy. The vessel is surgically opened, and the atheromatous plaque substance is removed. Once hemostasis is achieved, the vessel is closed. The disadvantage of this procedure over stenting is that it typically requires general anesthesia and there is a chance that the blockage may reappear, requiring another surgical procedure. Neurological assessment is a priority post-endarterectomy.

Angioplasty

Angioplasty is used in conjunction with the stenting procedure for carotid artery occlusion. Angioplasty is dilatation of the vessel via a balloon catheter inserted via a major vessel, typically in the groin or arm. Occasionally, simply the opening of the vessel via the balloon angioplasty is enough to provide adequate blood flow through the vessel, and the vessel remains open. More commonly, however, the stent is placed to allow for long-term recovery. These procedures are fairly new for carotid blockages, even though they have been used for some time with coronary artery occlusion.

Peripheral Stenting

As with coronary artery and carotid artery stenting, new techniques are being developed with the use of the balloon catheter, angioplasty, and insertion of stenting for peripheral vessel occlusion. The most common sites are the iliac, femoral popliteal artery, and renal arteries.

INTERVENTIONAL CARDIOLOGY

Cardiac Catheterization (Percutaneous Coronary Intervention, PCI)

Cardiac catheterization can be performed on an elective basis to diagnose coronary artery disease and blood flow, or it can be done emergently in conjunction with PTCA to open a coronary vessel when an obstructive atherosclerotic lesion is causing acute coronary ischemia and infarction. PTCA requires advancement of a balloon-tipped catheter through a percutaneous insertion site such as the femoral artery and vein. The catheter is threaded into the coronary artery system, and dye is injected to evaluate the patency of these vessels. If there is an observed obstruction, a guidewire can be inserted through the introducer, and the balloon catheter can be threaded to the site of the lesion and inflated to open the vessel. Stents may be placed in the vessel to assure continued patency. The patient does require systemic anticoagulation.

Intracoronary thrombolytics can also be injected through the catheter to the site of the lesion. There is a strong likelihood (30–40 percent) of restenosis of the vessel within the first six months of the procedure. Access to a surgical suite with open heart capability should always be available during this time due to the potential complication for acute coronary occlusion resulting from dissection, acute bleeding at the insertion site, or perforation of a coronary vessel.

There are multiple pressure or closure devices that can be used after the removal of the catheter. Manual pressure at the site of insertion should be held for a minimum of 15 minutes and frequently checked and observed for evidence of hematoma. However, newer closure devices are being used to prevent the need for manual pressure, which is not always effective. These include Fem-Stop, C-clamps, and other similar arterial closure devices (Angio-Seal, Perclose, StarClose, and Boomerang). The affected leg should remain straight and immobile for the next six to eight hours. Continuous cardiac and vital sign monitoring and CMS checks on the affected extremity should be done as a standard of care.

Complications that may occur after arterial cannulation/cardiac catheterization may include the following: hematoma, AV fistula, pseudoaneurysm, retroperitoneal bleed, and acute loss of distal circulation. Typically, a hematoma is the result of inadequate or early release of pressure on the insertion site. Care should be taken to ensure the artery has closed sufficiently and there is no evidence of subcutaneous bleeding. The patient should be assessed for bruit over the site of sheath insertion at least every eight hours. A positive bruit over the site, in combination with localized pain and a pulsatile mass, is indicative of a pseudoaneurysm—which requires immediate notification to the physician and surgical intervention or ultrasound-guided compression.

Cardiac Mapping—Identification of Localized Cardiac Potentials

Patients who have been diagnosed with irregular heart rhythms that may be caused by irritable or abnormal heart tissue can potentially be treated with ablation or an implantable cardiac pacemaker once the areas are localized and the cause of the arrhythmia determined. A procedure called cardiac mapping uses electrophysiology to create a three-dimensional "map" of the heart tissue; a specialized catheter has multiple miniature electrodes that are inserted percutaneously and serve similarly to a radio antenna receiving electrical signals from the various heart tissues or as a stimulator of electrical activity. These electrical signals are forwarded to a computerized software system, which creates the map. Once the area(s) have been identified as the cause of the arrhythmia, the interventional cardiologist must then make a decision as to what treatment approach is best for the patient. These approaches can include medication, implantable cardioverter defibrillator (ICD), pacemaker, or ablation therapy. Ablation therapy appears to be most effective for unstable ventricular tachycardias or complex atrial rhythms.

Newer electrophysiology systems have better resolution than older systems, which has provided increased insight into the mechanisms of cardiac arrhythmias. They have both contact and noncontact electrode catheters and more sophisticated computer systems to interpret the signals from these electrode catheters. In many facilities, these units are cost prohibitive and the skill required to perform the mapping is very specialized, which limits the ability to provide this service.

CARDIOTHORACIC SURGERY

After a brief period of reduction in the frequency of deaths due to cardiovascular disease from 1980 to 1990, deaths from cardiovascular disease have increased. As of 2014, heart disease is the leading cause of death in the United States. Even more troubling, there has been an increase in deaths in women from cardiovascular disease, while deaths in men have remained stable. Atherosclerosis remains the number one cause of coronary artery disease. Diet and genetic predisposition to the disease are contributing factors.

Acute coronary artery occlusion occurs as a result of the following:

1. The atherosclerotic plaque is an uneven surface where platelets form and fibrin is deposited. Red blood cells are attracted to this area, and a clot forms in the coronary

artery. Occasionally, this clot will break away and move to a more peripheral vessel of the coronary artery. The vessel may be partially or completely occluded. The patient experiences chest pain as a result, and coronary ischemia or infarction occurs from the point of the blockage and peripherally. ECG changes include ST elevation or depression in electrical leads that correspond with the ischemic tissue (see table 5.1 earlier for area of infarction and 12 lead ECG changes).

2. Additionally, local muscular spasm of the coronary artery can occur, which stimulates local nervous system reflexes and, in turn, wall contraction. Theories exist that this, too, may cause secondary thrombosis in the vessel.

3. Collateral blood flow develops, which sustains the coronary tissue health. It is felt that this may occur as soon as seconds after the primary occlusion and may provide up to 50 percent of the coronary blood flow to that area. This initial development does not change significantly until approximately two to three days after the injury, when there is a significant increase in the blood flow from the collaterals.

Coronary Artery Bypass Grafting (CABG)

The first coronary artery bypass was performed in 1967. In CABG, the myocardium is revascularized using grafts to bypass the blockage in the obstructed coronary arteries. It has been accepted as a safe and effective means in relieving medically uncontrolled angina pectoris and for revasculature of left main coronary artery, triple vessel disease, double vessel disease involving the LAD, or coronary artery disease with EF < 35 percent. There are cases where additional vessels will be grafted based on quality of circulation to the myocardium; however, the outcome may not be as successful in the prevention of mortality compared to coronary artery stenting. The length of an acute hospital stay for CABG has decreased considerably over the recent past with the length of stay now five to six days or nine for Medicare patients.

On-Pump CABG

Cardiopulmonary bypass is a mechanical device used for diverting and oxygenating the patient's blood away from the heart and lungs during CABG surgery. The patient must be heparinized during the period on pump. Incorporated into the pump is a means to chill the blood to approximately 28 °C and then to warm it prior to discontinuance of bypass. This reduces tissue oxygen requirements during the surgical procedure.

The sites for securing the graft vessels include the saphenous veins, internal mammary arteries, gastroepiploic artery, and radial artery. At this point, long-term patency is better with the mammary arteries. In addition, using mammary arteries prevents the need for leg incisions.

Postperfusion Syndrome

Postperfusion syndrome, or "pumphead" as it is more commonly called, is a neurocognitive syndrome that is evidenced in postoperative on-pump CABG patients. The symptoms of this include memory impairment, stilted speech, depression, confusion, and decreased hand–eye coordination. This syndrome is considered transient, and most patients resume normal cognitive function within a short period after surgery. Most functions return within 3 months, and after 12 months there is negligible evidence of the syndrome. There are varying theories as to the potential causes of this syndrome. One theory is that there are microemboli that are showered during the pump time. As a result of the research, which has demonstrated this syndrome is at minimum worrisome, and its etiology has not been clearly identified, surgeons promote the use of the minimum cardiopulmonary bypass time as needed for the procedure and are doing "off-pump" procedures if possible. Recent studies indicate that the underlying cause of "pumphead" is cardiac disease itself, and not the use of a heart-lung machine or pump.

Off-Pump CABG

Approximately 20–25 percent of the CABG procedures performed in the United States are done without the use of the cardiopulmonary bypass pump device. This procedure was implemented with the goal of reducing mortality and morbidity related to the on-pump procedure, particularly in high-risk groups. Thus far, studies have demonstrated that the graft patency rates are equal.

This procedure appears to be more successful in patients with focal stenosis versus diffuse disease. It also prevents the "pumphead" syndrome that develops in the postoperative period from the on-pump procedure. In contrast to the cooling of the patient's blood during the period when it is out of the patient, the off-pump procedure warms the patient with warming mattresses, warmed fluids, and warmed anesthesia gases. Off-pump CABG requires very specific positioning of the patient to maximize the visibility and access to the coronary arteries that are to be bypassed, specifically displacement of the heart to the right, and the use of mechanical stabilizers by compression or suction to control the constantly moving heart. Medications such as beta-blockers or calcium channel blockers are used to slow the heart to reduce movement as well. The sequence of the grafting of the vessels is from the easiest graft to the most difficult. It is felt that this helps with perfusion of tissues while the more difficult vessels are being repaired.

Long-term studies will provide additional support for this procedure over the on-pump procedure, with more data on long-term survival and graft patency.

Endoscopic Vein Harvesting

One of the most uncomfortable parts of the recovery from CABG in the past has been the healing of the wounds from where the graft vessels were harvested, particularly in the legs. This process was often hampered in diabetic patients, who occasionally would have prolonged healing times and the development of infections. A new technique in harvesting graft veins using an endoscopic approach is now being used. The benefits of this approach are smaller incisions required to remove an appropriate length of the vein, decreased pain, fewer wound-healing complications, reduced scarring, and faster recovery time.

Robotic-Assisted Surgery

Another new technique in cardiovascular surgery is using a robotic surgery system, which combines the traditional approach with laparoscopic techniques. The most common cardiovascular procedure for which this device is used is mitral valve replacement (MVR). Some of the benefits of this type of surgery are that sternotomy and rib spreading are not required—there is a shorter recovery period, less opportunity for infection, less blood loss, and potentially a better outcome.

One of the drawbacks of this procedure is that the surgeon has to be specially trained on the device and become efficient with hand-to-eye coordination, which is quite different than that required by traditional surgical instruments. Another deterrent for many organizations is the cost of the device, which exceeds $1 million.

Valve Replacement

Insufficient, prolapsed, or stenotic valves often require replacement in order to eliminate the hemodynamic dysfunctions that are associated with these problems.

However, medical management is used as long as the patient is asymptomatic. The goal is to maintain as much left ventricular function as possible during this phase. The assessment of ventricular function is most often done with the TTE (transthoracic echocardiogram). With surgical valve replacement, there are inherent risks with the use of both prosthetic and biological tissue valves.

Valvular Defects

Not all valvular defects require surgical intervention. The most common valves replaced in a surgical intervention are the aortic and mitral valves. The nursing interventions that should be undertaken with patients who have valvular defects include the following: a thorough assessment of hemodynamic stability and adequacy of tissue perfusion, evaluation of dysrhythmias, assuring diagnostic studies are carried out in a timely and efficient manner, standardized postoperative care, education based on assessed needs, and administration of medications that are pertinent to the patient's care.

Aortic Stenosis

In aortic stenosis, the inability of the valve to open effectively is due to the obstructive narrowing of the valve. Over time, the valve becomes thickened and calcified. As a result, there is impedance of blood flow to the aorta. To adapt to the increased pressure gradient, it has to push against the left ventricle hypertrophies and so becomes stiff and noncompliant. Left atrial and pulmonary artery pressures subsequently increase as the stiffened left ventricle works to eject the blood. Pulmonary congestion and right heart failure will then develop. Currently, the only effective surgical intervention for aortic valve disease is aortic valve replacement (AVR). The goal of AVR is to preserve ventricular function.

Valve replacement is done with either a mechanical valve made from a combination of metal alloys, such as pyrolite carbon, Dacron, and Teflon, or a bioprosthetic valve, such as a bovine, porcine, or human heart valve. This procedure requires open heart surgery and carries the risks associated with an interventional procedure such as infection, bleeding, hemodynamic instability, etc. In addition, as a result of the risk of stroke intra- or postoperatively due to emboli that originate from a calcified valve, cannulation of the aorta, hypoperfusion, or prosthetic valve thrombosis, the post-valve-replacement patient will need to be placed on anticoagulation such as intravenous heparin or enoxaparin. *Warfarin* may be used when the patient is stabilized and being prepared for discharge.

The normal International Normalization Ratio (INR), a measure of the effects of warfarin, without anticoagulation is 1.0. The expected therapeutic range for patients who have undergone valve replacement is 2.5 to 3.5. There are special diet modifications for patients who are on anticoagulants, including avoidance of foods high in vitamin K (broccoli, lettuce, spinach, and liver). Additionally, medications that can alter bleeding times should be avoided as well (e.g., aspirin, ibuprofen, birth control pills, and certain antibiotics).

Mitral Stenosis

The definition of mitral stenosis is a progressive narrowing (not opening properly) of the mitral valve opening to less than 1.5 cm. This can be caused simply by the aging process, but it may also develop as a result of inflammation and rheumatic fever. Fibrosis of one or more leaflets of the valves can cause fusion of one or both commisures. The chordae tendineae may also become thickened and shortened and decrease the mobility of the valve. As with aortic stenosis, the blood flow is impeded, and chamber pressures increase. If the orifice of the valve diminishes to less than 1 cm², pulmonary hypertension occurs, and increased pulmonary pressures cause an increase in right ventricular pressures, which could ultimately cause right-sided heart failure.

With mitral stenosis, the choices for correction are commissurotomy and valve replacement. During a commissurotomy, the fused leaflets of the stenotic valve are incised and debrided to improve valve mobility. Reconstruction avoids the potential complications that come with valve replacement surgery and prosthetic valves. Commissurotomy may eliminate the need for long-term anticoagulation.

Aortic Regurgitation

Regurgitation occurs when the cardiac valve becomes incompetent or weakened (not closing properly) by damage or degeneration of the cusps of the valves. The valves become "floppy," and blood flows backward during diastole as a result of the lack of complete closure of the valve. In turn, forward flow of blood is inhibited, peripheral vasoconstriction occurs, and aortic diastolic pressure decreases. The body attempts to compensate for the reduced blood flow by increasing heart rate, and as a result, oxygen myocardial demand increases and can potentially lead to ischemia and sudden death. *Widening pulse pressures* also occur and demonstrate low aortic diastolic pressures in the presence of high systemic pressures. The etiology of aortic regurgitation can be infection, idiopathic calcifications, congenital malformations, hypertension, trauma, and aneurysms.

Transcatheter Aortic Valve Replacement (TAVR)

Surgical aortic valve replacement (SAVR) is the gold standard treatment for aortic stenosis (AS); it reduces symptoms and improves survival. However, a large number of patients present a prohibitive risk for SAVR. Transcatheter aortic valve replacement (TAVR), or transcatheter aortic valve implantation (TAVI), is minimally invasive—surgical procedure repairs the valve without removing the old, damaged valve. Instead, it wedges a replacement valve into the aortic valve's place. The native aortic valve remains and is displaced against the aorta by the new valve implantation. Once in place, the new prosthetic valve begins to function. TAVR is indicated for use in senile degenerative calcification of the aortic valve (not for use in congenital bicuspid AS).

Somewhat similar to the placement of a stent in an artery, the TAVR approach delivers a fully collapsible replacement valve to the valve site through a catheter. This procedure is fairly new and is FDA-approved for people with symptomatic aortic stenosis who are considered an intermediate or high-risk patient for standard valve replacement surgery. The differences in the two procedures are significant. The benefits of TAVR include reduction in all-cause mortality, cardiovascular mortality, and repeat hospitalizations. Improvements in mean gradient and valve area, NYHA functional class, 6-Minute Walk Test, and quality of life are also noted with TAVR procedure.

Potential adverse effects and complications from TAVR procedure include: stroke, conduction disturbance, the need for a permanent pacemaker, bleeding, acute MI, valve dysfunction, paravalvular leak, urgent need for surgery, thrombosis, perforation, tamponade, and infection.

Mitral Valve Regurgitation

Mitral valve regurgitation (valve not closing properly) can occur chronically or acutely. Causes of chronic mitral valve disease of this nature can be infectious or autoimmune, congenital malformations, dilation of the left ventricle from other causes, and connective tissue diseases such as Marfan's syndrome. Acute disease can be caused by rupture of the chordae tendineae from endocarditis or rheumatic heart disease, traumatic injury, or papillary muscle dysfunction.

In mitral valve regurgitation, blood flows back into the left atrium (regurgitation) as a result of the incompetent valve. Left atrial diastolic pressures suddenly increase when this occurs acutely. As a result of the rapid onset, the left atrium cannot compensate for the change, and cardiac output falls dramatically, causing pulmonary edema and cardiogenic shock. Often the patient requires an intra-aortic balloon pump (IABP) and vasopressors for support until the patient is stabilized for surgical intervention.

Most Common Congenital Repairs

When caring for patients with congenital or acute defects of the heart, it is imperative for the critical care nurse to be observant for hemodynamic stability and changes that occur as a result of the increase in the ventricular and atrial pressures. This includes assessing the patient for evidence of shunting and the possible direction of the shunt, monitoring for atrial and junctional rhythms and conduction blocks, pre- and postoperative care, and administration of antibiotics to prevent infection.

Septal Defects

Structural defects may occur as a result of acute myocardial infarction in adults or may be congenital in infants and children. With these defects, blood most often is shunted from the areas of high pressure to low pressure, which is typically left ventricle to right ventricle. If the shunt is severe, the patient may develop acute heart failure, shock, and death. When the left to right shunt is long-standing, the right ventricular pressures may increase and surpass that of the left ventricle, causing peripheral cyanosis, referred to as Eisenmenger's syndrome (see Ventricular Septal Defect below).

Atrial Septal Defect

A defect may occur in the septum at the level of the atrium that allows shunting of blood to occur between left and right atria. There are typically three types of atrial septal defects: sinus venosus, ostium secundum, and ostium primum defects. These are named based on the location of the defect. A sinus venosus occurs where the right atrium and superior vena cava join. The ostium secundum occurs around the area of the foramen ovale. This type of defect is the most common of the three. The final defect, ostium primum, occurs at the lower end of the septum.

Most often the blood is shunted from the area of higher pressure to the lower pressure, in this case, left atrium to right atrium. Fluid overload subsequently occurs due to increased blood flow to the right heart. A systolic murmur is audible as blood flow increases across the pulmonic valve. Echocardiography and cardiac catheterization can assist with the diagnosis of atrial septal defect.

The exact cause of this type of defect is not known but may be related to maternal and fetal infections early in the pregnancy, medications, or genetic factors. Surgical intervention is recommended to avoid long-term pulmonary hypertension. A pericardial or Dacron patch is used to repair the defect. With repair of septal defects, there is a chance that the patient may develop conduction blocks due to injury of the bundle of His. In these situations, the patient may require a temporary pacemaker.

Ventricular Septal Defect

The ventricular septal defect (VSD) occurs between the ventricles within some portion of the membranous or muscular septum. The VSD is the most common type of congenital defect in children and occurs along with other types of defects. In addition to the membranous or muscular types, there are three additional types: supra-cristal, AV canal type, and crista superventricularis.

Smaller defects may close spontaneously and do not cause significant hemodynamic instability. Larger defects will cause shunting from left to right and an increase in the pulmonary venous return to the left atrium and, subsequently, the left ventricle. As pressures increase on the left, pulmonary congestion occurs and over time can lead to pulmonary hypertension. The pulmonary hypertension may then become irreversible, and systemic pressures can increase so that the shunt becomes right to left. This condition is called Eisenmenger's syndrome.

The repair of these defects requires open heart surgery with a sternotomy and cardiopulmonary bypass. A patch will be applied to the defect. Similar to the atrial septal defect, conduction arrhythmias can occur due to potential injury to the AV node or bundle of His. Patients will also be treated prophylactically with antibiotics to prevent infections such as endocarditis.

Patent Ductus Arteriosus

During fetal development, there is a patent connection between the descending aorta and the pulmonary artery to bypass the underdeveloped lungs. On occasion, this patency does not seal off as it should at the time of birth, and there remains a ductus (hole) between those two vessels. Since the aorta has a higher pressure flow, oxygenated blood will flow from the aorta through the patent ductus to the pulmonary artery and subsequently to the lungs. Symptoms of left-sided heart failure develop due to the increased fluid load on the lungs and left side of the heart. If the pressures begin to increase on the right side and within the pulmonary artery, the blood will begin to shift right to left. As a result, right-sided heart failure and cyanosis will occur. In large shunts, deoxygenated blood will be fed to the left arm and lower parts of the body below the ductus, while the upper body continues to receive oxygenated blood without problems. These patients are more prone to endocarditis and may have vegetative valvular growths which may embolize to the lungs. The end result is infarction and death.

Surgical intervention would be required when the patient experiences heart failure or, in children, if the ductus remains open after six months of life. The patent ductus should be closed and on occasion a patch may be required to successfully accomplish this. In severe cases where pulmonary hypertension and right to left shunting occur, the patient would need a heart–lung transplant. If the patient is unstable and cannot undergo open heart surgery, a transcatheter closure might be performed as an alternative. These procedures may not be successful but pose a lesser risk than a thoracotomy with closure.

Coarctation of the Aorta

This congenital defect typically is described as a narrowing or infolding of the lumen of the aorta. The result is increased resistance to the ejection of blood from the left ventricle proximal to the narrowing and decreased pressures and diminished blood flow distal to the narrowing. The defect most often occurs just past the branching of the third large vessel from the arch of the aorta, the left subclavian artery.

Similar to other defects, the ventricle enlarges as a result of the increased pressure gradient and can fail due to the increased afterload. Prolonged hypertension can lead to other conditions that result from cardiovascular disease such as strokes, CAD, heart failure, and possibly aortic dissection or rupture. Collateral circulation develops and helps to feed the lower body and extremities with oxygenated blood.

One of the distinct radiological findings of coarctation of the aorta is something called the "3" sign. This triad of findings is a dilated ascending aorta, constriction of the aorta, and a poststenotic dilation. A cardiac catheterization would be required to identify the degree of coronary artery disease and to assess the depth of the pressure gradients. An aortogram can also be done to assess the narrowing itself.

Surgical correction is required to excise the coarctation, either by an end-to-end anastomosis or an aortoplasty. The approach is via a thoracotomy incision. Complications of this type of surgery are typical for a thoracotomy and include hemothorax, chylothorax, paradoxical hypertension, and transient abdominal pain. Spontaneous aortic rupture can occur in an older patient prior to surgical intervention and most often leads to death.

Myxoma Removal

A cardiac myxoma is a benign neoplasm of the heart, most commonly located in the left atrium (75 percent of the cases) along the septum. The myxoma's origin is not known for certain, although it is thought to be a true tumor that originates from an infectious response from an organism such as herpes simplex, human papillomavirus, Epstein-Barr virus, or an inherited autosomal trait.

A triad of symptoms is demonstrated in a patient with myxoma, including heart failure (due to obstruction caused by the size of the tumor), evidence of embolism, and systemic illness involving fever and weight loss or fatigue. The patient may also experience general malaise or arthralgias.

Surgical resection of the tumor is the only current treatment available for this type of tumor. This is done via a sternotomy incision; the patient must be placed on cardiopulmonary bypass so that the area can be visualized and manipulated to ensure adequate resection of the tumor. Often the mitral valve will have to be replaced due to proximity to the tumor and the need to resect a portion of the myocardial wall. Recurrence of the tumor has a low probability even with a predisposition to the tumor due to genetic linkages.

Transmyocardial Laser Revascularization

The transmyocardial laser revascularization procedure is often done in conjunction with other open heart procedures, but it may be performed independently in a patient who continues to have unrelieved chest pain. The procedure requires a thoracotomy or sternotomy incision to access the heart tissue, although it can be accomplished via minimally invasive surgery. A specialized instrument that uses a carbon dioxide laser to create small channels in the exposed myocardium is used for this procedure. The external exposed openings close, while the internal openings assist in creating channels or bloodlines for the blood to circulate. The expected outcomes of these procedures are reduced angina chest pain, success in long-term pain control, and improved quality of life.

Thoracic Aneurysm Repair

Thoracic aneurysms are a significant health risk and can cause immediate death if the aneurysm ruptures and there is massive bleeding. Aneurysms do not typically manifest themselves until the patient reaches approximately 60 years of age or older, and they primarily occur in men. Thoracic aneurysms can occur in the ascending, transverse, or descending aorta or in the iliac, popliteal, or femoral arteries. Patients describe the pain with a dissection or rupture as a sudden ripping pain that radiates into the shoulders, neck, and back. There may be evidence of change in the patient's voice such as hoarseness or weakness, and a cough may be produced. As the blood accumulates in the thoracic cavity, there may be pressure placed on the trachea, which can cause dysphagia, dyspnea, and physical shifting of the trachea.

The nurse may observe other manifestations of the aneurysm in addition to those listed above. There may be audible bruits over the aorta or other related arteries. The patient may experience hypertension if intrathoracic pressure increases or severe hypotension if bleeding occurs. *Pulse pressures* (the difference between systolic and diastolic pressures) *widen,* and there may be a significant difference in blood pressures from one arm to the other. Pressure differences of greater than 10 mm Hg indicate the potential for dissection or occlusion of major arteries in the thorax. Shock symptoms may also appear such as cool, pale, diaphoretic skin; absence of central pressures and peripheral pulses; and sluggish capillary refill.

The patient requires immediate surgical intervention for dissection or rupture, as well as fluids and vasopressors to support blood pressure while preparing for surgery. An IABP is *contraindicated* due to the damage to the aorta.

MAZE Procedure for Treatment of Atrial Dysrhythmias/Radiofrequency Ablation for Intractable Supraventricular or Ventricular Dysrhythmias

The MAZE procedure is named for the appearance of an electrical "maze," which occurs as a result of a series of cuts made into the atrial tissues. It is indicated for patients who have *atrial fibrillation* or *atrial flutter* refractory to medical therapy. The goal of the "maze" is to disrupt reentry pathways and direct the impulse of the sinus node to the AV node. The end result is restoration of sinus rhythm and AV synchrony. If there is evidence that the sinus node is nonfunctional, a pacemaker will be implanted to restore AV rhythm. The MAZE procedure requires open heart surgery and, therefore, has the same risks as a CABG, including bleeding, infection, and cardiac dysrhythmias.

CARDIAC TRAUMA

Cardiac trauma occurs as a result of either blunt trauma (motor vehicle injuries, cardiac contusions, falls, or deceleration injuries) to the chest or penetrating trauma (stabbing, gunshot injury, or fractures of the ribs). The injury may be limited to the pericardium, one or more chambers of the heart, or the major arteries/veins, or it may be more diffuse such as in cardiac contusions. Obtaining an accurate history of the injury is critical for ascertaining the interventions to be implemented. If the patient is unconscious, attempt to obtain a history from direct observers or the emergency personnel who attended the patient at the site of injury. The nurse should be somewhat of a skeptic when obtaining the history from other sources and maintain a high degree of suspicion for cardiac injury in any of these types of events.

Blunt Trauma

One of the most common causes of blunt nonpenetrating injury to the heart is from the steering wheel of a motor vehicle. Other causes of blunt cardiac trauma include falls, physical crushing assault, direct blows to the chest, kicks from large animals, blasts, and electrical injuries. Patients who are injured in this manner require a 12-lead ECG and continuous cardiac monitoring to observe for myocardial damage. In addition to this type of global injury, blunt trauma can cause shearing or tearing of major vessels, resulting in massive hemorrhage, cardiac tamponade, and potentially cardiogenic shock.

The patient should be hemodynamically monitored for changes in blood pressure, CVP, or PAOP. In addition, continuous cardiac monitoring will allow the nurse to observe for dysrhythmias that may result from muscle damage. Serial cardiac markers (CK, CKMB, and troponin) should be done.

Penetrating Trauma

In penetrating injuries, open wounds can bleed into the pericardial space, or there may be actual damage to the myocardium, heart chambers, or major vessels of the heart. Hypovolemic shock will develop if the bleeding is severe and uncontrolled. Pericardial tamponade occurs in the greatest percentage of stab wounds involving the heart. Additionally, with gunshot wounds there may be extensive myocardial damage, cellular damage to areas adjacent to the myocardium, and emboli that develop due to remnants such as bullets or metal fragments in the chambers of the heart. Injuries to the coronary arteries can cause pericardial tamponade, acute MI, or death.

The nurse should also be prepared for emergency procedures that may be required in the event of serious complications of cardiac injury. These would include a periocardiocentesis, chest tube insertion, needle thoracotomy, or surgical thoracotomy at the bedside. It is critical to maintain hemodynamic stability with fluid infusion, blood transfusion, and vasopressors, if needed, prior to surgical intervention. The basic ABCs of trauma management should be the first priority with the unstable patient.

CARDIOMYOPATHIES

If the term *cardiomyopathy* is broken down into word parts and defined, the result is "disease/condition of the cardiac muscle." The etiologies of cardiomyopathy vary but include viral infections, autoimmune disorders, CAD, valvular heart disease, hypertension, and alcohol abuse. Nursing implications for care of the patient with cardiomyopathy incorporate maintaining appropriate fluid balance by monitoring the status of the patient's heart failure, administering medications and monitoring outcomes for improving cardiac function, and individualizing activity for patient's tolerance. For severe cardiomyopathy in the appropriate patient, a heart transplant may be indicated.

Dilated Cardiomyopathy

This type of cardiomyopathy is characterized by dilated ventricles (although it may only be left-sided dilation) without muscle hypertrophy. The result is more global left ventricular dysfunction, a low cardiac output, atrial and ventricular dysrhythmias, and venous pooling that leads to emboli. In severe cases, advanced heart failure and death can occur. Symptoms may also include *narrowing pulse pressures* and *pulsus alternans*.

The goals of therapy in dilated cardiomyopathy are to improve pump function, maintain fluid balance, and control heart failure. Medications that will assist with these goals are diuretics, beta-blockers, anticoagulant and antiplatelet therapy, and antidysrhythmics. In severe cases, where the patient meets criteria, a heart transplant may be indicated.

Hypertrophic Obstructive Cardiomyopathy (HOCM)

In contrast to dilated cardiomyopathy, the ventricles are stiff and noncompliant in hypertrophic cardiomyopathy. In addition, the ventricular septum becomes hypertrophied on a cellular level, resulting in obstruction of the aortic valve outflow tract. This stiffened ventricle also pulls the papillary muscles out of alignment and causes mitral valve dysfunction.

The symptoms of HOCM vary slightly from dilated cardiomyopathy. The patient experiences dyspnea upon exertion, myocardial ischemia, SVT, VT, syncope, and heart failure. Medication management is used to initially treat these symptoms. These include diuretics, beta-blockers, calcium channel blockers, and antidysrhythmics. Physical activity is limited by the patient's ability to tolerate mobility. In some cases, an implantable cardioverter defibrillator (ICD), surgical myectomy, or a mitral valve replacement may be required.

Restrictive Cardiomyopathy

This is the least common form of cardiomyopathy. Restrictive cardiomyopathy is characterized by ventricular wall rigidity and diastolic dysfunction. It often occurs as a result of myocardial fibrosis. In these cases, ventricular filling is obstructed by the rigid muscular wall. Symptoms are similar to those of constrictive pericarditis and therefore may be initially treated incorrectly. Right-sided heart failure (backward heart failure), low cardiac output, dyspnea, orthopnea, and liver engorgement are all symptoms of this type of cardiomyopathy. Some of the treatment modalities are similar to those for the other types of cardiomyopathies and include removal of excess fluid, modification of diet, and improvement of pump function.

It is important for the patient to be engaged and participate in her care, as these conditions have to be managed long-term; they require diligent attendance to symptoms and adherence to medications and dietary restrictions to achieve stabilization. The disease most commonly is not reversed, but the patient may live a reasonable quality of life with appropriate management of signs and symptoms of the disease.

CARDIAC DYSRHYTHMIAS

As a rule, the Advanced Cardiac Life Support (ACLS) guidelines should be used in the critical care unit when dysrhythmias occur. Continuous cardiac monitoring is the standard of care for critically ill patients. In most ICUs, the patient is monitored with 5 lead wires, which allows for a variety of lead options for the nurse. The primary lead by which the patient is monitored can be affected by the patient's clinical condition. In most cases, the two primary leads used for monitoring are Lead II and MCL_1. For patients with specific heart injury patterns identified on the 12 lead ECG, the primary continuous monitoring lead can be changed accordingly.

For the purposes of this chapter, dysrhythmias will be referred to as either too slow, too fast, regular, or irregular and by whether they generate a pulse. Specific pharmacological agents will be discussed in the section on Cardiovascular Pharmacology.

Symptomatic Bradycardia—Too Slow

Dysrythmias that result in symptoms that clearly evidence a change in the patient's condition are known as symptomatic dysrythmias. Examples of these symptoms include cool, moist skin, chest pain, hypotension, syncope, fatigue, weakness, decreased level of consciousness, and dyspnea. Bradycardias can be further broken down into dysfunction of the pacemaker for the heart, escape rhythms, drug-induced rhythms, or parasympathetic nervous system stimulation.

Conduction defects are the result of dysfunction of the primary or secondary pacemakers of the heart, specifically the SA and AV nodes in the right atrium. Etiologies of these defects can include coronary ischemia, myocardial infarction, degeneration due to age or illness, metabolic disorders, and drug effects. The most common medications that slow heart rate include beta-blockers, calcium channel blockers, and cardiac glycocides (e.g., digoxin). The rhythms that would be observed with these defects are SA exit blocks, sick sinus syndrome, sinus arrest/pause, first-degree heart blocks, second-degree heart blocks Type I and II, and third-degree (i.e., complete) heart block.

Treatment of symptomatic bradycardia is *atropine 0.5 mg IV,* which may repeat in 5-minute intervals up to 3 mg, and transcutaneous pacemaker. Care should be given not to administer atropine in doses less than 0.5 mg due to the potential for *paradoxical bradycardia.* Patients with second-degree heart block Type II or complete heart block will most likely require a permanent pacemaker. See bradycardia algorithm.

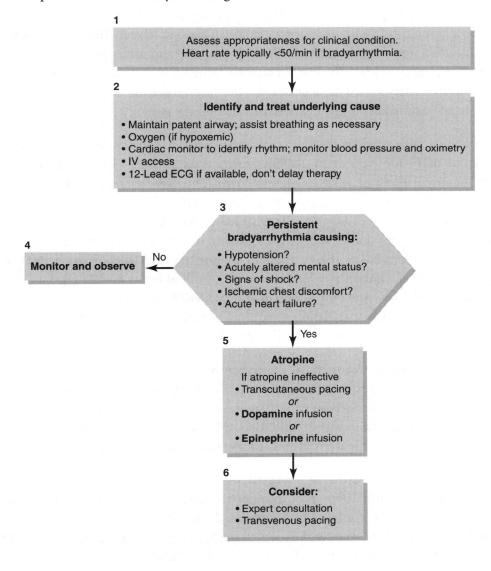

1

Assess appropriateness for clinical condition.
Heart rate typically <50/min if bradyarrhythmia.

2

Identify and treat underlying cause

- Maintain patent airway; assist breathing as necessary
- Oxygen (if hypoxemic)
- Cardiac monitor to identify rhythm; monitor blood pressure and oximetry
- IV access
- 12-Lead ECG if available, don't delay therapy

3

Persistent bradyarrhythmia causing:

- Hypotension?
- Acutely altered mental status?
- Signs of shock?
- Ischemic chest discomfort?
- Acute heart failure?

4 No

Monitor and observe

5 Yes

Atropine

If atropine ineffective
- Transcutaneous pacing
or
- **Dopamine** infusion
or
- **Epinephrine** infusion

6

Consider:

- Expert consultation
- Transvenous pacing

The critical care nurse must monitor the patient with bradycardia to ensure adequate tissue perfusion to vital organs. For severe bradycardia with hemodynamic compromise, it is likely that vasosuppressor support will also be required. If the bradycardia is drug related, discussion should be undertaken with the physician regarding dosage and necessity of continued treatment with this medication. Purposeful or accidental overdosages of drugs that cause bradycardia will require reversal agents or, if none are available, hemodynamic support until metabolized and excreted including, potentially, dialysis.

Symptomatic Tachycardia—Too Fast

Tachycardia is typically a symptom of another condition and in most cases should be investigated for its etiology prior to intervention with rate-controlling medication. Normally, it is the body's attempt to compensate for a change in cardiac output. However, symptomatic tachycardia with hemodynamic instability will require an immediate conversion either electrically or pharmacologically. It must also be recognized that the loss of atrial kick will result in approximately 15–20 percent drop in the cardiac output. Tachycardias can be generated by most pacemakers in the heart, depending on the etiology.

Atrial fibrillation with rapid ventricular response (referred to by some as "Rapid Atrial Fibrillation") is one of the most common sustained tachycardic rhythms. The immediate goal is to lower the ventricular response rate. Calcium channel blockers such as IV *diltiazem (Cardizem) or beta-blockers (esmolol, metoprolol, labetalol)* can be administered to treat this dysrhythmia. Cardiac glycosides (such as digoxin) have been used in the past, but they are not the standard of care for patients who acutely present with this tachyarrythmia; they may be useful on an outpatient basis. The IV calcium channel blocker works more rapidly at converting the rhythm. *Diltiazem* is administered in an initial bolus of 0.25 mg/kg given over 2 minutes and can be followed by a second dose if needed. A continuous infusion should then be started at 10 mg/hr. Anticoagulation is required in patients with atrial fibrillation or flutter due to the propensity for clot formation. The INR should be kept between 2 and 3.

In the monitored setting, treatment of the patient with a *narrow complex supraventricular* tachycardia is *adenosine.* The dosage for this drug is a 6 mg rapid bolus, followed by a 12 mg dose after one to two minutes. When effective, the drug causes a brief asystolic period as the SA or AV node is "reset" from reentry and followed by a return to sinus rhythm. It may also slow conduction briefly so the dysrhythmia can be identified more clearly.

Ventricular or wide tachycardias are treated with an *amiodarone* bolus of 150 mg over 10 minutes followed by initiation of a continuous infusion at 1 mg/min. The physician may choose to attempt a synchronized cardioversion if the patient remains hemodynamically stable. If the patient deteriorates and becomes unconscious or hemodynamically unstable, immediate defibrillation is required. Torsade de pointes (literally, twisting of the points) is a specific type of ventricular tachycardia that shows a classic polymorphous origination. Treatment for torsade is IV *magnesium sulfate* 1–2 grams over 30–60 seconds, which may be repeated in 5–15 minutes. A continuous infusion can be started at 3–10 mg/min if required.

Other tachycardias include multifocal atrial tachycardia (MAT), junctional tachycardia, paroxysmal SVT, and Wolfe-Parkinson-White syndrome (WPW). Vagal maneuvers can be attempted in the stable patient; however, *adenosine and calcium channel blockers* are given for symptomatic rhythms. Care must be used in identification of the rhythm prior to administration of these drugs, as they can cause wide ventricular tachycardias, such as refractory VT and VF, and death. See tachycardia algorithm.

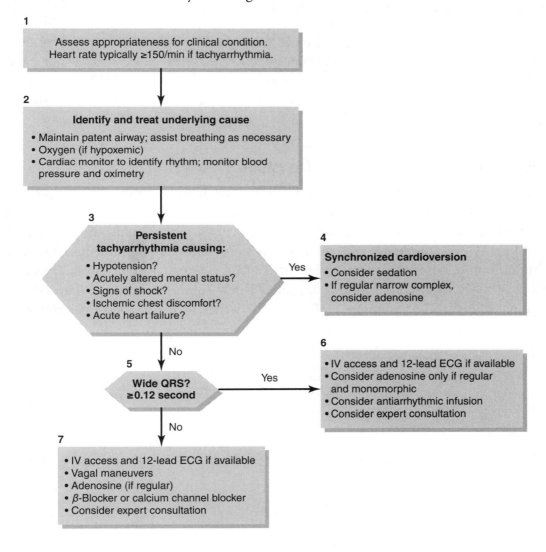

Ventricular Fibrillation (VF) and Ventricular Tachycardia (VT)

Ventricular tachycardia is a run of three or more PVCs. It occurs when an ectopic focus or foci fire repetitively and the ventricle takes control as the pacemaker. VT is a life-threatening dysrhythmia because of decreased CO and the possibility of deterioration to ventricular fibrillation, which is a lethal dysrhythmia. VT is associated with myocardial infarction (MI), CAD, significant electrolyte imbalances, cardiomyopathy, mitral valve prolapse, long QT syndrome, digitalis toxicity, and central nervous system disorders. VT can be stable (patient has a pulse) or unstable (patient is pulseless). Precipitating causes must be identified and treated (e.g., electrolyte imbalances, ischemia). Treatment involves drug therapy and/or synchronized cardioversion for a stable patient and rapid defibrillation for an unstable patient.

Ventricular fibrillation is characterized on ECG by irregular undulations of varying shapes and amplitude. VF results in an unresponsive, pulseless, and apneic state. If not rapidly treated, the patient will die. Treatment consists of immediate initiation of CPR and advanced cardiac life support (ACLS) measures with the use of defibrillation and definitive drug therapy.

Pulseless Electrical Activity (PEA)/Asystole

All of the above dysrhythmias are considered life threatening and should be treated as a medical emergency with immediate CPR and/or defibrillation. Rhythm should be confirmed and pulses checked. The drug of choice in asystole is *epinephrine*. Epinephrine is administered 1 mg IV every 5 minutes until spontaneous return of rhythm. Continuous CPR should continue with pulse checks every 2 minutes to ensure adequate compressions. The patient will most likely require intubation if not immediately converted to ensure adequate oxygenation. Efforts should continue until deemed effective or the physician determines the measures are futile. See adult cardiac arrest algorithm.

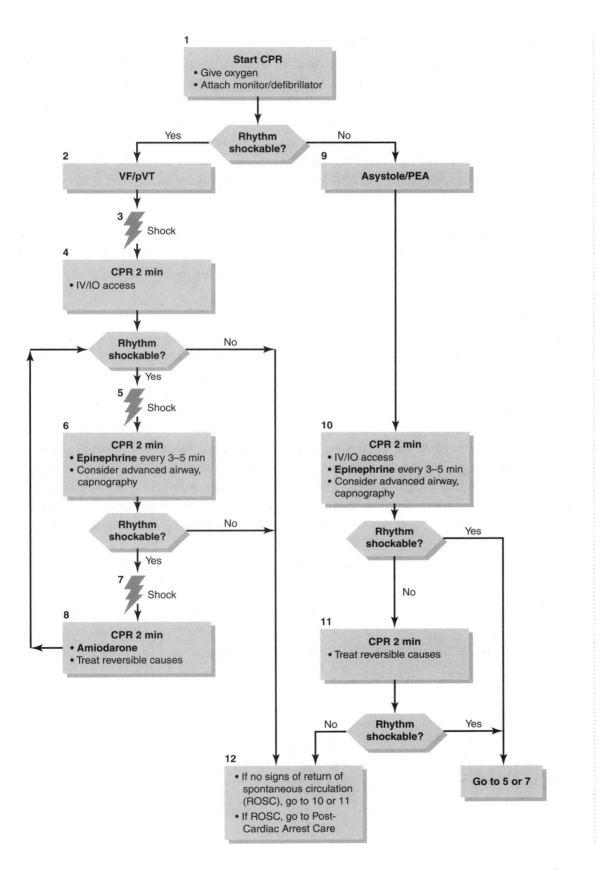

Automatic Implantable Cardioverter/Defibrillator (AICD)

The AICD is an implantable device that consists of sensing leads and defibrillator patches attached to the endocardium and to a pulse generator (all implanted internally). The procedure can be done through a thoracotomy incision or transvenously through an incision in the subclavian vein. These devices have the capability of detecting life-threatening dysrhythmias such as ventricular tachycardia or ventricular fibrillation and provide defibrillation, or they can pace the heart in bradycardic rhythms. The device can be interrogated to ascertain the frequency of delivered shocks, rhythm at the time of shock, and battery life.

When educating patients on these devices, the nurse should explain that there is up to a 75 percent likelihood of spontaneous discharges in the first year. They should also be informed that there is no potential harm to their family or medical staff. Patients still will require antiarrhythmic therapy to limit the potential need for the AICD.

Pacemakers

Cardiac pacemakers have become very sophisticated over time and have the ability to pace and sense either or both chambers, and they can defibrillate and deliver a shock when appropriate. Pacemakers can be inserted transcutaneously, transvenously, or via permanent placement based on the patient's clinical condition and stability. The primary purpose is to treat bradycardia in patients unable to sustain an adequate cardiac output.

Pacemakers are described by the following parameters: chamber paced, chamber sensed, response to sensing, programmability, and antitachyarrhythmia capability. Sensing and pacing occur in either one chamber (atrium or ventricle) or both chambers. When a pacemaker senses the rhythm, it can be either triggered, inhibited, or both. Programmability can be simple, multi-, or rare modulation. Finally, the pacemaker can pace, shock, or do both.

PACEMAKER TERMINOLOGY AND NOMENCLATURE					
Position/ Category	I	II	III	IV	V
	Chamber(s) Paced	Chamber(s) Sensed	Response to Sensing	Programmability Rate Modulation	Antitachyarrhythmia Function(s)
Letter Codes	0 = None	0 = None	0 = None	0 = None	0 = None
	A = Atrium	A = Atrium	T = Trigger	P = Simple Programmable	P = Pacing (antitachyarrhythmia)
	V = Ventricle	V = Ventricle	I = Inhibited	M = Multiprogrammable	S = Shock
	D = Dual (A + V)	D = Dual (A + V)	D = Dual (T + I)	C = Communicating	D = Dual (P + S)
				R = Rate Modulation	

The basic components of a pacemaker are the battery, lead system, and pulse generator. These components are found in both temporary and permanent pacemakers. A transcutaneous pacemaker is placed externally on the skin via external electrodes that adhere to the skin and are connected to the pulse generator, or in most cases, a combination portable defibrillator/monitor/pacing unit. The patient will most likely require analgesia and sedation if the pacemaker is to be required for any length of time, particularly at high mA (milliampheres or output voltage) due to the discomfort the shock causes. Higher mAs will often be required to pace successfully through the thoracic cavity. The rate and mA are set to ensure the most effective pacing to produce an adequate cardiac output. The patient's skin must be frequently evaluated for burning.

The transvenous pacemaker leads are inserted via a percutaneous approach through a large vein, typically subclavian or internal jugular, into the right ventricle and/or right atrium for dual chamber pacing. The lead wires are then connected to an external pulse generator. Upon initial insertion, the rate is set between 60–80/min while the mAs are set to the point where capture occurs. Complications of this type of pacing include migration of the lead wires or perforation of the myocardium. During cardiac surgery, the lead wires can be inserted in the epicardium and fed externally via the sternotomy incision for the potential need for postoperative pacing.

There are three conditions that the critical care nurse must observe while caring for the patient with a pacemaker: failure to pace, failure to capture, and failure to sense. Some of the most common troubleshooting interventions can be accomplished by checking the generator battery, verifying lead placement, checking for inadequate voltage to stimulate conduction, and examining the generator for general failure.

Therapeutic Hypothermia Post–Cardiac Arrest

Induced hypothermia was first described in the literature in the late 1950s and was initially used during neurosurgical or cardiovascular surgeries to reduce the incidence of neurological injury during these procedures.

Studies in early 2000 comparing patients treated with therapeutic hypothermia to 33 °C for 12 hours, initiated within 2 hours of cardiac arrest vs. standard treatment, reported that 49 percent survived to be discharged to rehab or home, compared with 26 percent of the patients treated with standard care. The main benefit of lowering temperature to 32–34 °C during the first few hours post-arrest is that it decreases brain injury.

Inclusion Criteria for Therapeutic Hypothermia

- Nontraumatic, out-of-hospital cardiac arrest with return of spontaneous circulation (ROSC) ≤45 minutes

- Patients with witnessed shockable rhythms (VF or VT)

- Patients with non-shockable rhythms (PEA or asystole) may be considered under exceptional circumstances

- Arrest took place less than 6 hours prior to start of therapeutic hypothermia

- Mean BP >60 with or without vasopressor support

- Age >18 and <75

- Coma, GCS <6

- Patient not following commands, no purposeful movement to stimuli

- Reflexes and pathological/posturing movements are permissible

Hypothermia is most effective when the cooling occurs within 6 hours of the return to spontaneous circulation. The patient must be cooled to a core temperature of 32–34 °C and must have this core temperature sustained for 12–24 hours. The patient requires sedation and, in most instances, paralytic agents to eliminate the shivering effects of the cooling. Monitoring of temperatures must be continuous, and rewarming is done slowly, typically 1 degree every hour until return to normothermic state.

SHOCK

Shock is defined as a general state where decreased tissue perfusion results in a variety of conditions that impact body functions on the cellular, organ, and system level. It is a complex pathological process that can eventually involve all major organs and systems within the body. The mortality from decompensated shock is extremely high despite aggressive treatment therapies.

Types of Shock

The classifications for shock are based on the type of etiology or pathology. There are four classifications of shock: hypovolemic, cardiogenic, obstructive, and distributive, which includes septic, anaphylactic, and neurogenic shock. Hypovolemic and cardiogenic shocks will be discussed in this chapter; distributive shock will be discussed in chapter 12: Multiorgan System.

Hypovolemic Shock

Hypovolemia is the result of loss of blood or fluid volume primarily in the intravascular space. Etiologies can include hemorrhage, surgery, gastrointestinal bleeding, severe vomiting and diarrhea, massive diuresis, or shifting of fluid volume with the intravascular and extravascular space.

The loss of circulating volume results in a decrease in venous return to the heart (preload). Stroke volume and cardiac output correspondingly decrease. Ultimately tissue perfusion and cellular oxygen supply are diminished, resulting in organ failure. The heart attempts to maintain cardiac output by increasing heart rate in response to sympathetic nervous system stimulation, which occurs as a result of the decreased volume. Vasoconstriction occurs to force more volume to the heart and preserve tissue perfusion. The lungs attempt to compensate for decreased oxygen by increasing respiratory rate, and respiratory alkalosis develops. Ultimately, the kidneys preserve fluid volume by slowing renal perfusion. Peripheral perfusion decreases, and the patient's skin becomes cool, clammy, and pale. Cerebral perfusion will also decrease, causing a change in neurological status. In the refractory stage, the patient's compensatory mechanisms deteriorate, and organ failure occurs.

The most appropriate treatment for the patient is to receive rapid fluid volume replacement in the form of red blood cells, crystalloids, or colloids, depending on the type of fluid loss. Hemodynamic monitoring of indicators of cardiac output such as HR, blood pressure, CVP, and PAWP is critical to ensuring the proper balance is achieved. Accurate documentation of intake and ouput and any further fluid loss is also important. The patient may require vasopressor support; however, agents which increase heart rate and myocardial demand should be avoided. These agents will be discussed in the pharmacological section of this chapter.

Cardiogenic Shock

Cardiogenic shock results from pump failure and the inability to move blood effectively. Right or left ventricular heart failure and inadequate pumping action lead to decreased tissue perfusion. It has a very high mortality rate in patients who have had an acute MI with subsequent heart failure. The etiology of this type of shock is typically cardiac dysfunction such as valvular problems, myocardial infarction, open heart surgery, cardiomyopathies, and dysrhythmias. The pathophysiology of this condition is fairly clear. When the heart is unable to push blood volume forward, there is a decrease in stroke volume and cardiac output. These processes cause a backup of volume into the right side of the heart, causing increased pulmonary pressures and pulmonary edema. Oxygenation decreases, and in turn oxygen supply to the cellular level also decreases, resulting in impaired tissue perfusion.

Clinically the patient demonstrates hypotension; tachycardia; cool, clammy skin; decreased urine output; chest pain; and evidence of lung congestion. Management of these symptoms requires identification of the cause of the pump failure. Inotropic medications will improve contractility of the heart muscle, while vasodilators will help reduce afterload. Hemodynamic monitoring via pulmonary artery catheter will provide several valuable measurements, such as central venous pressure (CVP), right atrial pressure, and pulmonary artery occlusion pressure (PAOP), to use for titration of medications and evaluation of the patient's clinical status. An arterial line is beneficial for directly monitoring arterial blood pressure. Ventilator support and potentially IABP and VAD devices might be needed for cardiac support. These temporary measures may be undertaken to support the heart and allow healing to occur or to serve as a bridge if heart transplant is an alternative for the patient.

The IABP is a mechanical device that augments diastole and coronary blood flow and reduces afterload. A vascular catheter with a balloon that wraps around the distal end is inserted percutaneously via the femoral artery. The balloon inflates during ventricular diastole concurrent with aortic valve closure. As a result, the blood in the aorta is displaced backward toward the aortic root, thus improving blood flow to the coronary arteries. The blood volume below the balloon is forced peripherally, which enhances renal perfusion. When the balloon deflates, the blood in the ventricle is ejected against less resistance, unimpeded, and facilitates ventricular emptying. IABP therapy is referred to as counterpulsation because the timing of balloon inflation is opposite to ventricular contraction. The IABP assist ratio is 1:1 in the acute phase of treatment. That is, 1 IABP cycle of inflation and deflation for every heartbeat. Complications of IABP therapy may include vascular injuries such as dislodging of plaque, aortic dissection, thrombus and embolus formation, and compromised distal circulation.

CARDIOVASCULAR PHARMACOLOGY

Medication administration is a key role of the critical care nurse, and drug titration is often required to stabilize the patient's hemodynamic condition. This section of the chapter will be approached by discussing the classifications of drugs that are used to treat cardiovascular disorders. (Note that some medications have been discussed in previous portions of the chapter and will not be duplicated here.)

Preload Reduction Agents

Reduction of preload in the critically ill patient is accomplished through medications that cause *venous dilation,* which will decrease filling pressures in the failing heart. *Diuretics* are the most common form of preload reduction medications. There are several types of diuretics, which are categorized by site of the kidneys affected by the drug. **Mannitol** is an osmotic diuretic. Loop diuretics include **furosemide** and **ethacrynic acid** and act in the loop of Henle. Thiazides such as hydrochlorothiazide inhibit sodium reabsorption in the distal convoluted tubule. Finally, potassium-sparing diuretics promote sodium secretion in the distal tubule and potassium reabsorption. Examples of these include **spironolactone, triamterene,** and **amiloride hydrochloride**.

Nitrates and **morphine** are vasodilators and are discussed in the section on treatment for chest pain associated with MI. Direct smooth muscle relaxants that are direct-acting vasodilators include **nitroglycerin** and **nitroprusside**. Nitroglycerin is used for treatment of heart failure because it reduces cardiac filling pressures and dilates coronary arteries. Initial dosage is 10 mcg/min and it is titrated until chest pain is relieved and blood pressure remains stable. Nitroprusside is more suitable for reduction of acute hypertension in hypertensive emergencies or afterload reduction in heart failure.

Beta-blockers such as **atenolol, metoprolol, esmolol,** and **labetalol** decrease heart rate and contractility, while increasing diastolic filling pressures. Care should be taken not to withdraw these drugs rapidly to prevent rebound effects such as unstable angina, hypertension, and MI. *Digoxin* is a cardiac glycoside, regulates heart rate, and is classified as a weak inotrope.

Afterload Reduction Agents

Angiotensin-converting enzyme inhibitors (ACEIs) cause vasodilation and afterload reduction, which results in decreased left ventricular workload. These drugs block the conversion of angiotensin I to angiotensin II. Examples of these medications include **captopril** and **enalapril**. One of the complications of these drugs is hypotension, particularly in volume-depleted patients. Patients taking ACEIs should be monitored for hyperkalemia and nagging dry cough.

ARBs (angiotensin II receptor blockers) work similarly to ACEIs. However, their primary function is to block the effects of angiotensin II, which is a potent chemical that causes the vessels to contract. The result is that the vessels then dilate, which in turn decreases blood pressure. The most common ARBs are **losartan, irbesartan, and valsartan**. These medications work well in patients who cannot take ACEIs. Heart failure and hypertension are conditions that respond well to ARBs. They may also be used to prevent renal failure. The side effects are similar to those of ACEIs.

Nitroprusside is classified as a smooth muscle relaxant and can have both arterial and venous vasodilator effects. The dosage is titrated to the desired effect and is typically infused at 0.25–6.0 mcg/kg/min via IV infusion.

Hydralazine is a potent arterial smooth muscle dilator. It is given via slow IV push in dosages of 5–10 mg every 4 to 6 hours. The most significant side effect is reflex tachycardia. It can be given intermittently to bridge the period during weaning of IV antihypertensives.

Vasopressor Agents

Dopamine was discussed earlier in the section on heart failure. **Norepinephrine, phenylephrine,** and **vasopressin** are the other vasopressors used in the care of the critically ill patient. Vasopressors are primarily sympathomimetic agents that mediate peripheral vasoconstriction. Care must be undertaken when administering these medications in patients with cardiac conditions, as they significantly increase afterload by the actions of peripheral vasoconstriction and increased systemic vascular resistance. However, in some shock states, tissue perfusion may be significantly reduced, and organ failure is likely to occur without adequate cardiac output and systemic perfusion. The risk must be evaluated against the benefits of the drugs. Vasopressin is useful in patients with gastrointestinal bleeding, as it is a vasoconstrictor and decreases blood flow to the visceral bed. It is administered with a loading dose of 20 units over 20 minutes IV and followed by a continuous infusion at 0.2–0.8 units/min.

Inotropic Agents

The function of inotropic agents is to improve cardiac contractility. The end result is improved cardiac output by decreased filling pressures. **Digoxin** is a mild inotrope. Sympathomimetic agents stimulate adrenergic receptors, thus stimulating the sympathetic nervous system. **Dobutamine** has been discussed earlier. Phosphodiesterase 3 inhibitors are inotropic agents given to treat acute HF. This drug group inhibits the enzyme phosphodiesterase, promoting a positive inotropic response and vasodilation. **Milrinone** is an example of this. This drug directly relaxes vascular smooth muscle and increases myocardial contractility. It is given in a loading dose of 50 mcg/kg over 10 minutes and followed by an infusion of 0.375 to 0.75 mcg/kg/min. Most inotropes do cause tachycardia.

Lipid-Lowering Agents

Some of the most commonly prescribed drugs in the United States are lipid-lowering agents. Elevated cholesterol and triglycerides are risk factors for cardiac disease. American Heart Association guidelines recommend these agents when levels for total cholesterol are > 200 mg/dL and for triglycerides > 150 mg/dL. Examples of these agents are the following:

- Atorvastatin (brand name: Lipitor)
- Fluvastatin (brand name: Lescol)
- Lovastatin (brand names: Mevacor, Altoprev)
- Pravastatin (brand name: Pravachol)
- Rosuvastatin calcium (brand name: Crestor)
- Simvastatin (brand name: Zocor)

Anti-Arrhythmic Agents

Anti-arrhythmics are a diverse category of medications that are used to treat abnormal heart rhythms. These drugs are classified as Class I–IV and an unclassified grouping. Class I is sodium channel blockers, Class II is beta-adrenergic blockers (beta-blockers), Class III is drugs that slow the rate of phase 3 depolarization, and Class IV is calcium channel blockers. Some examples of specific drugs are listed below.

Class	Drug name
I A	Quinidine
I A	Procainamide
I B	Lidocaine
II	Metoprolol
II	Propranolol
III	Amiodarone
IV	Diltiazem
IV	Verapamil
Unclassified	Adenosine
Unclassified	Magnesium

Anti-Anginals

Anti-anginal drugs, as the name implies, are medications that reduce the pain associated with angina pectoris. Angina is typically a reflection of diminished blood or oxygen supply to the myocardium. Examples of these drugs include multiple forms of nitroglycerin, isosorbide dinitrate or mononitrate, nicardipine, amlodipine, and felodipine. Other agents that are in other categories already listed above may also have anti-anginal effects.

Antihypertensives

Antihypertensives function to reduce blood pressure as a protective mechanism after strokes, renal failure, and coronary artery disease. The general effects of antihypertensives are reduced adrenergic nerve stimulation to the vasculature, vasodilation by relaxing vascular smooth muscle, and reduction of afterload. Examples of antihypertensives and the site of primary action include clonidine hydrochloride (central nervous system), reserpine (peripheral nerve endings), labetalol (beta receptor sites), and prazosin hydrochloride (alpha receptor sites).

Calcium Channel Blockers

Calcium channel blockers are considered negative inotropic, negative chronotropic, and dromotropic agents on SA and AV conductive tissue. They are successful in reducing ischemia by increasing the anginal threshold. They also can treat coronary vasospasm. One of the most potent vasodilators in this category of drugs is dihydropyridines, of which nifedipine is an example. Nicardipine and felodipine are examples of second generation dihydropyridines. The other two types of calcium channel blockers are phenylalkylamines (verapamil) and benzothiazepines (diltiazem).

Thrombolytics

Thrombolytics are used to treat acute coronary ischemia as a result of blockage of the coronary arteries and acute myocardial infarction. These can be given peripherally via IV lines or intracoronary via cardiac catheterization and angiography procedures (PTCA). Criteria for treatment with thrombolytics is specific and requires screening of the patient for history for time of onset of symptoms (goal is administration at less than 6 hours after onset of chest pain and symptoms), any evidence of bleeding, recent surgery or CVA, and evidence of persistent ST elevation despite sublingual nitroglycerin or nifedipine.

There are currently five thrombolytics available for use for treatment of acute coronary ischemia: streptokinase, urokinase, alteplase, reteplase, and anistreplace. The most common drug used at the present time is tPA (alteplase). It is administered 100 mg first hour and 20 mg over the second and third hours.

With any thrombolytic, it is imperative for the critical care RN to monitor the patient for any signs of acute bleeding. Neurological checks should be done minimally every 1 hour for the time of administration and every 2 hours for the next 24 hours. Other observations should be done as for any patient receiving anticoagulant therapy. Should serious bleeding occur, the infusion should be stopped and the patient treated symptomatically for blood loss. Intravenous lines must be placed before the infusion is started, and venipunctures should be limited to those only absolutely necessary. Stress ulcer prophylaxis should be given, especially if the patient complains of epigastric pain.

Evidence of coronary reperfusion can be profound, including reperfusion dysrhythmias, ventricular tachycardia, bradycardias, conduction defects, and, occasionally, ventricular fibrillation. ST segments should be normalized during reperfusion, and CK, CKMB, and troponins should also stabilize.

Anticoagulants

Warfarin, heparin, and enoxaparin have been previously discussed in the section on treatment for atrial fibrillation. CBC, aPTT, PT, and INRs should be checked daily while the patient is hospitalized for therapeutic levels and as per primary care physician once patient has been discharged.

Antiplatelets

Two of the most commonly used antiplatelet medications are aspirin (81 mg dose) and clopidogrel (Plavix). Research has demonstrated that these drugs have protective effects and reduce the potential for platelet aggregation at the site of atherosclerotic plaque.

Review Questions

1. A 72-year-old patient is in the CCU after undergoing angioplasty for an obstructive lesion in the right coronary artery. The patient suddenly complains of severe chest pain, then becomes bradycardic and hypotensive. Which of these diagnostic studies should be obtained immediately?

   A. cardiac enzymes

   B. pulse oximetry

   C. 12-lead ECG

   D. chest x-ray

2. While caring for a patient requiring a temporary transvenous pacing wire, the critical care nurse notices that the pacer is intermittently losing capture. After ensuring that the cables are correctly connected to the pulse generator (pacemaker) and pacing wire, the nurse should do which of these?

   A. Immediately apply external pads and begin transthoracic pacing.

   B. Gently advance the pacing wire until capture is obtained.

   C. Increase the mA output until consistent capture is obtained.

   D. Replace the battery in the pulse generator (pacemaker).

3. A patient is admitted to the ICU from the Emergency Department for further management of hypertensive crisis. Upon arrival at the ICU, the patient is receiving a sodium nitroprusside infusion (Nipride, Nitropress) at a high dose. The critical care nurse recognizes the need for and requests the health care provider to place

   A. a central venous catheter.

   B. an arterial line.

   C. a pulmonary artery catheter.

   D. an additional peripheral IV.

4. The critical care nurse is caring for a patient with a pulmonary artery catheter. After repositioning the patient, she notices the patient is experiencing frequent ectopy and observes the following waveform on the PA tracing. What action should be taken to prevent further complications?

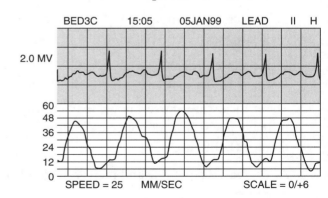

   A. Administer IV lidocaine.

   B. Flush the PA lumen of the catheter.

   C. Notify the health care provider immediately.

   D. Slowly withdraw the catheter until a CVP waveform is observed on the PA tracing.

5. The critical care nurse is caring for a patient with a history of tricuspid valve regurgitation who has a pulmonary artery catheter in place. The nurse knows that which of these hemodynamic values will be distorted because of the patient's condition?

   A. central venous pressure

   B. pulmonary artery pressure

   C. pulmonary artery occlusion pressure (wedge pressure)

   D. arterial pressure waveform

6. After receiving tPA for an acute myocardial infarction, a 65-year-old patient is admitted to the ICU from the Emergency Department. The patient currently denies chest pain, and the ECG has returned to normal. Shortly after arriving, the patient complains of a severe headache and then begins to have mental status changes. Which of these complications of tPA therapy for myocardial infarction is likely occurring?

   A. migraine headache

   B. intracranial hemorrhage

   C. meninigitis

   D. ischemic stroke

7. The critical care nurse knows that the two primary goals of intra-aortic balloon pump therapy (IABP) are

   A. decreased heart rate and increased blood pressure.

   B. increased heart rate and decreased blood pressure.

   C. afterload reduction and improved coronary perfusion.

   D. preload reduction and decreased coronary perfusion.

8. The critical care nurse is caring for a patient immediately following a cardiothoracic surgical procedure. The patient is experiencing frequent episodes of ventricular ectopy. The nurse knows that the most likely cause of dysrhythmia following cardiothoracic surgical procedures is

   A. hypoxia.

   B. presence of mediastinal chest tubes.

   C. myocardial ischemia.

   D. electrolyte abnormalities.

9. The critical care nurse is caring for a patient following coronary artery bypass grafting and aortic valve repair. The patient arrived to the ICU from the operating room 2 hours ago and has experienced total chest tube output of >400 mL per hour since then. The critical care nurse should

   A. notify the surgeon and prepare the patient for re-exploration.

   B. do nothing, as this is normal chest tube output.

   C. elevate the head of the bed to promote drainage.

   D. place the chest drains to water seal to reduce the amount of drainage.

10. The critical care nurse is caring for a patient who underwent coronary artery bypass graft surgery yesterday. The patient experiences sudden onset of a rapid dysrhythmia, and the nurse is unable to interpret the rhythm fully; however, the patient has stable hemodynamics. The nurse should consider obtaining which of these diagnostic studies?

    A. blood samples for electrolyte analysis

    B. arterial blood gas

    C. chest x-ray

    D. atrial electrogram

Review Answers and Explanations

1. C

The patient has known coronary disease, as he has just undergone angioplasty. Sudden onset of chest pain along with hypotension and bradycardia is associated with occlusion (in this case reocclusion) of the right coronary artery. Answer (A) is incorrect because obtaining cardiac enzymes is not the priority, as they do not reflect damage to heart muscle as quickly as an ECG would. Answer (B) is incorrect because there is no indication that the patient is hypoxic. Although pulse oximetry would be obtained at some point, it is not the priority here. Answer (D) is incorrect because the likely cause of the patient's chest pain is reocclusion of the right coronary artery, which will not be revealed on chest x-ray. A chest x-ray may be obtained later, but again, it is not the priority in this situation.

2. C

Increasing the mA output until consistent capture is obtained is the best nursing action in the scenario described. Answer (A) is incorrect because transthoracic pacing is not required unless other methods of troubleshooting the transvenous wire have failed and the patient is in distress. Answer (B) is incorrect because it is not appropriate for the critical care nurse to advance the pacer wire, as this may result in ventricular perforation. Answer (D) is incorrect because a low battery is not likely to be the cause of intermittent loss of capture.

3. B

Sodium nitroprusside is a potent vasodilator and can cause rapid changes in blood pressure. Therefore, an arterial monitoring line is essential for safe use of this medication. Answer (A) is incorrect because there is no indication for central venous access, and this would predispose the patient to infection. Answer (C) is incorrect for the same reasons. Answer (D) is incorrect because there is no mention of the need for additional IV access and it is within the scope of practice and autonomy for the bedside ICU nurse to perform peripheral IV access, whereas the other procedures are placed by a physician or an advanced practice nurse.

4. D

The waveform indicates that the PA catheter has migrated to the right ventricle. The provider has to be notified immediately to reposition the catheter. Ventricular irritation is what caused the ectopic beats noted by the nurse. Answer (A) is incorrect because the administration of lidocaine will not correct the underlying problem causing the ventricular ectopy. Answer (B) is incorrect because flushing the PA lumen will not correct the misplacement of the catheter. Repositioning of the PA catheter is not a nursing responsibility. The provider has to be notified at once, and a credentialed provider can adjust the catheter.

5. A

Patients with tricuspid regurgitation have altered central venous pressure readings due to turbulent blood flow backward through the right atrium and into the vena cava. Answers (B) and (C) are incorrect because tricuspid regurgitation will not alter pulmonary artery or pulmonary artery occlusion pressures. Answer (D) is incorrect because there is no mention of an arterial line and tricuspid regurgitation will not affect the arterial pressure waveform.

6. B

The patient's symptoms and history of tPA therapy support this scenario. Answers (A), (C), and (D) are incorrect because these are not complications of tPA therapy. All the other choices are not the goals of IABP therapy.

7. C

Afterload reduction and improved coronary perfusion is the only answer that is also a relevant goal of IABP therapy.

8. D

Patients experiencing dysrhythmias following cardiac surgical procedures often have electrolyte abnormalities (specifically in magnesium and potassium), which should be assessed and treated. While hypoxia (A) is a common cause of ventricular dysrhythmias, it is not the likely cause in cardiac surgery patients. The presence of mediastinal chest tubes (B) is not mentioned in the question. Myocardial ischemia (C) is a possible cause of dysrhythmias but is not likely to occur after cardiothoracic surgery.

9. A

The patient is experiencing severe bleeding after the surgical procedure and will need to return to the operating room for the source of bleeding to be identified and repaired. Answer (B) is incorrect because this amount is far higher than the acceptable amount of chest tube output. Answer (C) is incorrect because while elevating the head of the bed will promote chest tube drainage, it will not correct the underlying problem. Answer (D) is incorrect because this action will not allow the chest tubes to drain properly and may lead to clotting of the tubes and/or the development of tamponade, as the blood will not exit the chest.

10. D

This form of temporary ECG monitoring is particularly helpful when the rhythm is difficult to interpret in postoperative cardiac patients who have epicardial pacing wires in place. The other answers are incorrect because they will not assist the nurse with cardiac rhythm interpretation.

The Pulmonary System

Airway management is one of the most important functions of the critical care nurse. Oxygenation of tissues is foremost in ensuring end organ viability and prevention of complications that arise from lack of adequate oxygenation and airway management. This can be done simply by providing supplemental oxygen and suctioning of a patient or by more complex tasks, such as managing a ventilator dependent patient. Knowledge of acid-base balance is also critical to identifying appropriate interventions. The section of the CCRN exam on the pulmonary system, is secondary in percentage of total exam questions only to the cardiovascular system, with approximately 17 percent of the exam related to this system.

ACUTE PULMONARY EMBOLUS (PE)

An embolus is an object that occludes a vessel. An embolus can be composed of a detached thrombus or vegetation (mass of bacteria), foreign body, or fat. However, the term *pulmonary embolus* (PE) generally refers to either a detached thrombus or fat.

Pathophysiology

The exact pathophysiology of fat emboli is not completely understood, but it generally occurs approximately *three to four days after the patient experiences a trauma.* Although there are competing theories regarding the pathophysiology, the basic mechanism is that the trauma (generally a long bone fracture, such as a femur) results in the release of fat droplets and/or free fatty acids/chylomicrons in the venous circulation that embolize to the pulmonary vasculature, occluding a pulmonary vein.

Likewise, thromboemboli also generally originate from the extremities from deep vein thrombi (DVT). Essentially, a DVT forms in an extremity, generally the legs, and then a portion of the thrombus detaches and embolizes to the pulmonary vasculature.

Despite the character of the emboli, the effects are similar. There will be an acute increase in the pulmonary vascular resistance and extra strain on the right heart. This may manifest as a *new right bundle branch* on an ECG or *new onset atrial fibrillation.* Other, relatively more minor effects are decreased perfusion to the peripheral lung tissue and mismatch of the ventilation and perfusion of the lung tissue.

Risk Factors

The most common risk factors for pulmonary embolism are immobility or reduced mobility, surgery within the last 3 months, history of deep vein thrombosis, and malignancy. On the history and physical, patients will often state that they have "just returned from a long vacation and were in an airplane for a long period of time," or they are truck drivers and their symptoms began after they had been driving for several hours. Hence, one of the biggest risk factors for an acute pulmonary thromboembolism is long-term (generally more than 3–4 hours) immobilization, otherwise referred to as venous stasis. However, other risk factors are *medications* (such as oral contraceptives), *hypercoagulable states* due to anticoagulant deficiencies (such as proteins C and S), the presence of autoantibodies (such as lupus anticoagulant), presence of a *malignancy* (such as breast, lung, colon, etc.) that releases procoagulant hormones, and *damage to the endothelium* of the vasculature (such as inflammation from a vasculitis).

Inpatient Prophylaxis

When patients are admitted to the critical care units, they will generally receive gastric ulcer prophylaxis with a proton pump inhibitor or histamine-2 receptor blocker. Likewise, they also receive prophylaxis for DVT since they are likely to be immobile for a prolonged period. This can be done with *"Ted" hose* (e.g., compression stockings), either alone or in combination with *sequential compression devices* (SCDs), which are pneumatic cuffs that wrap around the distal lower extremity and intermittently inflate and decompress to prevent venous stasis. If there is no contraindication to anticoagulation, then patients may also be placed on twice daily subcutaneous injections of heparin, once daily subcutaneous injections *of low molecular weight heparin* (LMWH) (e.g., enoxaparin and dalteparin), or *antithrombin III binder* (e.g., fondaparinux). If patients are already on anticoagulation with warfarin, then as long as their INR is maintained between 2.0 and 3.0, no other prophylaxis is required. The goal of warfarin therapy for the treatment of PE is to keep the INR between 2.5 to 3.5, although variations may be noted depending on the specific clinical scenario, such as risk for bleeding.

Symptoms, Diagnosis & Treatment

When patients are present with PE, they will be present with *tachypnea, tachycardia, hypotension,* and, sometimes, *diaphoresis.*

A detailed description of each test that can be used to diagnose a PE is beyond the scope of this book and the CCRN. However, a critical care RN must understand the reasoning behind certain tests. Hence, here we will briefly list the tests used to diagnose PEs. Generally, the easiest test to order is a *CT of the chest with IV contrast,* sometimes referred to as a "spiral CT" based on the protocol used by the radiologist. However, if the patient has renal failure or cannot receive IV contrast due to access or allergy, then a *ventilation/perfusion*

(V/Q) scan is preferred. In difficult cases where the results of studies are ambivalent, the gold standard is *pulmonary angiography,* which again requires contrast administration. Some physicians may order a *"D-dimer" blood test.* This test is highly sensitive but has poor specificity, because many inflammatory conditions other than PE result in elevations of the D-dimer. Hence, this test is useful only in healthy patients with few to no other comorbidities. If this is negative, it is highly unlikely that the patient has a PE.

The treatment of acute pulmonary emboli depends on whether the patient is hemodynamically stable. If hemodynamic stability is not a concern, then either a *heparin drip* (unfractionated heparin) intravenously, subcutaneous injections twice daily of *LMWH* (e.g., enoxaparin, dalteparin, tinzaparin), or antithrombin III binder (e.g., fondaparinux). Patients are generally maintained on anticoagulation for three months after their first acute pulmonary thromboembolism once they are discharged from the hospital. However, recurrent episodes may require more invasive treatment such as an *inferior vena cava filter* (IVC filter, aka "Greenfield filter").

ACUTE HYPOXEMIC RESPIRATORY FAILURE

Respiratory failure is generally categorized as defects in either oxygenation or ventilation. If infiltrates are present, the respiratory failure can be further categorized as **cardiogenic** or **noncardiogenic**.

Cardiogenic Respiratory Failure

Cardiogenic pulmonary edema is the result of *failure of the left side of the heart to maintain forward flow through the left ventricular outflow tract.* This can occur for a number of reasons that are beyond the scope of this section. However, suffice it to say that failure of the left-sided cardiac function results in volume overload in the pulmonary vasculature, which can be measured as *an increase in the pulmonary artery occlusion pressure (PAOP).* Once the pulmonary capillary wedge pressure is decreased with diuresis, the pulmonary edema resolves.

Noncardiogenic Respiratory Failure: Acute Respiratory Distress Syndrome (ARDS)

Noncardiogenic respiratory failure is due to "leaky" pulmonary capillaries, which result in fluid leaving the vasculature and entering the lung parenchyma/interstitial compartment. Acute respiratory distress syndrome (ARDS) is a sudden, progressive form of acute respiratory failure in which the alveolar capillary membrane becomes damaged and more permeable to intravascular fluid, causing the alveoli to fill with fluid. The latest definition and clinical diagnosis of ARDS is based on the 2012 consensus guidelines by ARDS Definition Task Force, and it is known as the Berlin definition (the conference was held in Berlin, Germany).

Pathophysiology

It is believed that ARDS results from *damage to the pulmonary endothelium* with or without insult to the epithelium. ARDS exists on a continuum. Progression of ARDS varies among patients, and several factors determine the course of ARDS, including the nature of the initial injury, extent and severity of coexisting diseases, and pulmonary complications. The most common cause of ARDS is sepsis. It may also develop as a consequence of the systemic inflammatory response syndrome or multiple organ dysfunction syndrome. The pathophysiologic changes of ARDS are divided into three phases: injury, reparative or proliferative, and fibrotic or chronic. Diagnostic findings in ARDS include noncardiogenic pulmonary edema that progresses to multifocal consolidation, appearing as a "whiteout" on the x-ray film. These insults and damage can come about from *direct toxin exposure, medication side effects,* and/or *inflammation.* Toxic insult can occur from inhalation of aerosolized chemicals, smoking tobacco, etc. Systemic inflammation in sepsis results in widespread release of inflammatory cytokines, which causes epithelial damage. Medications such as amiodarone, methotrexate, and carbamazepine (brand name: Tegretol) have also been associated with ARDS. Some comorbidities may make patients susceptible to the acquisition of ARDS. The Berlin definition of ARDS is listed in table 6.1.

TABLE 6.1 *Berlin Definition of ARDS*

ACUTE RESPIRATORY DISTRESS SYNDROME	
Timing	Within 1 week of a known clinical insult or new or worsening respiratory symptoms
Chest imaging[a]	Bilateral opacities—not fully explained by effusions, lobar/lung collapse, or nodules
Origin of edema	Respiratory failure not fully explained by cardiac failure or fluid overload Need objective assessment (e.g., echocardiography) to exclude hydrostatic edema if no risk factor present
Oxygenation[b]	
Mild	200 mm Hg $<PaO_2/FiO_2 \leq 300$ mm Hg with PEEP or CPAP ≥ 5 cm H_2O[c]
Moderate	100 mm Hg $<PaO_2/FiO_2 \leq 200$ mm Hg with PEEP ≥ 5 cm H_2O
Severe	$PaO_2/FiO_2 \leq 100$ mm Hg with PEEP ≥ 5 cm H_2O

Abbreviations: CPAP, continuous positive airway pressure; FiO_2, fraction of inspired oxygen; PaO_2, partial pressure of arterial oxygen; PEEP, positive end-expiratory pressure

[a] Chest radiograph or computed tomography scan

[b] If altitude is higher than 1,000 m, the correction factor should be calculated as follows: $[PaO_2/FiO_2 \times$ (barometric pressure/760)].

[c] This may be delivered noninvasively in the mild acute respiratory distress syndrome group.

Management and Treatment

The goal in ARDS management is to *maintain oxygenation and provide symptomatic support,* allowing the lungs to recover from the insult. Hence, first treat the cause (e.g., sepsis). This should occur simultaneously with administration of oxygen and mechanical ventilation, if necessary (almost always). Again, a detailed discussion regarding ventilators is beyond the scope of the CCRN, but a critical care RN should know that the lungs are generally "stiffer" in noncardiogenic respiratory failure. As a result, the ventilation parameter that will be important is the positive end-expiratory pressure (PEEP). *Increasing the PEEP* will help keep the alveoli open and available for oxygenation. The general standard for O_2 administration is to give the patient the lowest concentration that results in a PaO_2 of ≥60 mm Hg. Alternative modes of ventilation may be used and include airway pressure release ventilation, pressure control inverse ratio ventilation, high-frequency ventilation, and permissive hypercapnia. Positioning strategies to improve oxygenation that can be considered for patients with ARDS include prone positioning, continuous lateral rotation therapy, and kinetic therapy. Complications from ARDS include ventilator-associated pneumonia (VAP), barotrauma or volutrauma (e.g., pneumothorax), stress ulcers, and renal failure.

RESPIRATORY INFECTIONS

"Pulmonary infection" is a broad topic. However, for the CCRN, the scope of this section will be limited to **community-acquired pneumonia** (CAP), **aspiration pneumonia**, and **healthcare-associated pneumonia** (HAP).

Symptoms

The presenting symptoms of all respiratory infections are similar: *dyspnea* with or without a *cough.* The cough may or may not be productive. The patient may report *fever, chills,* and/ or *night sweats.* The latter should raise suspicion for either septicemia or tuberculosis (TB). Other constitutional symptoms such as body aches and rhinorrhea (runny nose) may be present in viral upper respiratory infections (URI). In the elderly, mental status changes and headache may also be present.

Community-Acquired Pneumonia (CAP)

CAP is defined as pneumonia in a patient who has not recently been hospitalized. The risk factors associated with community-acquired pneumonia are age greater than 65; comorbidities such as asthma, diabetes, or renal failure; a weakened immune system such as with HIV (human immunodeficiency virus); or antibiotic resistance. Diagnosis is made by physical examination, chest x-ray, complete blood count, and cultures of sputum if available. A host of organisms can cause CAP. They can be categorized as typical and atypical. Typical bacterial pathogens include *Streptococcus pneumoniae, Haemophilus influenzae,* as well as *Moraxella catarrhalis* (previously called *Branhamella*). Atypical organisms include *Legionella* species,

Mycoplasma species, and *Chlamydophila pneumoniae* (formerly called *Chlamydia pneumoniae*). Organisms that are considered rare, unless the clinical picture is appropriate, are *Klebsiella pneumoniae* (aspiration in chronic alcoholics), *Staphylococcus aureus* (post-viral pneumoniae), and *Pseudomonas aeruginosa* (in patients with cystic fibrosis or bronchiectasis). The antibiotic regimen chosen can vary for CAP. Patients who are treated on an outpatient basis will most likely be treated with one of three agents: macrolides, fluroquinolines, or doxycycline. Patients who have been diagnosed as moderate to high risk will be treated with a combination of antibiotics to include a beta lactam such as cefotaxime (Claforan) or ceftriaxone (Rocephin) and either a macrolide or fluoroquinolone (Levaquin).

Aspiration Pneumonia

Aspiration pneumonia generally develops in those patients with dysphagia, either due to intrinsic musculoskeletal/nervous system disease or ingestion of medications that cause drowsiness and/or intoxication. Hence, the patient with aspiration pneumonia may be an elderly patient with mild dysphagia or a young patient who is intoxicated and whose state of mental alertness is depressed. In either case, the mechanism and organisms are essentially the same. There will be *multiple oropharyngeal organisms* found in the sputum culture and tracheal aspirate. Further, in aspiration pneumonia, the physicians will often add clindamycin or metronidazole to cover for anaerobes.

Healthcare-Associated Pneumonia (HAP)

When patients develop pneumonia during a hospital admission, it can be difficult to determine whether it was a developing preexisting condition or acquired as a result of the hospital stay. As a result, the definition of hospital or nosocomial pneumonia is a pneumonia that *develops at least 72 hours after being admitted.* Further, since the pathogens within the in-patient setting are much different than those in the community, the antibiotic choices may also vary and include vancomycin, third- and fourth-generation cephalosporins, carbapenems, fluoroquinolones, and aminoglycosides (e.g., gentamycin). Currently, the recommendations are to *treat with a double or triple antibiotic regimen in the setting of hospital-acquired pneumonia.* A form of HAP is ventilator-associated pneumonia (VAP).

Ventilator-Associated Pneumonia (VAP)

Ventilator-associated pneumonia is defined as a pneumonia where the patient is on mechanical ventilation for >2 calendar days on the date of the event, with day of ventilator placement being day 1 *and* with the ventilator in place on the date of the event or the day before. Diagnosis of VAP also includes clinical evidence of:

- Fever and/or elevated white blood cell count

- Purulent or odorous sputum

- Crackles or rhonchi on auscultation

- Pulmonary infiltrates on chest x-ray

Multiple episodes of healthcare-associated pneumonia may occur in critically ill patients with lengthy hospital stays. Excluded organisms that cannot be used to meet the VAP definition are as follows: normal respiratory flora, normal oral flora, mixed respiratory flora, mixed oral flora, altered oral flora, or other similar results indicating isolation of commensal flora of the oral cavity or upper respiratory tract. The following organisms, unless identified from lung tissue or pleural fluid, are not used in the diagnosis of VAP: *Candida* species, coagulase-negative *Staphylococcus* species, and *Enterococcus* species.

Care "Bundle" to Prevent VAP

The following nursing interventions are part of the care "bundle" to be implemented to prevent VAP:

- HOB elevation at least 30 to 45 degrees unless medically contraindicated

- No routine changes of ventilator circuit tubing

- DVT prophylaxis

- H2 blockers and proton-pump inhibitors (PPI)

- Use of an ET that allows continuous suctioning of secretions in subglottic area

- Drain condensation that collects in ventilator tubing

PULMONARY DISEASES AND ABNORMAL CONDITIONS

Many different diseases and conditions can affect the pulmonary system. For the CCRN exam, we will concentrate on reviewing chronic obstructive pulmonary diseases (COPDs), including asthma, emphysema, and chronic bronchitis; pulmonary hypertension; "air leaks"; thoracic surgery; and trauma.

Chronic Obstructive Pulmonary Disease (COPD)

Chronic obstructive pulmonary disease (COPD) is a class of lung disease that includes emphysema and chronic bronchitis. Within this group, these are the diseases most likely to appear on the CCRN. All of these diseases share common pathophysiology. Namely, they all result in "air-trapping" within the lungs. The etiology behind this "air-trapping" can vary, depending on the disease. In some cases, it is loss of pulmonary elasticity and recoil (e.g., emphysema), narrowing of the airways that may or may not be due to inflammation, thus limiting the amount of expired air (e.g., chronic bronchitis).

Risk Factors

The risk factors for COPD can be thought of as environmental and genetic. Environmental risk factors include tobacco use, secondhand smoke exposure, and occupational exposure (coal, gold, cadmium, isocyanates, silica, and asbestos). Air pollution is also believed to play a role in triggering, and possibly initiating, COPD. Genetic risk factors include, classically, alpha-1-antitrypsin deficiency. This enzyme helps protect the lung from a self-made digestive enzyme (trypsin). The lack of this protein results in unbalanced activity of this digestive enzyme and destruction of lung parenchyma, leading to emphysema (see below). Further, there is evidence that some COPD may be caused by an autoimmune reaction in those with a certain immunological profile. Hence, COPD may also partly be an autoimmune disease.

Symptoms

As one would imagine, the most obvious symptom of COPD is that of dyspnea. *Dyspnea* will gradually worsen over time, to the point that it begins to limit activities of daily living (ADL). A *cough* may or may not be associated with the dyspnea. Likewise, not all patients with COPD have copious *sputum production,* although sputum production increases with time. In the advanced stages, *cyanosis* may be apparent, indicating significant aberration in gas exchange. Finally, in the end stages, cardiovascular circulation in the pulmonary vasculature will be compromised and lead to right-sided heart failure in the absence of left-sided heart failure, otherwise known as **cor pulmonale**. On exam, there may be expiratory *wheezing* (often best heard in the anterior and lateral lung fields), *tachypnea, chest protrusion, use of accessory muscles for breathing* (in exacerbations), breathing with *pursed lips,* and/or the presence of *rales* (crackles) on posterior lung field auscultation.

Chronic Bronchitis

Chronic bronchitis is defined clinically and is characterized by productive *cough on most days for three months of a year and over the course of two consecutive years.* As the name implies, chronic bronchitis results from long-standing inflammation of the airways. As a result, there is hyperplasia and hypertrophy of the mucus-producing cells (goblet cells). Inflammation is histologically dominant. The chronic inflammation also leads to scarring and thickening of the airway, resulting in limited ability to fully expire air. Over time, the chronic obstruction places the patient at increased risk for pulmonary infections, primarily pneumonia.

Emphysema

Emphysema is histologically defined as the *destruction of airspace distal to the terminal bronchioles.* There is also destruction of the walls of the alveoli in the absence of fibrosis. On imaging, these airspaces are referred to as *bullae.* In emphysema, the patient loses elastic recoil of the lung due to the destruction of the parenchyma, and as a result, there is limited ability to expire the inhaled air. Furthermore, there will be gas-exchange abnormalities, since the alveoli are no longer present.

Asthma

Classically, asthma has been defined as *hyperresponsive airways*. There is some overlap with chronic bronchitis. However, there is almost complete reversibility of airway constriction in asthma. Furthermore, the etiology behind asthma is felt to be environmental, and interestingly, each person with asthma may have a different *environmental trigger*.

COPD and Asthma Exacerbations

Often a "trigger" will cause an exacerbation of preexisting pulmonary disease. When this occurs, the patient will often be placed in an intensive care setting due to *tachypnea, dyspnea,* and possibly *hypoxemia.*

In COPD exacerbations, the trigger is a bacterial infection 70–75 percent of the time. Hence, therapy needs to be targeted toward inflammation, airway constriction, oxygenation, and infection. Often, these therapeutic regimens will include *beta agonists* (e.g., albuterol), *anticholinergics* (e.g., ipratropium), *intravenous corticosteroids* (e.g., methylprednisolone), and *antibiotics.* The antibiotic(s) chosen vary(ies) based on each clinical situation and the organism suspected, but they include quinolones (e.g., levofloxacin), doxycycline, trimethoprim-sulfamethoxazole, macrolides (e.g., azithromycin), cephalosporins (e.g., ceftriaxone), antipseudomonas (e.g., piperacillin-tazobactam), and/or aminoglycosides (e.g., tobramycin).

Asthma exacerbations (status asthmaticus) are treated in a similar manner to COPD exacerbations. Understanding that bronchodilation and controlling inflammation is the primary focus of treatment in asthma exacerbations, it comes as no surprise that therapy consists of beta-agonists (inhaled metered dose inhalers or nebulizers) and intravenous corticosteroids (e.g., methylprednisolone). Treatment with antibiotics should take place only in the context of strong clinical suspicion, in contrast to COPD exacerbations, that the trigger is an infection.

Pulmonary Hypertension

Increased blood pressure to the pulmonary vasculature, known as pulmonary hypertension (PH), is generally caused by tightening of pulmonary arteries, fibrosis of pulmonary vessels, or blood clots restricting blood flow in the pulmonary vessels, therefore increasing pressure. In individuals with PH, pressure in the pulmonary arteries is greater than 25 mm Hg at rest and 30 mm Hg under exertion, whereas normal at-rest pressure is 15 mm Hg. Symptoms generally worsen as the individual exerts himself and include shortness of breath during normal tasks, dizziness and fainting, fatigue, nonproductive cough, and peripheral edema. PH can be severe, inhibiting exertion tolerance and often leading to heart failure.

Five types of PH have been classified:

1. *Pulmonary arterial hypertension* is associated with a tightening of blood vessels leading to and inside the lungs. The etiology may be idiopathic, inherited, drug/toxin induced, or associated with other conditions such as connective tissue diseases, HIV infection, or chronic hemolytic anemia.

2. *Pulmonary hypertension caused by left heart disease* occurs when the left side of the heart pumps blood inefficiently, leading to pulmonary edema and pleural effusions. This condition is associated with left ventricular systolic dysfunction, left ventricular diastolic dysfunction, and valvular disease.

3. *Pulmonary hypertension caused by lung diseases and/or hypoxia* arises when lung diseases such as COPD, breathing sleep disorders, and lung abnormalities lead to low levels of oxygen in the blood.

4. *Chronic thromboembolic pulmonary hypertension* is caused by blood clots in the pulmonary blood vessels.

5. *Pulmonary hypertension with unclear multifactorial mechanisms* may be caused by hematologic, systemic, or metabolic disorders; tumor obstruction; or chronic renal failure.

Depending on the type of PH, treatment may include drug therapy, such as diuretics, beta-blockers, and blood thinners; surgical procedures, including mitral or aortic valve repair or replacement; and lifestyle changes.

"Air Leaks"

The phrase *air leaks* is not a medical or clinical term. Instead it is a functional term used here to help you remember syndromes where there is *abnormal air collection in the thorax cavity.* For the most part, if you remember that air should be in the airways, lungs, esophagus, and stomach, then if you see air any place else, it is abnormal. For example, air between the chest wall and the lung periphery is referred to as a **pneumothorax** ("collapsed lung"); air in the space around the heart is referred to as **pneumopericardium**; air in the space between the two lungs (mediastinum) is known as **pneumomediastinum**; and air in the space around the alveoli is referred to as **perivascular interstitial emphysema** (PIE).

Pneumothorax and Pneumopericardium

The most significant of the "air leak" syndromes are pneumothorax and pneumopericardium since these can be fatal. Generally, there is no air in the pleural space. However, when air enters the pleural space, it is referred to as a pneumothorax. As a result, the underlying lung may "collapse." If this occurs, the underlying lung cannot be involved in ventilation, and the patient may present with *dyspnea* if the area involved is large. The treatment for a pneumothorax depends on the size, but in cases where the patient will be admitted to the intensive care unit, the rim of air between the lung and chest wall on a radiograph will likely be more than 2 cm. If this is the case, and the patient is short of breath, then a *needle thoracostomy* is performed, and a *chest tube* may need to be inserted.

Likewise, a pneumopericardium is air in the pleural space around the heart. The consequences of a pneumopericardium will be the same as a pericardial effusion. Thus, if there is only a small amount of air, then the patient may be asymptomatic. However, if there is a larger amount of air, then there may be compromise of the filling of the heart and, subsequently, the cardiac output, referred to as *cardiac tamponade*. The treatment is similar to that for a large pericardial effusion: needle decompression (pericardiocentesis).

Perivascular Interstitial Emphysema

Normally there is no air between the wall of the alveoli and the surrounding vasculature. However, when air leaks from an alveoli or the alveoli bursts, air can be seen in this perivascular space and is referred to as perivascular interstitial emphysema (PIE). In the majority of cases, this is not fatal and patients are asymptomatic. However, the air in this space has the potential to "dissect" through tissues if there is large alveolar pressure. If this air spreads, it has the potential to lead to a pneumothorax and/or pneumopericardium, where the patient may be symptomatic and require immediate intervention, as outlined above.

Pneumomediastinum

The space in the thorax demarcated by the medial borders of the lung laterally, the sternum anteriorly, and the spine posteriorly is known as the mediastinum. A pneumomediastinum refers to air in this space. Generally, there is no emergency in a pneumomediastinum, since this space is more than able to accommodate air without compromising pulmonary or cardiac function. However, the patient may feel some discomfort if the pneumomediastinum is large. Further, if there is compromise of the visceral pleura that lines this space, then the patient may develop a pneumothorax and/or a pneumopericardium and require intervention. Hence, pneumomediastinum is not fatal, but it should not be taken lightly and needs close follow-up. The critical care RN should be aware of tachypnea, tachycardia, hypoxia, and hypotension—signs that may suggest that there is hemodynamic compromise.

Thoracic Surgery

Thoracic surgery may include removal of one or more lobes (*lobectomy*) or an entire lung (*pneumonectomy*) for malignancy, abscesses, or trauma. Removal of wedge-shaped section of the lung (*wedge resection*) is used for small lesions or pulmonary blebs, while resection of damaged tissue (*lung volume reduction*) is used to achieve a more normal chest wall. The critical care RN should be aware of pulmonary hygiene and chest physiotherapy; DVT prophylaxis; and fluid, electrolyte, and pain management.

Trauma

Trauma to the thorax cavity can be categorized as **nonpenetrating (blunt)** or **penetrating**. Further, trauma can also be categorized by site of injury (e.g., airways, cardiac, pulmonary, esophagus, chest wall, diaphragm). The signs and symptoms of trauma to the thorax will generally be the same and may include respiratory distress, subcutaneous emphysema, pneumothorax, hemoptysis, mediastinal emphysema, hypotension, and tachycardia. Hemoptysis will generally occur in penetrating trauma, but if there is compromise of a structure, such as a great vessel or airway in nonpenetrating trauma, these patients may also present with hemoptysis.

Nonpenetrating trauma to the thorax can occur during motor vehicle accidents, other accidents, fights, etc. The force of the trauma, if large enough, will often be transmitted to the internal organs: heart and lungs. This can result in a cardiac or pulmonary contusion. Generally, the patient may be mildly dyspneic and may or may not have oxygenation issues, depending on the severity of the contusion and percentage of the lung involved. The other important structures within the thorax cavity are the great vessels (vena cavae, aorta, pulmonary veins, and pulmonary artery). Depending on the nature and direction of the nonpenetrating force, these vessels may experience shearing forces and may rupture. In these cases, it is important that the patient be stabilized immediately and emergent thoracotomy performed. In addition to symptoms of dyspnea, tachypnea, and, possibly tachycardia, the patient may also experience pulmonary hemorrhage with hemoptysis in extensive pulmonary contusions and/or pulmonary vasculature rupture.

It is important always to look and assess for fractured ribs, as these may compromise the patient's ability to ventilate. Specifically, the most serious condition that can result from multiple fractured ribs is "**flail chest**." Some sources state that at least two adjacent ribs must be broken in a minimum of two places, while others state three or more ribs must be fractured in two or more places. Either way, there are multiple rib fractures in multiple places. The rib fractures compromise the patient's ability to control the expansion of the thorax cavity, and the "flail segment" moves in the opposite direction as the rest of the chest wall (i.e., it moves inward when the chest expands and moves out when the patient exhales). There will most likely be an accompanying pulmonary contusion as well. The pulmonary contusion will compromise the oxygenation, as stated above. The degree to which the oxygenation is compromised will be a determining factor in survival. The treatment of flail chest is positive pressure ventilation, analgesia, supplemental oxygenation, and chest tube placement.

Penetrating trauma compromises the integrity of the thorax cavity. An example is a stab wound. In these cases, the risk of bleeding is high. As a result, the possibility of a hemothorax is likely. A hemothorax is similar to a pneumothorax, but instead of air in the thorax cavity (which may also occur with penetrating trauma), there is blood in the pleural space. The treatment is evacuation and chest tube placement, similar to pneumothorax. If more than 1,500 mL of blood are removed from the thorax cavity, it is important to consider injury to a major vessel and pursue thoracotomy. In penetrating trauma, if an impaled object is present, it is important to remember: DO NOT REMOVE THE IMPALED OBJECT until the patient is in the operating room and the proper measures have been taken to stabilize the patient as much as possible. This will help deal with the consequences of removing the impaled object (e.g., massive hemorrhage) under controlled circumstances and allow for an immediate thoracotomy.

Tracheal perforation can result from nonpenetrating and penetrating trauma. Tracheal perforation or compromise is more often cervical (above the carina) in penetrating trauma and within 2–3 cm of the lower aspect of the carina in nonpenetrating trauma. The symptoms are similar to penetrating trauma in that there is a compromise in the structure of the airway. The treatment of choice is bronchoscopy, if possible, and primary closure with end-end anastomosis.

MECHANICAL VENTILATION

When patients need assistance with ventilation or are unable to ventilate themselves, mechanical ventilation may be utilized. Mechanical ventilation is categorized as noninvasive and invasive. Noninvasive ventilation is also referred to as **noninvasive positive pressure ventilation** (NPPV). The goal of mechanical ventilation is to provide adequate oxygenation (PaO_2) and ventilation ($PaCO_2$).

Noninvasive Positive Pressure Ventilation (NPPV)

NPPV is generally used when the patient has a sufficient respiratory drive to breathe on their own but may need assistance in helping keep the airways open. The theory behind NPPV is that positive pressure delivered through a mask can help keep the airways open while a patient is breathing and that this can decrease the work of breathing. There are generally two types of NPPV: **continuous positive airway pressure** (CPAP) and **biphasic positive airway pressure** (BIPAP). In both types of NPPV, the patient wears a mask with a seal. In CPAP, the patient receives a constant amount of pressure that is delivered throughout inspiration and expiration. In contrast, in BIPAP, the patient receives a different pressure during inspiration (inspiratory positive airway pressure, **IPAP**) and during expiration (expiratory positive airway pressure, **EPAP**).

The types of clinical situations in which NPPV should be considered as a first modality of ventilation are COPD exacerbations, cardiogenic pulmonary edema, acute respiratory failure in immunosuppressed patients, and patients with COPD who are being extubated. The institution of NPPV in the above clinical scenarios has been studied and shown to reduce the need for intubation, decrease mortality, and decrease the length of hospital stay in the intensive care setting. NPPV may also be considered for patients with status asthmaticus, but there are limited numbers of studies looking at the benefit of NPPV with regard to the above endpoints or improvement in pulmonary function (e.g., FEV_1). When instituting NPPV, there are a variety of masks to choose from: full face, oronasal, and nasal.

Who are **not** good candidates for Bi-PAP machines?

Exclusion criteria for the use of NPPV include:

- Those who require immediate intubation (what's the patient's ABG?)
- Those who cannot protect their airway and are at high risk for aspiration
- Respiratory failure with hemodynamic instability (what are the patient's vitals?)

- Uncooperative patients

- Recent craniofacial trauma, surgery, or burns

- Patients with extreme anxiety, agitation, or excessive secretions

Complications of NPPV therapy include:

- Mucus plugging and atelectasis in patients with excessive secretions due to lack of access to the upper airway

- Facial ulcerations and eye irritation due to mask pressure

- Gastric insufflation and distention

- Feelings of claustrophobia and anxiety

- Dryness of the oral cavity

Invasive Mechanical Ventilation

Invasive mechanical ventilation refers to patients in whom an endotracheal tube (ET) has been placed and a ventilator is being used to ventilate the patient. As with NPPV, there are certain indications to use invasive mechanical ventilation. The obvious cases are where patients are unconscious, cannot protect their airway, or are in acute respiratory distress with or without hemodynamic instability. More specifically, clinical scenarios where invasive mechanical ventilation should be seriously considered are when a patient fails a trial of NPPV, is in acute respiratory distress (as evidenced by oxygenation/ventilation and/or the use of accessory muscles for breathing or a respiratory rate of 35 breaths/minute or greater), or in shock.

Ventilators can be confusing, and although this section is not designed to transform the reader into an expert, it should provide you with the tools as a critical care RN to understand the basic terminology and modes of ventilation. There are two modes of invasive mechanical ventilation used in the intensive care units: **volume** and **pressure control**. In *volume control*, the machine simply controls the amount of tidal volume inspired by the patient. Currently, the trend is to use "low-volume ventilation" (also referred to as lung protective ventilation), which is believed to minimize barotrauma to the lung. In volume control, the operator can set the respiratory rate, tidal volume, and the positive end-expiratory pressure (the amount of pressure remaining in the lungs after all the tidal volume has been expired [PEEP]). You should note that the PEEP can also be thought of as EPAP. In *pressure control*, the ventilator allows the patient to determine the tidal volume. However, the ventilator is set to control the IPAP and PEEP or EPAP, as well as the respiratory rate. Whichever mode of ventilation the physician is using, the ventilator will always allow control over the percentage of inspired oxygen that the patient receives (FiO_2). Normally the FiO_2 is 21 percent at room air. Hence, if a patient is requiring the ventilator, it is common for the

FiO_2 to be set anywhere from 30–100 percent. Complications of PEEP include barotrauma, pneumothorax, and hypotension. It is important to monitor the patient's BP closely, especially when using PEEP greater than 10 cm.

Volutrauma and Barotrauma

When using mechanical ventilation, primarily invasive mechanical ventilation, the patient may experience pulmonary trauma. The simple theory behind the trauma is that the lungs are being overventilated (i.e., overexpanded). The two ways in which this occurs are by delivering very *high tidal volumes* (resulting in volutrauma) and by delivering *high airway pressures* (resulting in barotraumas). These forms of trauma damage the parenchyma and may result in pulmonary edema from "leaky" perialveolar capillaries. Hence, using minimal pressures and volume is preferred in invasive mechanical ventilation. Although institutions vary on which mode (volume or pressure control) they prefer, there seems to be a tendency to use volume control to minimize the risk of barotraumas.

TROUBLESHOOTING MAJOR VENTILATOR ALARMS		
ALARMS	**CAUSES**	**TROUBLESHOOTING**
Low Pressure Alarms (low volume)	• Leak in the ET tube or tubing • Disconnection of tubing • Self-extubation	• Change tubing PRN • Connect all tubing • Assess if patient no longer needs intubation, place patient on 100% non-rebreathing mask, suction and prepare for re-intubation, sedate PRN, restrain PRN
High Pressure Alarms (increased airway resistance and decreased pulmonary compliance)	• Secretions • Water accumulation in tubing • Kink in the tubing or patient biting the tube • Pneumothorax • Pain/anxiety • Bronchospasm	• Suction ET/tracheostomy and mouth • Remove water or change filter • Unkink tubes, bite block, sedation PRN • CXR, prepare for chest tube insertion, check ABGs, sedation • Give pain meds and/or sedation PRN, emotional support to patient and family • Bronchodilators and sedation PRN, check ABGs, and change settings PRN

ARTERIAL BLOOD GAS ANALYSIS

In managing patients in the intensive care setting, it will be important to monitor the arterial blood gases (ABG) and be able to interpret the results. For the purposes of the CCRN, the discussion will be focused on the steps necessary to interpret an ABG. However, a preliminary review of the physiology is important prior to undertaking this discussion.

The body generally has a normal pH in the bloodstream of approximately 7.4 and will attempt to maintain this pH through a number of mechanisms. The key components/organ systems involved in the maintenance of normal blood pH are the bicarbonate (HCO_3^-) buffer system in the blood, the lungs, and the kidneys. The lungs and kidneys can respond to the changing pH of the blood to help correct disturbances in the pH. For example, the lungs can breathe faster and/or increase the tidal volume to make the blood alkaline in response to an acidic change. Conversely the lungs can breathe more slowly and/or decrease the tidal volume to make the blood more acidic in response to an alkaline change in the blood. Likewise the kidneys can reabsorb more or less bicarbonate (HCO_3^-), depending on whether there is an acidic or alkaline change in the blood.

In order to understand acid-base balance, it is important to know the relationship between CO_2 and HCO_3^- (e.g., the chemical equation for the bicarbonate buffer system):

$$CO_2 + H_2O \leftrightarrow H_2CO_3 \leftrightarrow H^+ + HCO_3^-$$

Next, in order to interpret blood gases, it is important first to know the components of an ABG and their normal values. The five measurements on an ABG are pH, arterial partial pressure of carbon dioxide ($PaCO_2$), arterial partial pressure of oxygen (PaO_2), HCO_3^-, and base excess (BE). There are four primary acid-base disorders: respiratory acidosis, respiratory alkalosis, metabolic acidosis, and metabolic alkalosis. The normal values for these measurements are listed next.

Normal ABG Values

pH	PaCO$_2$	PaO$_2$	HCO$_3^-$	BE
7.35–7.45	35–45 mm Hg	80–100 mm Hg	22–26 mEq/L	−2 to +2 mEq/L

Respiratory Acidosis: Low pH and High PaCO$_2$

Respiratory acidosis occurs when the lungs are not sufficiently ventilating. In other words, CO_2 is building up in the bloodstream. Based on the bicarbonate buffer equation above, a build up of CO_2 will lead to an increase in the concentration of H^+, making the blood acidic. Based on this understanding, respiratory acidosis is defined as a pH below 7.35 and a $PaCO_2$ greater than 45 mm Hg. Common causes of respiratory acidosis are cardiac arrest, COPD, sedation/drug overdose, and lactic acidosis (e.g., sepsis).

Respiratory Alkalosis: High pH and Low PaCO$_2$

Respiratory alkalosis occurs when the lungs are "overbreathing" and releasing too much CO_2 from the bloodstream. Hence, the CO_2 concentration is decreasing in the bloodstream. Based on the previous bicarbonate buffer equation, a decrease in the concentration of CO_2 will lead to an decrease in the concentration of H^+, making the blood alkalotic. Based on this understanding, respiratory alkalosis is defined as a pH above 7.45 and a $PaCO_2$ less than

35 mm Hg. Common causes of respiratory alkalosis are hyperventilation (e.g., panic attacks, anxiety), hypermetabolic states (e.g., hyperthermia), high mechanical ventilation, and CNS disorders affecting patterns of respiration.

Metabolic Acidosis: Low pH and Low HCO_3^-

Metabolic acidosis occurs when the pH of the bloodstream is less than 7.35 and there is a decrease in the HCO_3^- (below 22 mEq/L). The decrease in the HCO_3^- can occur as a result of gastrointestinal disorders (e.g., diarrhea), endocrine disorders (e.g., diabetic ketoacidosis), nutritional deficiency, and/or renal disorders (e.g. renal tubular acidosis, acute kidney injury, chronic renal insufficiency, etc.).

Metabolic Alkalosis: High pH and High HCO_3^-

Metabolic alkalosis occurs when the pH of the bloodstream is greater than 7.45 and there is an increase in the HCO_3^- (above 26 mEq/L). The increase in the HCO_3^- can occur as a result of gastrointestinal disorders (e.g., prolonged emesis), prolonged gastric suctioning with a nasogastric (NG) tube, hypochloremia, administration of diuretics (e.g., furosemide), and/or elevated levels of aldosterone.

Compensation

Compensation is an effort of the body to correct the pH by either respiratory or metabolic changes (depending on the primary impairment). Compensation is present when both parameters ($PaCO_2$ and HCO_3^-) are out of normal range. Both parameters have to be going opposite directions (one indicating alkalosis and the other acidosis). If the pH is within normal range then compensation is full. If the pH is not within normal range but both parameters are out of normal range and going opposite directions, then compensation is partial. To identify the primary impairment in a fully compensated ABG result, match the parameters with the pH. A pH below 7.40 indicates an acidotic process; a pH above 7.40 an alkalotic process.

Simple Steps to Interpreting ABG

Step 1: Look at the pH and determine whether it is acidic or alkalotic:

If the pH is < 7.35, there is an acidosis.

If the pH is > 7.45, there is an alkalosis.

Step 2: Assess the $PaCO_2$:

If the $PaCO_2$ is > 45 mm Hg, the primary disorder is respiratory acidosis.

If the $PaCO_2$ is < 35 mm Hg, the primary disorder is respiratory alkalosis.

Step 3: Assess the HCO_3^-:

If the HCO_3^- is > 26 mEq/L, the primary disorder is metabolic alkalosis.

If the HCO_3^- is < 22 mEq/L, the primary disorder is metabolic acidosis.

	Respiratory Acidosis	Respiratory Alkalosis	Metabolic Acidosis	Metabolic Alkalosis
pH	↓	↑	↓	↑
PaCO$_2$	↑	↓	Normal / ↓	Normal / ↑
HCO$_3^-$	Normal / ↑	Normal / ↓	↑	↑

Review Questions

1. Which of these conditions is a nonpulmonary cause of hypoxia?

   A. ARDS

   B. pneumonia

   C. atrial septal defect with shunt

   D. fat embolus

2. A 50-year-old patient is admitted to the ICU with a diagnosis of liver failure. The nurse notices that the patient's respiratory rate has been progressively increasing. An arterial blood gas (ABG) is obtained and reveals pH 7.35, PCO_2 28, PO_2 93, HCO_3 8. The critical care nurse interprets this clinical picture as

   A. respiratory acidosis with metabolic compensation leading to tachypnea.

   B. metabolic acidosis with respiratory compensation leading to tachypnea.

   C. metabolic acidosis with hypoxia leading to tachypnea.

   D. respiratory acidosis with hypoxia leading to tachypnea.

3. The nurse cares for a client with Acute Respiratory Distress Syndrome (ARDS) on mechanical ventilation who is on 100 percent FiO_2 and positive end-expiratory pressure (PEEP) of 10 cm H_2O. The oxygen saturation is 88 percent and blood pressure is 82/40. Which provider order would the nurse anticipate?

   A. Discontinue PEEP and observe O_2 saturation.

   B. Place the client in Trendelenburg position.

   C. Repeat arterial blood gases (ABG) in 8 hours.

   D. Give the client 1 liter normal saline IV bolus.

4. While caring for a patient receiving mechanical ventilation, the critical care nurse notices that the patient suddenly becomes hypoxic and the ventilator begins to alarm. The nurse is unable to identify quickly why the ventilator is alarming. Which of these is the priority action for the nurse to take to prevent further complications?

   A. Press the "Alarm Silence" button on the ventilator and continue troubleshooting.

   B. Administer 100 percent oxygen via the ventilator.

   C. Detach the patient from the ventilator and deliver manual ventilations.

   D. Call for a respiratory therapist to evaluate the problem.

5. The critical care nurse hears a ventilator alarm coming from a patient's room. The nurse determines that the alarm is for "low pressure." Which of these is a likely cause of a "low-pressure" ventilator alarm?

   A. The ventilator circuit has a kink in it.

   B. The patient is biting down on the ET tube.

   C. The ventilator circuit has become disconnected.

   D. The ventilator alarms need to be adjusted.

6. A patient is transferred to the ICU after spending a week on the medical/surgical floor recovering from a right total hip replacement. She has developed a fever and dyspnea, with increasing oxygen requirements and a cough that produces thick green sputum. The critical care nurse knows that the patient will likely be treated for which of these conditions?

   A. aspiration pneumonia

   B. hospital-acquired pneumonia

   C. healthcare-associated pneumonia

   D. fungal pneumonia

7. A patient is admitted to the ICU with a diagnosis of COPD exacerbation. The respiratory status declined, and required endotracheal intubation and mechanical ventilation. A few minutes after the patient is intubated, the patient becomes tachycardic and severely hypotensive. Pulse oximetry readings also decrease significantly. Which of these life-threatening conditions must be immediately identified and treated?

   A. The patient is agitated and needs sedation.

   B. The ventilator settings are inappropriate and need to be adjusted.

   C. The patient is exhibiting signs of a potential tension pneumothorax.

   D. The patient is experiencing increased preload due to positive pressure ventilation.

8. The critical care nurse is caring for a patient with acute respiratory distress syndrome (ARDS). The ventilator settings include low tidal volumes and high levels of PEEP (positive end expiratory pressure). The nurse knows that the goal of this ventilation strategy is to

   A. prevent trauma to the lungs while keeping the alveoli open to improve oxygenation.

   B. prevent pneumothorax while improving removal of carbon dioxide.

   C. prevent high airway pressures while improving removal of secretions.

   D. prevent trauma to the lungs while mimicking normal breathing patterns.

9. The nurse reviews the medical records of a client with acute respiratory distress syndrome (ARDS). Which statement accurately describes an ARDS diagnostic criterion?

   A. Symptoms appear within 1 week of mechanical ventilation.

   B. Symptoms develop within 1 week of a known clinical condition.

   C. Symptoms worsen within 1 week of hospital admission.

   D. Symptoms accompanied by 1 week of productive cough.

10. A patient is in the ICU awaiting lung transplantation. The patient is dependent on BiPAP therapy continuously for oxygenation and "work of breathing" support. The critical care nurse notices that the patient frequently takes off the mask to eat snacks during the day. The critical care nurse should understand that these actions increase the patient's risk for

    A. aspiration.

    B. pneumothorax.

    C. dehydration.

    D. hypotension.

Review Answers and Explanations

1. C

Patients with intracardiac shunts experience mixing of oxygen-rich and oxygen-poor blood, which leads to systemic hypoxia. Such patients will often continue to be hypoxic despite increasing levels of supplemental oxygen. ARDS (A) and pneumonia (B) are classic pulmonary causes of hypoxia, as both cause alveolar obstruction leading to ineffective gas exchange. Fat embolus (D) prevents blood from reaching the alveoli in the lungs, thereby obstructing gas exchange from within the pulmonary vasculature.

2. B

Answer (A) is incorrect because the ABG values are not indicative of respiratory acidosis, as the PCO_2 is far below normal. Answer (C) is incorrect because the patient is not hypoxic, as a PO_2 of 93 is normal. Answer (D) is incorrect because there are no respiratory acidosis and no hypoxia present.

3. D

Blood pressure of 84/40 needs immediate intervention such as fluid boluses. (A) is incorrect because the PEEP is required and cannot be discontinued due to severe hypoxia. (B) is incorrect because Trendelenburg positioning puts the client at risk for aspiration. (C) is incorrect because an ABG might be required sooner than 8 hours—the client has severe hypoxia.

4. C

If the critical care nurse is unable to correct a ventilator alarm quickly and the patient is experiencing negative effects, the nurse should deliver manual ventilations until the problem can be fully evaluated and corrected. The nurse should never press the alarm silence button (A) unless the problem is fully corrected, as the patient may be placed in a dangerous situation. Administering 100 percent oxygen via the ventilator (B) will not ensure that the patient is receiving adequate ventilations, nor will it correct the underlying issue with the ventilator. Answer (D) is incorrect because the critical care nurse must be able to provide appropriate care for patients receiving mechanical ventilation, including basic troubleshooting and emergency procedures. Calling for a respiratory therapist to evaluate the problem is prudent, but the nurse must take action to prevent harm to the patient in the meantime.

5. C

Answer (A) is incorrect because kinking of the ventilator circuit would cause a "high-pressure" alarm. Answer (B) is incorrect because occlusion of the ET tube would also cause a "high-pressure" alarm. Answer (D) is possibly correct, but not likely. The most common cause of a "low-pressure" ventilator alarm is disconnection of the ventilator circuit at any point from the ventilator to the patient.

6. B

The patient has been hospitalized for more than 24 hours and has signs/symptoms consistent with pneumonia. Answer (A) is incorrect because there is no mention of any actual or potential aspiration risks. Answer (C) is incorrect because community-acquired pneumonia is defined as pneumonia that is contracted outside of the hospital or develops before 72 hours of hospitalization. Answer (D) is incorrect because fungal pneumonias are atypical and not usually contracted unless the patient has significant risk factors such as severe immune compromise.

7. C

This potential complication of positive pressure ventilation will occur relatively quickly after intubation. Tachycardia and hypotension result from decreased cardiac output, and hypoxia results from ineffective air exchange. This condition is life threatening and must be treated immediately. Answer (A) is incorrect because agitation is rarely life threatening by itself and the patient would be hypertensive, not hypotensive. Answer (B) is potentially correct, but inappropriate ventilator settings are rarely life threatening in the short term. Answer (D) is incorrect because patients experience decreased preload due to positive pressure ventilation, not increased preload.

8. A

The most common and recommended ventilation strategy for patients with ARDS includes low tidal volumes to prevent volutrauma and high levels of PEEP to keep alveoli open and improve oxygenation. Answer (B) is incorrect because preventing pneumothorax and removal of carbon dioxide are not goals of ARDS treatment. In fact, patients with ARDS often are allowed to retain carbon dioxide to prevent the use of higher tidal volumes. Answer (C) is incorrect because improving removal of secretions is not a goal of ventilation strategies for ARDS. Answer (D) is incorrect because ventilation strategies for ARDS do not mimic normal breathing patterns and, in fact, are often very uncomfortable for patients.

9. B

A clinical precipitating factor that takes place within 1 week of a new or worsening respiratory symptom is a diagnostic criterion for ARDS. (A) is incorrect because mechanical ventilation, by itself, is not a diagnostic criterion for ARDS. (C) is incorrect because the timing of hospital admission is not a diagnostic criterion for ARDS. (D) is incorrect because cough is not a diagnostic criterion for ARDS.

10. A

The combination of oral food intake and non-invasive positive pressure ventilation greatly increases the patient's risk for aspiration, as food may be forced into the pulmonary tree by the BiPAP airflow. The other choices are incorrect because they are not complications of BiPAP therapy or related to the scenario given.

The Endocrine System

7

The endocrine system is the essential regulator of the body's internal environment. It is important to delineate the difference between endocrine and exocrine glands. Endocrine glands secrete their hormones into the bloodstream, where exocrine glands secrete their hormones/enzymes into ducts. Together with the nervous system, the endocrine system regulates growth, reproduction, sex differentiation, metabolism, fluid and electrolyte balance, and internal homeostasis.

FIGURE 7.1 *The Endocrine System*

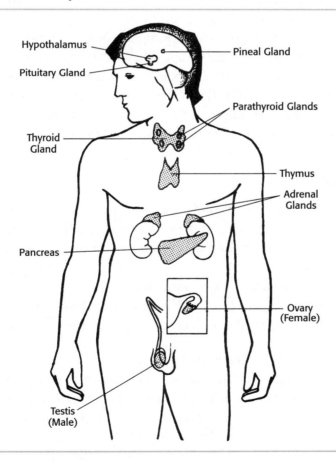

HORMONES

Hormones are chemical messengers that have an effect on target cells distant from the secreting cells. While most hormones travel in the blood, we also know more recently that some hormones never enter the blood and instead act locally in the area where they are released. Hormones that act more locally are described as paracrine (acting on neighboring cells) or autocrine (acting on the cell from which the hormone was secreted) messengers.

Hormones travel to target cells, where they act on specific receptors on the target cell. Some hormone receptors are located on the surface of the cell and act through second messenger mechanisms. Other receptors are located within the cell where they directly influence the synthesis of proteins. After acting on specific receptors on the target cells, hormones are metabolized or inactivated by the target tissues or by the liver. They are excreted by the kidneys to prevent excessive amounts from accumulating in the body over a period of time.

Types

Hormones modulate four broad categories of body function: growth and development, maintenance of homeostasis, energy production during metabolic processes, and reproduction. There are three categories of hormones: peptides, steroids, and amines. Peptides (also called protein hormones) include vasopressin (ADH), thyrotropin-releasing hormone (TRH), insulin, growth hormone (GH), follicle-stimulating hormone (FSH), luteinizing hormone (LH), corticotropin (ACTH), and calcitonin. The steroids include aldosterone, cortisol, estradiol, progesterone, and testosterone. Amines (amino acid derivatives) include norepinephrine, epinephrine, triiodothyronine (T3), and thyroxine (T4).

Feedback Mechanisms

Some hormones are needed in very small amounts and act for variable amounts of time, while other hormones have a prolonged period of cellular action; some interact with other hormones, producing a very complex and intricate system of control. The levels of many of the hormones are regulated by positive and negative feedback mechanisms, although the majority of hormones are controlled by negative feedback. The levels of many hormones are regulated by feedback mechanisms that involve the hypothalamic pituitary target cell system. The hypothalamus and pituitary provide a more complex control system for some hormones.

The hypothalamus secretes releasing or inhibiting factors such as thyrotropin-releasing factor (TRF), which acts on the pituitary gland to secrete thyroid-stimulating hormone (TSH). TSH then stimulates the thyroid gland to increase secretion of the thyroid hormones. The release of the thyroid hormones (T3, T4) into the circulation results in an increase in metabolism (the biological effect of thyroid hormone). High levels of the thyroid hormones *inhibit* secretion of TSH. This is an example of negative feedback and allows tight control over hormone levels.

ANATOMY AND PHYSIOLOGY

Pituitary Gland

The pituitary gland is located in the sella turcica of the sphenoid bone. It is connected to the hypothalamus by the pituitary stalk and links the nervous and endocrine systems. The two lobes of the pituitary gland are the adenohypophysis (anterior pituitary) and the neurohypophysis (posterior pituitary). Hormones of the anterior lobe (75 percent of gland) are controlled by hypothalamic releasing or inhibiting hormones from the hypothalamus issued in response to stimuli received in the central nervous system (CNS). These releasing and inhibiting hormones are delivered from the hypothalamus to the anterior pituitary by a portal circulation. Posterior lobe (25 percent of gland) hormones are controlled by nerve fibers beginning in the hypothalamus and ending in the neurohypophysis. The hormones are synthesized in the hypothalamus, stored in the posterior lobe, and then released after activation of the cell bodies in the nerve tract.

The anterior pituitary hormones can be remembered by the pneumonic "FLAT PEG." This acronym stands for **F**SH, **L**H, **A**CTH, **T**SH, **P**rolactin, **E**ndorphins, and **G**rowth Hormone. Posterior pituitary hormones are vasopressin (aka antidiuretic hormone, ADH) and oxytocin (not discussed in this chapter).

FIGURE 7.2 *Hypothalamus and Pituitary Gland*

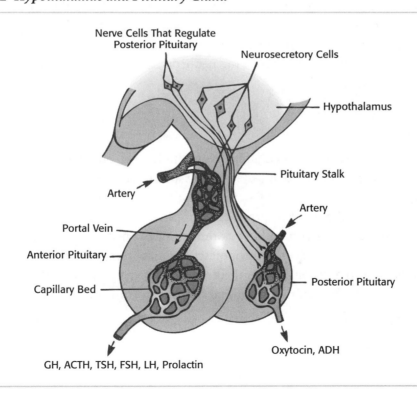

Growth hormone (GH), also called somatotropin, exerts powerful effects on growth and metabolism; it increases protein synthesis, elevates blood glucose levels, increases lipolysis, promotes positive nitrogen balance, and stimulates bone and cartilage growth. Disorders resulting from dysfunction are gigantism or acromegaly with excess and dwarfism with deficiency. Adrenocorticotropic hormone (ACTH) secretion is stimulated by corticotropin-releasing hormone (CRH) in response to physical and/or emotional stress, trauma, hypoglycemia, hypoxia, surgery, and decreased plasma cortisol level. It is inhibited by increased plasma cortisol levels, but stress can override this negative feedback. Disorders resulting from dysfunction are Cushing disease with excess and adrenal insufficiency or Addisonian crisis with deficiency. TRH stimulates TSH in response to low plasma concentration of thyroid hormones. TRH is inhibited by high plasma concentrations of thyroid hormones. Disorders resulting from dysfunction are hyperthyroidism and thyroid storm from excess thyroid hormones, hypothyroidism, and myxedema coma with deficiency.

Posterior pituitary hormones are ADH and oxytocin (not discussed in this chapter). ADH regulates water balance and plasma osmolality. The site of action of ADH is the collecting ducts and distal convoluted tubules of the nephron. ADH directly increases the reabsorption of water, causes vasoconstriction, and, in the CNS, acts to lower body temperature and facilitate memory. There may be excess ADH secretion or a deficiency of secretion in the body. In instances when ADH is being secreted secondary to causes other than serum osmolality or electrolyte concentration, this is referred to as a Syndrome of Inappropriate ADH secretion (SIADH). The lack of ADH activity is manifested as profuse dilute urination, because water is not being reabsorbed. This is referred to as diabetes insipidus and can be categorized as central (lack of secretion from the posterior pituitary or lack of secretion in the hypothalamus) or peripheral (lack of DH effect in the nephron due to lack of or inactivation of ADH receptors in the kidney).

Thyroid Gland

The thyroid gland is located immediately below the larynx, on either side and anterior to the trachea. There are two lobes connected by an isthmus. Three hormones are produced by the thyroid gland: triiodothyronine (T3), thyroxine (T4), and calcitonin. Follicular cells produce T3 and T4. Parafollicular cells produce thyrocalcitonin. T3 and T4 regulate the body's metabolic rate, influence growth and development, have positive chronotropic and inotropic effects on the heart, increase erythropoiesis, regulate temperature, and are needed for normal hypoxic and hypercapnic drive in the respiratory center. Disorders resulting from thyroid dysfunction are hyperthyroidism and thyroid storm from excess and hypothyroidism and myxedema coma with deficiency.

Thyrocalcitonin (calcitonin) affects bone metabolism. It decreases serum calcium by inhibiting calcium mobilization from bone and decreasing calcium resorption in the kidney. Phosphate levels are decreased by inhibiting bone remodeling and increasing phosphate loss in urine.

Parathyroid Glands

Four parathyroid glands are located on the posterior surface of the thyroid gland at the upper and lower ends of each lobe. They receive their blood supply from the thyroid gland and are often damaged by thyroid surgery. Parathyroid hormone (PTH) is released by the chief cells of the parathyroid gland. Stimulation of PTH increases serum calcium levels through direct action in the bone, small intestine, and kidney. Inhibition of PTH decreases serum calcium levels, decreases vitamin D metabolites, and may alter magnesium levels. Disorders resulting from parathyroid dysfunction are hypercalcemia from excess and hypocalcemia from deficiency.

Adrenal Glands

The adrenal glands are located on the upper lobes of each kidney. They are composed of two separate tissues: the adrenal cortex (outer layer) and the adrenal medulla (inner layer). The adrenal cortex (90 percent of the gland) produces three classes of hormones: mineralocorticoids (e.g., aldosterone), glucocorticoids (e.g., cortisol and cortisone), and androgens (e.g., DHEA). Aldosterone helps regulate electrolyte balance by promoting sodium reabsorption and potassium loss. Disorders resulting from dysfunction are primary aldosteronism from excess and Addison disease or adrenal crisis from deficiency.

FIGURE 7.3 *Adrenal Gland: Cortex and Medulla*

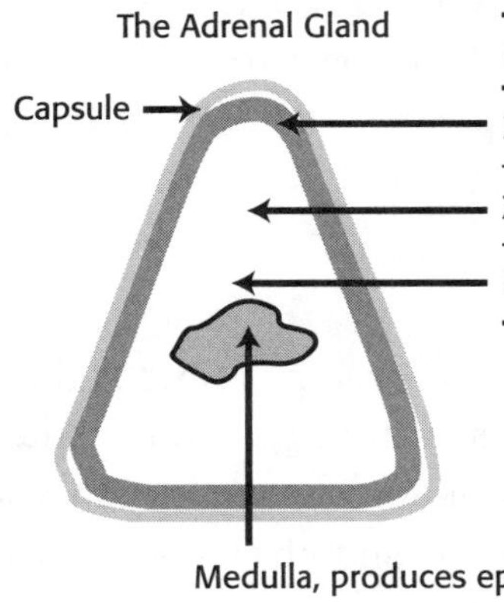

The Adrenal Gland

Capsule →

Region	Hormones	Control system
Zona Glomerulosa	Aldosterone	Angiotensin II, $[K^+]_{plasma}$
Zona Fasciculata	Cortisol	ACTH
Zona Reticularis	Androgens	ACTH (LH has no effect here)

Medulla, produces epinephrine, controlled by sympathetic nervous system

Cortisol influences carbohydrate storage, has anti-inflammatory effects, suppresses corticotropin secretion, and increases protein catabolism. Disorders resulting from adrenal cortex dysfunction are Cushing syndrome from excess and Addison disease or adrenal crisis from deficiency. Pheochromocytoma is due to excess hormone production by the adrenal medulla.

The adrenal medulla (10 percent of the adrenal gland) produces two catecholamines: epinephrine (e.g., adrenaline) and norepinephrine (e.g., noradrenaline). Epinephrine is a positive inotrope and a major insulin antagonist and is responsible for the fight or flight (stress) response. Norepinephrine is a potent peripheral vasoconstrictor. Disorder resulting from excess is pheochromocytoma, a tumor that produces epinephrine and/or norepinephrine causing labile hypertension.

Pancreas

The pancreas is located transversely in the left upper abdominal quadrant, behind the peritoneum and stomach. It has both exocrine and endocrine components. The endocrine functions originate from the islets of Langerhans (which constitute 2 percent of the total pancreatic volume). There are three types of specialized islet cells: alpha, beta, and delta. The beta cells (65 percent of the gland) produce insulin. Insulin decreases blood glucose; promotes synthesis of proteins, carbohydrates, lipids, and nucleic acids; facilitates active transport of glucose across cell membranes; increases glucose uptake by the liver; stimulates glycogen and fatty acid synthesis in the liver; inhibits gluconeogenesis and glycogenolysis by the liver; facilitates the intracellular transport of potassium; and stimulates protein synthesis by muscle cells. Disorders resulting from dysfunction are hypoglycemia from excess and type I diabetes mellitus (DM-I) from deficiency. Complications of DM-I include diabetic ketoacidosis and hyperosmolar hyperglycemia syndrome. The alpha cells produce glucagon. Glucagon increases blood glucose levels, increases lipolysis, increases amino acid transport to the liver for conversion to glucose precursors, and is a major insulin-antagonistic hormone. Delta cells produce somatostatin and gastrin. Somatostatin inhibits secretion of insulin, glucagon, growth hormone, TSH, and gastrin. Gastrin acts on the stomach and gallbladder and is not discussed in this chapter.

ASSESSMENT

The clinical assessment is primarily carried out by analyzing laboratory values and radiological studies, since most endocrine glands are seated deep within the body. However, the signs and symptoms of an imbalance or malfunctioning endocrine system can also be picked up during the history taking. Knowledge of the anatomy and physiology discussed in the previous section helps the critical care nurse with interpretation of the assessment findings. Assessment of the endocrine system begins with the history. The health history interview collects subjective data. The second portion is the physical examination of the endocrine system, which collects objective data. Since most of the endocrine glands are deeply encased in the body, direct examination is difficult. The use of indirect measures (laboratory, radiology) allows the critical care nurse to assess the physiology of the gland by monitoring the target tissue.

History of Present Illness

The initial patient presentation determines the urgency and direction of the interview. For patients in acute distress, the history involves questions focusing on the chief complaint and precipitating events. When presenting in a critical care setting, many patients will be in acute distress. This acute distress may or may not be due to a patient's known or unknown endocrine diseases. With this in mind it is important to ask questions, as with all organ systems, during the history-taking process that are directly related to the chief complaint. However, to identify potential endocrine issues, a thorough understanding of the anatomy and physiology is paramount. For example, patients that present with hypotension and tachycardia may have atrial fibrillation with rapid ventricular response. In such a case, the patient should be questioned about signs and/or symptoms that may be related to hyperthyroidism (e.g., weight loss, heat intolerance, menstrual cycle abnormalities in women, dry skin, hair loss, vision trouble, etc.). Questions in the history-taking process regarding prenatal history, such as exposure to drugs, alcohol, infections, radiation, and pregnancy complications, may be useful but should be reserved only for situations where the patient is not in acute distress and has been stabilized.

The patient's chief complaint is why he is seeking help and how long the problem has existed. Have the patient describe when the problem started, what symptoms were experienced, any treatments tried, and the effect of the treatments. This helps to focus the interview and physical examination. A review of the patient's past medical and surgical history helps to identify any preexisting or traumatic endocrine dysfunction. Next, a review of any medications taken regularly or as needed, including prescription, over-the-counter, and herbal remedies, may identify occult problems. Indicators of altered health patterns include the following:

- Cognitive changes (vision, personality, depression, memory)
- Nutrition/metabolism (weight change, GI upset, edema, heat/cold intolerance)
- Elimination (diarrhea, constipation, polyuria, nocturia, excessive sweating)
- Activity/exercise (fatigue, weakness, impaired activities of daily living)
- Sleep/rest (restlessness, insomnia, excessive sleeping)
- Sexual (decreased libido, impotence, menstrual irregularities, infertility)
- Coping/stress (past or present psychiatric history, coping mechanisms)

Then, determine the patient's perception and what behaviors he uses to manage his health. Next, review any family history of endocrine disorders and social history, including the use of tobacco products, alcohol, or illicit drugs.

Physical Examination

Inspection and palpation start with a general inspection of the patient including stature and posture; fat distribution; any gross deformities or asymmetry; hair distribution and texture; and any visible scars, goiter, or edema. Vital signs, including blood pressure (lying, sitting, standing); heart rate and rhythm; respirations (rate, depth, rhythm); temperature; and height and weight, should be obtained. Examination of the head and neck involves checking eyes for exophthalmos, strabismus, facial or periorbital edema, visual acuity, facial bone structure, and thyroid gland (enlargement, palpable mass, nodules, tenderness, and palpable thrill). Skin, hair, and nail examination includes color, texture, turgor, temperature, evidence of bruising, striae, thinning, edema, acne, spider angiomas, alopecia, brittle nails, and tongue enlargement or protrusion. In addition, cardiac point of maximal impulse; heaves; breath odor; mental status; pupil size, shape, and reactivity; and any visible tremors should be assessed. Ascultation area includes the following:

- Neck: Bruits over thyroid gland
- Heart: Distant heart sounds; third heart sound
- Lungs: Crackles or stridor
- GI: Hyperactive or hypoactive bowel sounds
- Tendon reflexes

Diagnostic Studies

Laboratory studies of blood and urine include the following: chemistry (electrolytes, renal panel, ketones, glycosylated hemoglobin), hormone levels (TSH, T3, T4, ACTH, random cortisol, ADH, activated PTH, FSH, LH, testosterone), CBC, arterial blood gases (ABGs), nutritional labs (vitamin D, B1, B6, B12, folate), plasma and urine osmolality/osmolarity, and urinalysis. Radiology studies include x-ray (chest and abdomen); scans (thyroid, pancreas); CT of abdomen (note: IVP dye may cause long-term issues with oral hyperglycemic drugs); MRI; angiography; and a bone mineral densitometry (DEXA scan). In addition, an ECG and visual field testing should be done.

PATHOLOGIES

Diabetes Insipidus (DI)

Diabetes insipidus is defined as either a deficiency of or insensitivity to ADH. This leads to an inability to concentrate urine with the resultant volume depletion. The presenting signs and symptoms are the result of dehydration and hypernatremia. DI can complicate the course of the critically ill patient and result in acute, life-threatening fluid and electrolyte disturbances.

Three types of diabetes insipidus have been identified: **neurogenic, nephrogenic and dipsogenic**. *Neurogenic* (hypothalmic or central) DI is due to damage of the posterior pituitary gland by tumors or trauma, causing insufficient amounts of ADH to be synthesized, transported, or released. *Nephrogenic* DI (peripheral) is an inadequate response by the kidneys to ADH, usually related to kidney disorders or drug toxicity, and is fairly uncommon. *Dipsogenic* DI (primary polydipsia) results from the oral intake of large amounts of water, which suppresses the release of ADH, causing polyuria. Impaired ADH activity causes rapid excretion of large amounts of dilute urine, increasing plasma osmolality and decreasing urine osmolality.

Causes of Diabetes Insipidus

Neurogenic (Central) Congenital	Nephrogenic Pyelonephritis	Dipsogenic Idiopathic
Idiopathic	Amyloidosis	Psychoses (compulsive water drinking)
Trauma	Sarcoidosis	Impaired thirst mechanism
Surgery	Polycystic kidney disease	
Primary/metastatic malignancies	Multiple myeloma	
Autoimmune diseases	Sickle cell disease	
Infections	Nephrotoxic drugs	

When DI is seen following brain surgery or head trauma, it usually occurs in the first one to three days after the inciting event. Trauma (including brain surgery) may lead to edema of the hypothalamus and/or the neurohypophysis, causing a decreased secretion of ADH. The reason this takes time to manifest is that the posterior pituitary often has reserve amounts of ADH stored and it takes some time to deplete these stores. If there is damage to the supra-optic nuclei in the hypothalamus and/or proximal end of the pituitary stalk, then permanent DI will ensue; however, in most cases it is transient and resolves with resolution of the edema. *Primary polydipsia* is the inappropriate drinking of water, despite normal hydration or even over-hydration. It can occur due to hypokalemia, hypercalcemia, or increased angiotensin II levels. It is usually **psychogenic** in origin and found, most often, in patients with a history of psychosis, hysteria, or depression. They often have irrational faith that more water will rid them of a real or imagined disease (hiccups, worms, poisons, or cancer). Dipsogenic patients have a plasma osmolality lower than normal.

Clinical manifestations include *polyuria, polydipsia, hypernatremia, hyperosmolality, hypotension,* and *mental status changes.* Initially urine output may exceed 300 mL per hour (2 to 20 liters per day), regardless of intake. Alert patients have excessive thirst and may consume as much as 5 to 20 liters of fluids per day. When the patient is unable to replace the fluid lost by responding to thirst, signs of hypovolemia will develop: hypotension, decreased skin turgor, hypernatremia, dry mucous membranes, tachycardia, low central venous (CVP), low venous oxygen saturation (SVO_2), and pulmonary artery occlusion pressures (PAOP, otherwise also known as wedge pressure). Hypernatremia results from hypovolemia due to concentration of the serum sodium from polyuria. Hyperosmolality is the increased concentration of solutes in the serum. Normal serum osmolarity is 275–295 mOsm/kg (mmol/kg). This will correspond with a decreased urine osmolality, since the urine should be correspondingly dilute. Mental status changes such as confusion, irritability, and seizures are related to the increased serum osmolality and hypernatremia, causing neural cells to shrink. Hypotension is secondary to volume depletion (polyuria).

Diagnostic Procedures

- Negative running fluid balance

- UA: Colorless, odorless, specific gravity < 1.005, sodium < 20 mEq/L, and osmolality < 300 mOsm/L.

- Serum osmolality > 295 mOsm/L, sodium > 145 mEq/L, increased BUN and creatinine.

- Water restriction test can help discriminate between neurogenic and nephrogenic DI (see table 7.1). Baseline values for serum ADH, serum and urine osmolalities, and serum sodium concentrations are obtained. Then measure the urine volume and urine osmolality every hour and the serum's sodium and osmolality every two hours. If the urine osmolality reaches 600 mOsm/kg, then the ADH secretion and response are both intact and there is no DI. However, the test should be stopped earlier to prevent harm to the patient. The criteria to stop the test are if a normal response is obtained as stated above, the urine osmolality remains the same on two to three consecutive hourly assessments despite rising serum osmolality, and the serum osmolality exceeds 295–300 mOsm/kg. In a normal patient, the urine osmolality can be concentrated upward of 1000–1200 mOsm/kg when deprived of water.

TABLE 7.1 *Interpreting the Results of Water Restriction Tests and Exogenous ADH*

Primary Polydipsia	• Urine osmolality > Plasma osmolality. • Urine osmolality increases minimally (<10%) after exogenous ADH.
Central Diabetes Insipidus	• Urine osmolality remains less than plasma osmolality after water restriction. • After ADH is given, urine osms increase 50–100% in complete CDI.
Nephrogenic Diabetes Insipidus	• Urine osmolality remains less than plasma osmolality. • After ADH, urine osms increase by less than 50%.

- Vasopressin test differentiates between neurogenic and nephrogenic DI. First give no fluids. Measure output hourly to get a baseline. Then give Pitressin (ADH) five units SQ, IM, or IV or desmopressin (DDAVP) 10 mcg nasal spray or 1 mcg SQ. Urine is measured at 30-60-90-120 minute intervals. If the urine volume decreases *and* the urine osmolality increases more than 50 percent, the test is positive for neurogenic DI. The patient with nephrogenic DI will either not respond or will respond with less than 50 percent increase in the urine osmolality.

- Serum osmolality can be estimated by the following formula:

$$\text{Serum osmolality} = 2(\text{serum Na}) + \text{BUN}/2.8 + \text{Glucose}/18 = (275\text{–}295 \text{ mOsm})$$

Treatment

The goals of treatment are to identify and correct the underlying cause and restore normal fluid volume, osmolality, and electrolyte balance. If the patient is alert and able to respond to thirst, she will generally drink enough fluids to avoid symptomatic hypovolemia. Patients in the critical care unit and the elderly with cognitive impairments are unable to respond appropriately to thirst, and fluid replacement is necessary. Volume replacement, especially if the patient is hypotensive, is rapid infusion of *hypotonic* (e.g., D5W) intravenous solutions and careful monitoring without a rapid reduction of serum sodium. Since the volume that is lost is simply extra water, we refer to this clinically as "free water," which means water without any solutes. The serum sodium (Na) is the marker that we use to measure the "free water deficit" in such patients. The amount of free water deficit can be estimated based on normal fluid stores and usual body weight, using this formula:

$$\text{Body water deficit in liters} = (0.6) \times (\text{weight in kg}) \times [(\text{serum sodium}/140) - 1]$$

The formula assumes that 60 percent of an individual's weight is fluid. The amount of estimated fluid deficit can be used as a guide for replacement fluids.

Medications used to treat DI successfully include desmopressin (DDAVP) and vasopressin (Pitressin) given as replacement for the decreased ADH. Pitressin is synthetic, but it is identical in structure to naturally occurring ADH. Desmopressin is a structural analog of ADH. Vasopressin has powerful vasoconstrictor actions and can cause adverse cardiovascular effects. By constricting arteries of the heart, it can cause angina pectoris or myocardial infarction. In addition, it may cause gangrene by decreasing the blood flow to the periphery. Desmopressin has very few vasoconstrictive (i.e., "pressor") effects and is the agent of choice because it has a long duration of action, is easy to administer, and lacks significant side effects. Potential adverse effects include abdominal pain, transient headache, nasal congestion, rhinitis, nausea, and water intoxication, especially young children and older adults. Caution patients to drink only enough to quench their thirst.

Nursing Responsibilities

Establish a baseline (weight, blood pressure, serum/urine osmolality, serum electrolytes, and strict intake/output) from which to monitor the effects of the drug and coordinate testing throughout therapy. Monitor for possible cardiac adverse effects and possible nasal septum ulceration. Remove/stop offending chemical(s) if patient has nephrogenic DI. Maintain accurate input and output records and perform the testing as ordered by the physician at the proper times, as the osmolality will change with time and timing is essential in interpreting the results of the water restriction and DDAVP administration.

Syndrome of Inappropriate Antidiuretic Hormone Secretion (SIADH)

Syndrome of inappropriate antidiuretic hormone secretion is the excessive release of ADH without regard to plasma osmolality or fluid volume status. The normal inhibition of ADH by the posterior pituitary is absent, resulting in excessive reabsorption of water by the renal tubules and collecting ducts of the kidney. The presenting signs and symptoms are the result of hypervolemia and dilutional hyponatremia. SIADH can complicate the course of the critically ill patient and result in acute, life-threatening fluid and electrolyte disturbances.

Etiology

There are multiple causes of SIADH, including ectopic ADH production, central nervous system disorders, and medications that increase or potentiate ADH secretion. Excess ADH production or utilization is seen in patients with malignant cancers (lung, pancreas, prostate, thymus, duodenum, Hodgkin's, and leukemia), nonmalignant pulmonary conditions (tuberculosis, pneumonia), CNS disorders (brain trauma, tetanus, meningitis, vascular lesions, Guillian-Barré syndrome), and medications (nicotine, TCAs, chemotherapeutic drugs, ADH therapy, lisinopril, metoclopramide, narcotics, SSRIs, anesthetics).

Clinical signs and symptoms of SIADH are related to the hypovolemia and hyponatremia and may present as mild to severe. Symptoms of mild hyponatremia (serum sodium level less than 135 mEq/L) include low urine output, dark concentrated urine, thirst, dulled sensorium, dyspnea on exertion, hypertension, weight gain without edema, headache, and nausea. Central nervous system symptoms are due to cellular swelling as a result of a reduction in the serum osmolality and hyponatremia. The severity and the rate of onset of the hyponatremia determine the extent of the mental status changes. As the water and sodium imbalance continue (sodium levels below 120 mEq/L), progressive neurological deterioration includes irritability, confusion, lack of concentration, apprehension, seizures, loss of consciousness, coma, and death.

Diagnostic Procedures

Laboratory values provide the diagnostic hallmarks of SIADH:

- UA: Dark, concentrated, specific gravity >1.025, sodium >20 mEq/L, and osmolality >300 mOsm/L

- Serum osmolality <275 mOsm/L; sodium <135 mEq/L; low BUN, creatinine, and albumin

- Water-loading test with elimination of less than 50 percent of the fluid challenge

Treatment

The goals of treatment are to identify and correct the underlying cause, eliminate excess water, and increase serum osmolality. In many instances, treatment of the underlying cause returns the patient's condition to normal. In mild to moderate SIADH (sodium 125 to 135 mEq/L), fluid restriction is calculated on the basis of individual needs and losses; a general criterion is 500 mL less than average daily output. Patients with severe hyponatremia (less than 115 mEq/L) or those experiencing seizure may be given hypertonic saline (3 percent or 5 percent). Hypertonic saline administration should be no faster than 1 to 2 mL/kg per hour to raise the serum sodium no more than 0.5 to 2 mEq/L per hour. Administration of a loop diuretic such as furosemide (brand name: Lasix) prevents urine concentration when given with hypertonic saline, increasing the removal of the excess fluid. Medications such as lithium, phenytoin sodium (Dilantin), and demeclocycline may be given to block secretion of ADH.

Nursing Responsibilities

Establish a baseline (weight, blood pressure, serum/urine osmolality, serum electrolytes, and strict intake/output) from which to monitor the effects of treatment and coordinate testing throughout therapy. Monitor for possible cardiac adverse effects, including distended neck veins. Remove/stop offending chemical(s). Correct electrolytes slowly.

Thyrotoxic Crisis (Thyroid Storm)

Thyrotoxic crisis is a rare, severe form of hyperthyroid disease often leading to systemic decompensation, and it can result in death within 48 hours without treatment. It occurs most often in patients with Graves disease that is either undiagnosed or undertreated and is precipitated by another illness, injury, or surgery. Theories regarding the occurrence of thyrotoxic crisis include a change in the binding of thyroid hormone to albumin, a change in the thyroid hormone receptors of the target tissues, or an exaggerated response to sympathetic activity. Hyperthyroidism can produce a hyperdynamic, hypermetabolic state that disrupts major body functions.

The most frequent clinical symptoms of thyrotoxic crisis are high fever, tachycardia, palpitations, arrhythmias, altered respirations, fatigue, tremors, delirium, stupor, coma. Temperature regulation is lost, and the patient's temperature may be as high as 106 °F (41.1 °C). The increased heat production and accumulated metabolic end products cause dilation of the blood vessels of the skin, the reason for warm moist skin. The increased metabolism and stimulation of catecholamines cause a hyperdynamic heart and may be severe enough to produce heart failure and cardiovascular collapse. Neurological disturbances are secondary to hypermetabolism, causing hyperactivity of the nervous system. The respiratory system responds to the hypermetabolism by increasing respirations to increase the oxygen supply. However, the increased protein catabolism reduces the muscle mass of the diaphragm and intercostal muscles, which can prevent the patient from meeting the increased oxygen demand, causing hypoventilation, carbon dioxide retention, and respiratory failure.

Diagnostic Procedures

There are no specific laboratory tests to differentiate thyrotoxic crisis from uncomplicated hyperthyroidism. TSH, T3, T4, and resin T3 uptake should be measured. Resin T3 uptake is an indirect measure of free T4 levels (free T4 is the portion that is biologically active) and is elevated in hyperthyroid states.

Treatment

Patients with suspected or diagnosed thyrotoxic crisis should be managed in the ICU. Goals of treatment are to inhibit thyroid hormone biosynthesis, block thyroid hormone release, antagonize the peripheral effects of thyroid hormone, provide supportive care, and treat the precipitating cause. Inhibition of thyroid hormone biosynthesis is accomplished with antithyroid medications. Propylthiouracil (PTU) is the preferred agent because it prevents the peripheral conversion of T4 to T3. The U.S. Food and Drug Administration (FDA) had added a boxed warning to the prescribing information for PTU. The warning emphasizes the risk of severe liver injury/failure and recommends reserving PTU for patients who cannot tolerate other treatments such as methimazole, radioactive iodine, or surgery. A loading dose of 600 mg is given and followed by 200 mg every four hours until production of thyroid hormone is blocked. PTU must be given orally, via a nasogastric tube, or rectally, since there is no parenteral preparation available in the United States. Patients not able to take PTU are given methimazole (brand name: Tapazole), 20 mg orally every four hours until inhibition is achieved. Since PTU and Tapazole lack immediate effect, iodine agents are administered to block the release of the thyroid hormones from the gland. Sodium iodine is given by slow IV drip, or Lugol's solution (saturated solution of potassium iodine) may be given orally. Serum T4 levels fall by 30–50 percent and stabilize in three to six days. Radiographic contrast media such as ipodate (brand name: Oragrafin) or iopanoic acid (brand name: Telepaque) may also be used. For patients with iodine allergy, lithium carbonate may be used, but it has worse side effects and must be monitored regularly to maintain therapeutic levels. It is given orally or via a nasogastric tube every six hours.

Hormone synthesis inhibition and blockade may take days or weeks. Therefore, antagonism of the peripheral effects is required to minimize injury to the major organ systems and decrease the signs and symptoms of beta-adrenergic stimulation. The mortality rate of thyrotoxic crisis (20 percent) has been significantly reduced with the use of beta-blockers. The most frequently used is propranolol (brand name: Inderal), but esmolol (brand name: Brevibloc) or atenolol (brand name: Tenormin) may also be used. Results, including reduction of tachycardia, restlessness, sweating, tremors, and agitation, may be seen within one hour when given by IV. Supportive care includes stress doses of hydrocortisone; acetaminophen (brand name: Tylenol), cooling blankets, or ice packs for fever; fluid replacement to prevent dehydration; and anticoagulation if necessary. Treatment of the precipitating cause will prevent the recurrence of thyrotoxic crisis.

Nursing Responsibilities

Nursing responsibilities include monitoring the effects of treatment and cardiovascular status; monitoring and treatment of hyperthermia; administering fluids, oxygen, and medications; and providing adequate nutrition and injury prevention.

Myxedema Coma

Myxedema coma is a life-threatening emergency, seen in *hypothyroid* patients, resulting from the addition of a stressor such as infection; trauma; exposure to cold; or intake of tranquilizers, barbiturates, or narcotics. These stressors increase the patient's metabolism and deplete any stored thyroid hormone from the body, causing a crisis. Myxedema coma occurs more often during the winter, is seen in women and the elderly, and has a mortality rate estimated at 20 percent to 50 percent.

Presenting signs and symptoms include hypothermia, hypoventilation, hypotension, bradycardia, hyporeflexia, hyponatremia, and generalized interstitial edema. The patient's hypothermia is due to the decreased metabolic rate and low thermal energy production. Of patients presenting with hypothermia, 80 percent have temperatures between 80 °F (26.7 °C) and 88.6 °F (32 °C) and have a grave prognosis. Depressed cardiac function causes bradycardia, decreased contractility, low stroke volume and cardiac output, and hypotension. Respirations are depressed causing hypoventilation and CO_2 retention, leading to decreased mentation. Slowed neuron conduction depresses the deep tendon reflexes. The hyponatremia is due to water retention. Fluid collects in the tissues of the face, joints, and muscles and can cause pericardial effusion.

Diagnostic Procedures

Laboratory testing should include thyroid function tests, complete blood count (CBC), biochemical profile (electrolytes, hepatic functions tests, renal indices), random cortisol, creatine kinase (CK), blood cultures, arterial blood gases (ABGs), and urinalysis (UA). Chest x-ray, electrocardiogram (ECG), abdominal ultrasound, and CT of the head may also be required. Serum T3, T4, and T3 resin intake levels will be low. TSH will be elevated if the patient has primary hypothyroidism, and it will be normal or low if the problem is in the hypothalamus or pituitary gland (secondary hypothyroidism). Serum glucose and sodium levels will be low. Cortisol levels may be low. If cortisol levels are low, then a cosyntropin stimulation test will be ordered to rule out the possibility of adrenal insufficiency. In a cosyntropin stimulation test, cosyntropin is injected parenterally, and the cortisol level is drawn before administration and 30–60 minutes after administration. If there is a rise in the cortisol levels following administration of the cosyntropin, then the patient does not have adrenal insufficiency; however, if there is not an adequate rise in the cortisol level, then the patient is diagnosed with adrenal insufficiency and needs exogenous steroid administration.

Treatment

Patients with suspected or diagnosed myxedema coma should be managed in the ICU. The goals of treatment include hormone replacement, correct fluid and electrolyte balance, supportive care, and identification and treatment of the precipitating cause. Thyroid hormone replacement should be started early. Whether to use T4 alone, combined T4 and T3, or T3 alone remains a subject of controversy. The loading dose of T4 (levothyroxine) is 500–800 mcg IV, followed by 50–100 mcg every 24 hours. Some practitioners advocate the use of additional IV T3 (liothyronine) 10–20 mcg IV every 12 hours until the patient responds with an elevation of body temperature, pulse, and blood pressure and improved mental status and ABGs. While the thyroid hormones are being loaded, the patient may require intubation and mechanical ventilation due to airway compromise. Patients with cardiac dysrhythmias may require continuous cardiac monitoring. Symptomatic bradycardia may require temporary pacing using transvenous or transcutaneous methods. Hyponatremia (serum sodium less than 120 mEq/L) may be treated with hypertonic saline and limited water using a central venous catheter. Hypothermia is best monitored with core temperature. Glucose may be added to the IV solution, and stress doses of steroids will help to increase both blood pressure and serum glucose. Hydrocortisone (brand name: Solu-Cortef) 100 mg IV is given every 8 hours for 48 hours.

Nursing Responsibilities

Nursing responsibilities include monitoring the effects of treatment and cardiovascular status; monitoring and treating hypothermia; administering fluids, oxygen, and medications; and providing adequate nutrition and injury prevention.

Acute Adrenal Insufficiency (Addisonian Crisis)

Addisonian crisis is the acute form of chronic adrenal dysfunction resulting in inadequate adrenal secretion of glucocorticoids (cortisol) and mineralocorticoids (aldosterone). Dysfunction of the adrenal glands may result from primary, secondary, or tertiary causes. Primary insufficiency may be due to idiopathic autoimmune disease, granulomatous disease (tuberculosis, sarcoidosis, histoplasmosis), metastatic cancer, trauma, sepsis, acquired immunodeficiency syndrome (AIDS), drugs (ketoconazole, trimethoprim, phenytoin, barbiturates, rifampin), or a developmental abnormality. At least 90 percent of the adrenal cortex must be destroyed before clinical signs and symptoms become evident. Secondary causes interfere with hormone secretion, including pituitary tumors, hemorrhage, radiation, Sheehan's syndrome (postpartum hemorrhage), trauma, surgery, and hypothalamic disorders. Tertiary adrenal insufficiency is iatrogenic, secondary to long-term use of steroids, causing failure of the adrenal glands to resume hormone production of cortisol when exogenous administration stops.

The lack of cortisol results in decreased glucose production, decreased metabolism of protein and fat, decreased appetite, decreased intestinal motility and digestion, decreased vascular tone, and diminished catecholamine effectiveness. When patients with deficient cortisol are stressed, profound cardiovascular collapse can result. Low levels of aldosterone cause decreased retention of sodium and water, decreased circulating blood volume, and increased potassium and hydrogen ion reabsorption.

Presenting signs and symptoms are often nonspecific and can be attributed to other medical disorders. Since acute adrenal insufficiency is a medical emergency, it must be considered in any patient with fever, vomiting, hypotension, shock, decreased sodium, increased potassium, or hypoglycemia unresponsive to standard therapy. The most common presentation in the ICU is hypotension refractory to fluids and requiring vasopressors. Other symptoms may include decreased cardiac output, dysrhythmias, cold/pale skin, headache, confusion, lethargy, anorexia, nausea, vomiting, vague abdominal pain, and decreased urine output.

Diagnostic Procedures

Laboratory testing should include complete blood count (CBC), biochemical profile (electrolytes, hepatic, renal), ABGs, cortisol, and aldosterone levels. Common laboratory results with acute adrenal insufficiency are hypoglycemia, hyponatremia, hyperkalemia, eosinophilia, elevated BUN, hypercalcemia, and hyperuricemia. A decreased serum cortisol level is suspicious for adrenal insufficiency. In acute adrenal crisis, there is no time to wait for the laboratory results to confirm the diagnosis before beginning treatment. If cortisol levels are low, a cosyntropin stimulation test will be requested by the physician to rule out the possibility of adrenal insufficiency. Failure of the cortisol level to rise adequately 30–60 minutes after parenteral administration of 250 mcg of cosyntropin is diagnostic of adrenal insufficiency.

Treatment

The treatment goals for acute adrenal crisis include hormone replacement, correct fluid and electrolyte balance, supportive care, and identification and treatment of the precipitating cause. Fluid deficit should be replaced with 5% glucose with 0.9% normal saline (D5.9NS), providing both volume replacement and enough glucose to minimize hypoglycemia. The patient may require as much as 5 liters of fluid in the first 12 to 24 hours. Glucocorticoid replacement is the most important hormone to be given first. Hydrocortisone (brand name: Solu-Cortef) is given as a bolus of 100 mg IV and followed by 100 mg every eight hours. Mineralocorticoid replacement may also be required with fludrocortisone (brand name: Florinef) 0.1 to 0.2 mg daily.

Nursing Responsibilities

Nursing responsibilities include monitoring the effects of treatment and cardiovascular status and administering fluids and medications.

Hypercorticism (Cushing Syndrome)

Hypercorticism is an increased production of mineralocorticoids, glucocorticoids, and androgen steroids. Causes include adrenal cortex tumor, pituitary tumor, ectopic ACTH-producing pulmonary neoplams, or long-term use of steroids. Adrenal cortex tumors (usually adenomas) produce excess cortisol. A pituitary tumor stimulates increased release of ACTH, causing hyperplasia of the adrenal cortex and increased hormone production. Ectopic ACTH-producing tumors (usually oat cell carcinomas) stimulate excess cortisol production. Long-term exogenous steroid administration for other medical diseases, such as chronic obstructive pulmonary disease or inflammatory bowel disease, may cause Cushing syndrome.

Presenting signs and symptoms include truncal weight gain with a pendulous abdomen; facial, supraclavicular, and dorsocervical deposition of fat (hump); purple striae on the abdomen and breast; acne; hirsutism and male pattern hair loss in women; extreme muscle wasting; hypertension; abnormal glucose intolerance; sodium and water retention, altered libido, and poor wound healing.

Diagnostic Procedures

A 24-hour urine free cortisol level is the gold-standard screening test. Serum cortisol and ACTH levels (drawn between 8 AM and 10 AM) help to differentiate between pituitary and adrenal sources. MRI of the head, chest and abdomen may identify a tumor source.

Treatment

Treatment of pituitary adenoma may include transsphenoidal resection of the pituitary adenoma or radiation therapy if surgery is not possible. Adrenal adenomas and ectopic ACTH-producing tumors are usually surgically removed.

Nursing Responsibilities

These patients may be cared for in the ICU after surgery and require stress doses of corticosteroids. Their immune systems will be depressed due to the high levels of steroids prior to surgery, and they will require close monitoring for signs of infection.

Pheochromocytoma

Pheochromocytoma is a rare cause of hypertension (0.3 to 1 percent), but it is malignant in 3 to 36 percent of the patients found to have this tumor. Fifty percent of the patients with malignant pheochromocytoma die within five years. The disease can be life threatening due to the possibility of cerebrovascular accidents (CVA) and heart failure. It is an encapsulated vascular tumor of neuroendocrine chromaffin cells of the adrenal medulla, and it secretes norepinephrine and/or epinephrine.

Presenting signs and symptoms include sustained or paroxysmal (intermittent) hypertension (90 percent), postural hypotension, chest pain, headache, sweating, palpitations, tremor, and hyperglycemia. The symptoms may last for just a few seconds to hours, and the episodes occur with irregular frequency. Triggers for the attacks may include diagnostic procedures, anesthesia, medications, or foods (chocolate).

Diagnostic Procedures

Measurement of serum and urine free metanephrines (catecholamine metabolites) is the first priority for diagnosis. The urine sample should be collected after a symptomatic episode. A second test, if the first is nonspecific, involves clonidine suppression (0.3 mg/kg), then measurement of norepinephrine levels in three hours. Failure to suppress the level of norepinephrine would suggest pheochromocytoma. Once the diagnosis is made, tumor localization is done using either CT or MRI imaging. The newest method uses the positron emission tomography (PET) for identifying both primary and metastatic lesions.

Treatment

Surgical excision of the tumor(s) is the best treatment method for pheochromocytoma. Two weeks prior to surgery, catecholamine blockade is started using alpha-adrenergic blockers [phenoxybenzamine (brand name: Dibenzyline)] and beta-adrenergic blockers [atenolol (brand name: Tenormin)]. Preoperative volume expansion is used to prevent hypotension from the alpha and beta blockade. When diagnosed and treated early, 90 percent of the cases are cured. Left untreated, pheochromocytoma is usually fatal from arrhythmias, myocardial infarction, or cerebrovascular accidents.

Nursing Responsibilities

These patients may be cared for in the ICU after surgery. Monitor closely for shock, hypotension, hemorrhage, and hypoglycemia.

Diabetic Ketoacidosis (DKA)

Recent epidemiological studies indicate that hospitalizations for DKA in the U.S. are increasing. In the decade from 1996 to 2006, there was a 35 percent increase in the number of cases, with a total of 136,510 cases with a primary diagnosis of DKA in 2006. DKA was diagnosed for patients between the ages of 18 and 44 years (56 percent) and 45 and 65 years (24 percent), with only 18 percent of patients <20 years of age. Two-thirds of DKA patients were considered to have type 1 diabetes and 34 percent to have type 2 diabetes; 50 percent were female, and 45 percent were nonwhite. DKA is the most common cause of death in children and adolescents with type 1 diabetes and accounts for half of all deaths in diabetic patients younger than 24 years of age. In adult subjects with DKA, the overall mortality is <1 percent; however, a mortality rate >5 percent has been reported in the elderly and in patients with concomitant life-threatening illnesses. The most common causes of DKA are failure to take sufficient insulin, stressful events, trauma, surgery, infections, pregnancy, alcohol intoxication, and undiagnosed DM. DKA is almost always the first presentation of type I diabetics, and although it is possible for type II insulin-dependent diabetics to present with DKA, DKA is almost exclusively limited to type I diabetes (also known as juvenile-onset diabetes).

DKA has four hallmark pathologies: hyperglycemia, hypovolemia, ketonemia, and anion gap metabolic acidosis. Hyperglycemia is caused by a lack of insulin, preventing cellular glucose utilization. Thus, although blood glucose rises, the negative feedback to the cells producing glucagons cannot be activated; hence, glucagon is released and breaks down glycogen and stimulates gluconeogenesis, releasing more glucose and further increasing the blood glucose. The high glucose level in the blood exceeds the renal threshold, spilling glucose into the urine. Ketonemia results from the accumulation of ketones (from fat metabolism, beta-oxidation) in the bloodstream, contributing to metabolic acidosis. To compensate, the lungs attempt to eliminate the excess carbonic acid by hyperventilation (Kussmaul respirations).

Excess serum glucose produces osmotic diuresis, extracting water from the vascular space and causing rapid dehydration. The body attempts to buffer the excess hydrogen ions, causing a decrease in bicarbonate levels. Excess cellular hydrogen ions cause the potassium ions to leave the cells, increasing the serum potassium levels. Altered consciousness is related to acidosis and dehydration.

Clinical signs and symptoms include acetone breath, altered sensorium, hypothermia, Kussmaul breathing, tachycardia, abdominal pain, nausea, vomiting, polyuria, polydipsia, weakness, weight loss, and fever. The patient with DKA may be lethargic, stuporous, or unconscious depending on the extent of dehydration and electrolyte imbalance. Physical examination reveals flushed, dry skin, dry mucous membranes, skin "tenting" greater than 3 seconds, hypotension, tachycardia, Kussmaul respirations, "fruity"-smelling breath, abdominal tenderness on palpation, and temperature alterations.

Diagnostic Procedures

Laboratory tests should include serum biochemical panel (lytes, renal, liver function), CBC, ABGs, serum ketones, serum osmolality, urine for glucose and ketones, and serum ketones (beta-hydroxybutyrate) and lactic acid. An ECG may show tachycardia. Blood sugar will be >300 mg/dL. Elevated sodium, potassium, and magnesium levels will be due to dehydration and acidosis. Serum ketones will be >3 mOsm/kg. BUN will be increased with a BUN/creatinine ratio greater than 20:1, which is strongly indicative of dehydration. Also present: Metabolic acidosis with pH less than 7.30, bicarbonate less than 15 mEq/L, $PaCO_2$ less than 35 mm Hg, and anion gap greater than 12–16 mEq/L. Ketones will be elevated in both urine and blood. Hematocrit and white blood cell count will be elevated. Serum osmolality will be 295–330 mOsm/kg.

Treatment

Treatment of the patient with DKA requires an aggressive approach. Management goals include correction/restoration of hypovolemia, hyperglycemia, acidemia, electrolytes, and the insulin-glucagon ratio. Volume replacement is accomplished with rapid infusion of 0.9% normal saline (NS) or lactated Ringer solution: 1–3 L during the first hour; 1 L during the second hour; 1 L during the following two hours; and then 1 L every four hours, depending on the degree of dehydration and CVP. When the serum glucose is 180 mg/dL, the IV solution is changed to 5% dextrose with 0.45% NS (D5/ ½ NS) to avoid hypoglycemia, hypokalemia, and cerebral edema caused by the glucose diuresis. Correction of hyperglycemia requires the administration of insulin. Regular insulin is administered at 10 to 20 units IV bolus and followed by a continuous infusion of 0.1 unit/kg/hr. Hourly blood glucose monitoring and insulin infusion rate adjustments should be done. When the blood glucose levels are between 100 and 200 mg/dL, begin subcutaneous insulin for one to two hours before stopping the insulin infusion. Replace potassium, phosphorus, and magnesium as needed.

Complications Associated with Treatment of DKA

- Hypoglycemia is reported in 10 to 20 percent of the patients during insulin therapy. Most common causes are failure to reduce the insulin infusion rate and failure to use dextrose-containing solutions when glucose levels reach 200 mg/dL.

- Hypokalemia occurs when insulin therapy and correction of acidosis decreases the serum potassium levels. Reduce the risk by using low-dose insulin protocols and aggressive potassium replacement.

- Relapse can occur with a sudden interruption of IV insulin, when patient is not given concomitant subcutaneous insulin, or with a lack of frequent monitoring.

- Treatment of acidosis includes frequent assessment of respiratory compensation and level of consciousness. It is usually corrected by fluids and insulin. Give bicarbonate if the pH is less than 6.9.

Nursing Responsibilities

These patients may be cared for in the ICU for cardiac, respiratory, and hemodynamic monitoring. Assessment of intake and output, skin turgor, mucous membranes, and neurologic status should be done hourly. Continuous cardiac monitoring may reveal U waves with hypokalemia, "peaked" or "tented" T-waves with hyperkalemia, and tachycardia that converts to bradycardia with increasing hyperkalemia. Maintaining a patient's airway, suctioning to prevent aspiration, and evaluating the ABGs will identify and prevent hypoxia. Frequent blood pressure, CVP, and SVO$_2$ monitoring will identify the effectiveness of fluid administration. Urine should be checked every one to two hours for glucose and ketones. Use of a diabetic flow sheet helps to identify changes, trends, and potential complications quickly.

General Comments Regarding Control of Hyperglycemia in the Acutely Septic Patient

The recommendations for glucose management in the critically ill patient with sepsis have been reevaluated based on recent evidence-based research in the NICE-SUGAR trial. At the present time, the recommendation from the Society of Critical Care Medicine and the Surviving Sepsis Campaign is to maintain the patient's blood sugar between 150 and 180 mg/dL, with a goal of 150 mg/dL, using a combination of the continuous insulin infusion and subcutaneous sliding-scale insulin regimens. Attempting to maintain the blood sugar in a normal range of 80–100 mg/dL with the use of continuous insulin infusions results in an increased frequency of hypoglycemia, which can cause metabolic complications and elevated mortality risks (refer to following section on hypoglycemia). This requires hourly blood sugar analysis via glucometer, and if results are <60 or >400, a confirmatory serum blood sugar level is recommended, as well as appropriate titration of the insulin therapy based on the results.

Hyperosmolar Hyperglycemic State (HHS)

Incidence rate is lower than DKA, accounting for approximately 1 percent of adult hospital admissions. Where DKA is generally an illness of type I diabetics, HHS is an acute illness primarily of type II diabetics. HHS is very rare in children; however, the recent increase of type II diabetes in children and adolescents may increase the incidence rate. Mortality attributed to HHS is considerably higher than that attributed to DKA, with recent mortality rates of 5–20 percent. It is often seen in geriatric patients with decreased compensatory mechanisms. The most common causes of HHS are stressful events, infections, medications, trauma, surgery, and undiagnosed or inadequately treated type II diabetes.

HHS has three hallmark pathologies: hyperglycemia, hypovolemia, and hyperosmolality. Hyperglycemia is caused by insufficient insulin production and decreased cellular glucose utilization. As blood glucose rises, glucagon is released and breaks down glycogen and stimulates gluconeogenesis, releasing more glucose and further increasing the blood glucose. The high glucose level in the blood increases the extracellular osmolality and exceeds the renal threshold, spilling glucose into the urine. Excess serum glucose produces osmotic diuresis, extracting water from the vascular space and causing profound dehydration. HHS develops more slowly than DKA, sometimes over weeks or months. Alterations in neurologic status are due to the cellular dehydration. The average total body deficit in HHS is 9 to 10 liters.

Clinical signs and symptoms include *altered sensorium* (paresthesia, paresis, plegia, aphasia, decreased deep tendon reflexes, seizure), *hypothermia, tachycardia, tachypnea, abdominal pain, nausea, vomiting, polyuria, polydipsia, weakness, weight loss,* and *fever.* The patient with HHS may be lethargic, stuporous, or unconscious depending on the extent of dehydration and electrolyte imbalance. Physical examination reveals warm, dry skin, dry mucous membranes, skin "tenting" greater than three seconds, hypotension, tachycardia, abdominal tenderness on palpation, and temperature alterations.

Diagnostic Procedures

Laboratory tests should include serum biochemical panel (lytes, renal, liver function), CBC, ABGs, serum osmolality, and urine for glucose and ketones. An ECG may show changes and tachycardia. Blood sugar is *600–2000 mg/dL* with average of 1100 mg/dL. Serum sodium is normal to slightly elevated. Decreased potassium, calcium, phosphorous, and magnesium levels are due to dehydration. Serum ketones are normal or slightly elevated. BUN is increased with a BUN/creatinine ratio greater than 20:1. ABGs have a normal or mildly acidotic pH. If acidosis is present, it is lactic acidosis related to hypoperfusion, not ketoacidosis. Ketones in urine are negative or trace. Hematocrit and white blood cell count are elevated. Serum osmolality is often greater than 330 mOsm/kg and may be as high as 450 mOsm/kg.

Treatment

Treatment of HHS requires an aggressive approach. Management goals include correct hypovolemia, correct hyperglycemia, replenishment electrolytes, and restoration of the insulin-glucagon ratio. Volume replacement is accomplished with rapid infusion of 0.9% normal saline: 1–3 L during the first hour; 1 L during the second hour; 1 L during the following two hours; and then 1 L every four hours, depending on the degree of dehydration and CVP. When the serum glucose is 250 mg/dL, the IV solution is changed to 5% glucose with 0.45% NS (D5/ ½ NS) to avoid hypoglycemia, hypokalemia, and cerebral edema caused by the glucose diuresis. Patients with HHS often respond to fluid alone; however, IV insulin in dosages similar to those used in DKA can correct hyperglycemia. Regular insulin is administered as needed at 10 to 20 units IV bolus and followed by a continuous infusion of 0.1 unit/kg/hr. Hourly blood glucose monitoring and insulin infusion rate adjustments should be done. When the blood glucose levels are between 100 and 200 mg/dL, begin subcutaneous insulin for one to two hours before stopping the insulin infusion. Replace potassium, calcium, phosphorus, and magnesium as needed.

Complications Associated with Treatment of HHS

- Hypoglycemia is reported in 10 to 20 percent of the patients during insulin therapy. Most common causes are failure to reduce the insulin infusion rate and failure to use dextrose-containing solutions when glucose levels reach 250 mg/dL.

- Hypokalemia occurs when insulin therapy and correction of acidosis decrease the serum potassium levels. Reduce the risk by using low-dose insulin protocols and aggressive potassium replacement.

- Relapse can occur with a sudden interruption of IV insulin, if patient is not given concomitant subcutaneous insulin, or with a lack of frequent monitoring.

Nursing Responsibilities

These patients may be cared for in the ICU for cardiac, respiratory, and hemodynamic monitoring. Assessment of intake and output, skin turgor, mucous membranes, and neurologic status should be done hourly. Continuous cardiac monitoring may reveal U waves with hypokalemia, peaked or tented T waves with hyperkalemia, and tachycardia that converts to bradycardia with increasing hyperkalemia. Maintaining a patent airway—suctioning to prevent aspiration—and evaluation of ABGs will identify and prevent hypoxia. Frequent blood pressure and CVP monitoring will identify effectiveness of fluid administration. Urine should be checked hourly for both glucose and ketones. Trending these values over time via a continuous medication and lab flow sheet in the electronic medical record or diabetic flow sheet in a written patient record can quickly identify changes and prevent potential complications.

Acute Hypoglycemia

Acute hypoglycemia can be a life-threatening event if left untreated. Hypoglycemia is a blood glucose level less than 60 mg/dL and is a common endocrine emergency. It is an imbalance between glucose production and glucose utilization. Glucose is the metabolic fuel of the brain, and since it is not synthesized or stored in the brain, the brain is dependent on blood glucose concentration. When the serum glucose concentration drops below normal levels, the physiologic effect on the brain can be profound, leading to coma or death.

The etiology of hypoglycemia includes endogenous, exogenous, and functional causes. Endogenous hypoglycemia is caused by tumors (pancreatic, insulinoma) or inborn metabolic errors. Exogenous low blood glucose is caused by insulin excess, insulin secretagogues, oral antidiabetic agents (sulfonylureas, meglitinides), alcohol use, and other drugs (salicylates, pentamidine). Functional hypoglycemia causes include dumping syndrome, spontaneous reactive hypoglycemia, other endocrine deficient states, and prolonged muscle use (exercise, seizures).

Clinical signs and symptoms are related to the activation of the sympathetic nervous system (epinephrine release) and neuroglycopenic indicators. Most commonly seen are palpitations, tachycardia, diaphoresis, anxiety, nausea, pallor, weakness, hunger, restlessness, difficulty thinking or speaking, visual disturbances, tremors, piloerection, slurred speech, staggering gait, seizures, and coma.

Diagnostic Procedures

Laboratory studies include electrolytes, renal panel, liver function studies, and serum drug screen. ECG is used to screen for cardiac causes. Blood glucose level less than 60 mg/dL (varies with individual patients) is diagnostic for hypoglycemia. Serum glucose of 20 to 40 mg/dL is associated with seizures. Less than 20 mg/dL is usually seen in comatose patients.

Treatment

Treat adult hypoglycemia with 15 g carbohydrate orally, if the patient is alert and able to swallow, or IV D50 (25 grams of dextrose in 50 mL water), if the patient is unconscious. Assess response. Recheck blood glucose in 20 to 30 minutes. Repeat treatment is necessary. Provide longer-acting carbohydrate source (cheese, crackers) or a meal to prevent recurrence. Identification and treatment of the cause of the hypoglycemia is done after the patient stabilizes. Monitor for complications such as myocardial ischemia or infarction, seizures, coma, or irreversible neurologic injury.

Emergency Foods for Hypoglycemia

- 4 oz apple or orange juice
- 4 oz carbonated cola
- 8 oz skim or 1% milk
- 4 cubes or 2 packets of sugar
- 2 oz corn syrup, honey, grape jelly
- 6 Life Savers or jelly beans

- 10 gumdrops
- 2 tablespoons of raisins
- ½ cup regular gelatin
- 2 to 3 graham cracker squares
- 3 glucose tablets (5 grams each)

These amounts have 10 to 15 grams of carbohydrates.

Review Questions

1. Arterial blood gas (ABG) results of a client with diabetic ketoacidosis (DKA) reveal the following: pH of 7.20, CO_2 of 35 mm Hg, HCO_3 of 17 mEq/L, PaO_2 of 92 mm Hg. Which provider order would require the nurse to intervene?

   A. Apply oxygen nasal cannula 2 liters per minute.

   B. Perform fingerstick every hour and notify provider.

   C. Give sodium bicarbonate 100 mmol in 400 mL H_2O.

   D. Repeat ABG readings in 2 hours.

2. In transitioning a diabetic ketoacidosis (DKA) client from receiving intravenous regular insulin to subcutaneous (SC) insulin, the nurse's priority action is to

   A. continue intravenous insulin for 1–2 hours after SC insulin is started.

   B. check the blood sugar every 30 minutes for 24 hours.

   C. turn off the insulin infusion as soon as the SC insulin is administered.

   D. monitor the client closely for signs of seizure activity.

3. Which of these is the best treatment for severe hypoglycemia in an unresponsive patient?

   A. 50 g of dextrose in 25 mL of water IV; reassess in an hour

   B. cheese and crackers; reassess in 15 minutes

   C. 25 g of dextrose in 50 mL of water IV; reassess in 30 minutes

   D. 10 gumdrops; reassess in 6 minutes

4. You are caring for an ICU patient suffering from psychosis. The nurse noticed that the patient drinks water excessively. The assistant has refilled the patient's water pitcher eight times within six hours. On the Intake and Output graph over the last 24 hours, the patient has had an excess of 20 liters per day in output. With the above information you contact the physician, and you both agree that this patient is showing signs of

   A. dehydration.

   B. diabetes insipidus.

   C. SIADH.

   D. acute adrenal insufficiency.

5. The nurse cares for a client with hyperglycemic hyperosmolar syndrome (HHS). In addition to hyperglycemia, which finding correlates with HHS?

   A. absence of ketonuria

   B. low serum osmolarity

   C. acetone breath

   D. no mental status changes

6. You are caring for a patient with malignant lung cancer who recently started chemotherapy. As an ICU nurse, you know that this combination of health status and treatment regimen could place this patient at a higher risk for developing

   A. Cushing syndrome.

   B. SIADH.

   C. Addison disease.

   D. thyroid storm.

7. Treatment and care of a patient suffering from SIADH could consist of which of these?

   A. close monitoring of dietary intake

   B. administration of demeclocycline, lithium, and dilantin

   C. infusion of hypotonic saline to help retain water

   D. monitoring of the BUN and creatinine

8. SIADH is an acute disorder that is defined by the excessive release of ADH resulting in which of these?

   A. hypovolemia

   B. hypervolemia

   C. hypocalcemia

   D. hyperuricemia

9. A blood glucose level of greater than 300 mg/dL with Kussmaul respirations and "fruity breath" is indicative of which of these?

   A. diabetes insipidus

   B. acute hypoglycemia

   C. hyperosmolar hyperglycemic state

   D. diabetic ketoacidosis

10. Which three pathologies are present with hyperosmolar hyperglycemic state (HHS)?

    A. bradycardia, serum glucose <300 mg/dL, serum osmolality <330 mOsm/kg

    B. tachycardia, serum glucose <300 mg/dL, serum osmolality >330 mOsm/kg

    C. bradycardia, serum glucose 600–2000 mg/dL, serum osmolality <330 mOsm/kg

    D. tachycardia, serum glucose 600–2000 mg/dL, serum osmolality >330 mOsm/kg

Review Answers and Explanations

1. C

Sodium bicarbonate is only given in DKA if pH is 6.9 or lower. (A) is incorrect because supplemental oxygen will help improve oxygen saturation in a patient with DKA. (B) is incorrect because hourly fingerstick is indicated to monitor blood glucose. (D) is incorrect because frequent and serial ABG is necessary to monitor acid-base imbalances.

2. A

Continuing the IV insulin for 1 to 2 hours after the SC insulin (long-acting) has been administered allows for the long-acting insulin to have its peak effect before discontinuing the short-acting (regular) IV insulin and to prevent hyperglycemia. (B) is incorrect because a client with DKA who is transitioning to SC insulin will require less frequent blood sugar checks, not every 30 minutes. (C) is incorrect because discontinuing the IV regular insulin before the long-acting SC insulin reaches its peak action will lead to hyperglycemia. (D) is incorrect because a client with DKA who is transitioning to SC insulin is stable and does not require monitoring for seizure activity.

3. C

Answer (C) is correct because it states the correct dose of IV dextrose, and it also includes the reassessment step to make sure the glucose level doesn't fall again. The dose in answer (A) is too concentrated. Voluntary oral intake is not possible because the patient is unresponsive, so answers (B) and (D) are incorrect.

4. B

In this case, diabetes insipidus is idiopathic. Because the patient has a compulsion to drink excessive amounts of water, this suppresses the release of ADH, causing polyuria.

5. A

In HHS, glucose is typically >400 mg/dL, with absent or minimal ketonuria. (B) is incorrect because serum osmolarity is elevated in HHS due to severe dehydration. (C) is incorrect because acetone breath is observed in DKA, not in HHS. (D) is incorrect because severe neurological abnormalities are typically seen in HHS, less in DKA.

6. B

Excessive ADH production or utilization is seen in patients with malignant cancers, with CNS disorders, and on medications used to treat these conditions.

7. B

Demeclocycline, lithium, and dilantin all work to increase serum osmolality, decrease risk of seizures, and prevent urine concentration when given with hypertonic solution, which increases removal of excess fluid.

8. B

Excessive release of ADH results in excessive retention or overload of fluid in the blood, known as hypervolemia.

9. D

Hyperglycemia is caused by the lack of insulin, preventing cellular glucose utilization. The blood glucose rises, and the negative feedback to the cells produces glucagon and cannot be activated. Glucagon is then released and breaks down glycogen, stimulating gluconeogenesis, which releases more glucose. This contributes to a metabolic acidosis. To compensate, the lungs attempt to eliminate the excess carbonic acid through hyperventilation.

10. D

Hyperosmolar hyperglycemic state (HHS) causes tachycardia, elevated glucose, and hyperosmolality.

The Hematologic and Immunological Systems

8

The hematology and immunology portion of the CCRN exam is approximately 2 percent of the total number of questions.

Critical care nurses need to be able to *identify alterations in the hematology and immunology systems* to manage appropriately patient conditions related to these systems and reduce unexpected outcomes. This requires a general knowledge of the processes related to the anatomy and physiology of those systems, including formation of cells, hemostasis, coagulation, oxygenation, immune responses, and antibody formation. In addition, the nurse must be able to plan for the care of the critically ill adult with abnormal conditions in these systems, including appropriate goals, interventions, and evaluation of those interventions.

This chapter will provide an overview of the basic hematologic components and anatomical structures, primary organs of the immunological system, pathophysiology, management of patients with hematologic and immunologic disorders, and care of patients receiving transfusions or undergoing organ transplantation. Generally, the hematologic and immunological systems provide support for the other major systems in the body (oxygenation and acid-base balance); however, when there is a malfunction of the normal processes in these systems, such as abnormal bleeding due to a coagulopathy or an anaphylactic response, significant complications can occur, and these patients are often treated in the critical care setting.

BASIC HEMATOLOGIC COMPONENTS/ANATOMICAL STRUCTURES

Human blood is comprised of several types of cells, which are responsible for a range of functions within the body. The primary precursor to the cells outlined below is the *pluripotent stem cell*. In the adult, this cell is produced in the bone marrow of the membranous bones within the body (vertebrae, sternum, ribs, and ilia) and moves through various stages of cell division to form the different cells in the circulating blood volume.

Red Blood Cells (RBCs)/Erythrocytes

The first of these are the *red blood cells* (RBCs) or erythrocytes. Typically RBCs remain alive and active for approximately *120 days*. Upon death of the cell, the spleen or liver filters out these products of the primary circulation. Iron is retained from the RBC, put back into circulation with transferrin as the transporter, and returned to the bone marrow for reuse. Normal RBC count in the blood for the male is $4.5–5.0 \times 10^6$/L and $4.0–5.0 \times 10^6$/L in the female. The pluripotent stem cell differentiates into three phases of colony-forming units: the colony-forming unit—spleen (CFU-S); the colony-forming unit—blast (CFU-B); and the colony-forming unit—erythrocyte (CFU-E), which transitions into the erythrocyte. The regulation of this process is guided by the glycoprotein *erythropoietin*. This protein is produced primarily in the kidneys. In the event there are decreased oxygen levels in the blood, the kidneys will stimulate the release of erythropoietin, which acts upon the bone marrow to produce more RBCs.

Blood and Rh typing is determined by antigens located on the RBC membrane. The two main antigens are named A and B. From these, the four major blood groups are created: A, B, AB, and O, which are based on the presence or absence of these antigens. For example, the A antigen is present in people with Type A blood. Conversely, since the B antigen is *not* present in Type A blood, a person with Type A blood will have antibodies *against* the B antigen. The Rh antibody develops if the Rh negative person is exposed to Rh positive blood, such as in pregnancy or in transfusion.

	Antigen	Antibodies	Donate To	Receive From
Type A	A	Anti-B	A, AB	A, O
Type B	B	Anti-A	B, AB	B, O
Type AB	AB	None (no antibodies are present)	AB only	All Blood Types (UNIVERSAL RECEIVER)
Type O	None (no antigens are present)	Anti-A & Anti-B	All Blood Types (UNIVERSAL DONOR)	O only

White Blood Cells (WBCs)/Leukocytes

Another primary type of cell is the *white blood cell* (WBC) or leukocyte. Unlike RBCs, there are several subtypes of WBCs, which are based on the developmental stage and function of the WBC. The precursor of the WBC is also the pluripotent stem cell and the CFU-S or colony-forming unit—spleen, which forms the *granulocytes (neutrophils, eosinophils,* and *basophils), monocytes, megakaryocytes,* and *platelets* and the *lymphoid stem cell (LSC),* which forms the T-lymphocytes and the B-lymphocytes. The average life span of a WBC is four to eight hours and another four to five days in the tissues. WBCs are formed partially in the bone marrow and partially in the lymph tissue. Leukocytes are considered mobile units as they are transported in the blood to various sites where they are needed; the most important function of this mobility is to provide defense against inflammation and infection. Complementary substances that assist in the function of these cells include the factors of the complement system (composed of serum proteins C1–C9), cytokines, and eicosanoids. These will be discussed later in this chapter.

When measuring WBCs in the complete blood count (CBC), two measurements are done: the total number of WBCs (4,500–10,000/mcL) and the differential, which includes the percentage of the following types of WBCs: bands, neutrophils, esosinophils, basophils, lymphocytes, and monocytes. These percentages total 100 percent. Leukocytosis is defined as an overall WBC count greater than 10,000. White counts greater than 30,000 typically indicate a massive infection unless there is an overproduction of immature cells, which can demonstrate conditions such as leukemia. In contrast, when a patient has a WBC less than 4,000, she is referred to as leukopenic. When analyzing the blood, the CBC will also be accompanied by a microscopic differential, where the approximate number of each of type cell will be estimated. If the neutrophils component of the WBC is less than 500, then the patient is referred to as leukopenic and also neutropenic. Since patients with leukopenia and/or neutropenia are susceptible to infections, they present with a fever. A febrile neutropenic patient is a clinical emergency and warrants immediate hospitalization. Unless she has hemodynamic compromise, such as signs of septic shock, she can generally be managed in reverse isolation on a general floor, but she should receive immediate broad spectrum antiobiotics such as Cefepime. Prior to antiobiotic administration, patients should have a chest radiograph, blood cultures × 2 from the periphery, blood cultures from each chronic IV or central line, urinalysis, and urine culture.

Hemoglobin/Hematocrit

Hemoglobin is a protein that is formed within the red blood cell. The heme molecule is a portion of the hemoglobin that is comprised of *iron* and *protoporphyin IX* (this is formed from pyrrole molecules generated during the Krebs cycle). The globulin portion of the molecule is a polypeptide synthesized by the ribosomes. The heme and the globulin form a chain, and in turn, *four chains* bind to form the hemoglobin. One of the most significant functions of the hemoglobin is oxygen transport. When the hemoglobin is concentrated in the cell fluid, it can be measured. The normal range for hemoglobin for men is 13.5 to 17.5 grams per deciliter. The normal range for hemoglobin for women is 12.0 to 15.5 grams per deciliter.

Hematocrit is a calculation of the percentage of hemoglobin in the blood. It is based on the hemoglobin and the volume of blood. This concentration varies with the age and sex of the individual, with the highest concentrations appearing in neonates and stabilizing as the person matures. In adult men, the hematocrit is 42–52 percent, while in adult women, it is 36–48 percent. The primary reason women have a lower hematocrit is related to menstruation.

Plasma/Platelets

Plasma is the substance in which blood cells are suspended, and it serves as a transporting media. It is comprised primarily of water but also contains other particles such as dissolved proteins, glucose, mineral ions, hormones, carbon dioxide, as well as the blood cells. Plasma also contains coagulation factors and proteins such as fibrinogen, which are critical to hemostasis in the body. Plasma that is taken via phlebotomy from a single donor may be frozen for future use. It is especially helpful to patients with coagulopathies related to blood loss or bleeding diathesis.

Platelets are fragments of megakaryocytes that are formed in the bone marrow. These thrombocytes are very small discs approximately 1–4 micrometers in diameter. Platelets have no nuclei and cannot reproduce. Their life span is fairly short at approximately 10 days. A unique characteristic of platelets is that their cell membranes have a coat of glycoproteins that reduces their adherence to normal endothelial cells but actually increases their ability to adhere to injured cells or vessel walls. Platelets are transported to the site of blood vessel or tissue injury and form a "plug" that adheres to the site of injury. At that site, the platelets release cytokines, which help to stimulate the recruitment of additional platelets and additional clotting factors. Upon death of platelets, macrophages in the spleen remove them from the circulation. Normal platelet count ranges from 150,000 to 450,000 platelets per microliter of blood.

Clotting Factors

Research has discovered more than 50 substances that may cause or affect coagulation either in the blood or tissue. Those that promote coagulation are called *procoagulants,* and those that prohibit coagulation are called *anticoagulants.* Not all of these substances will be discussed. Table 8.1 describes the most common of these factors.

Anatomical Organs of the Hematologic System

Bone Marrow

The majority of the blood cells originate in the bone marrow of the vertebrae, ribs, skull, pelvis, and proximal epiphyses of the long bones in the leg and arm, the femur and humerus. Bone marrow is the spongy interior of the bone. An infant's bones contain only red marrow where the blood cells are formed. As individuals age, fatty yellow marrow forms and replaces the red marrow. Amazingly, the bone marrow releases approximately 10–15 million erythrocytes *every second,* and the same amount are destroyed by the spleen as they become inactivated. Blood vessel membranes serve as a barrier to prevent immature blood cells from leaving the marrow.

TABLE 8.1 *Clotting Factors and Components*

Factor	Description/Function
Thrombin	A compound split from prothrombin
Fibrinogen Factor I	High molecular weight protein, formed in liver; essential factor in the coagulation process
Prothrombin Factor II	Plasma protein, formed in liver; assists in blood clotting
Tissue factor (Factor III)	Composed of phospholipids plus a lipoprotein complex; functions as proteolytic enzyme
Calcium	Required for promotion/acceleration of all blood-clotting reactions
Factor V	Combines with factor X to form a complex called prothrombin activator
Factor VII	Prothrombin conversion accelerator
Factor VIII	Participates in the intrinsic pathway for clotting
Factor IX	Component of plasma thromboplastin
Factor X	Activation of this factor results in formation of prothrombin activator
Factor XI	Second step in the intrinsic pathway for blood clotting
Factor XII	Converts to proteolytic enzyme when exposed to collagen
Factor XIII	Fibrin-stabilizing factor
Platelets	Assists in forming "plug" at the site of bleeding; abnormally low platelet count is called thrombocytopenia

Liver

The liver is the largest solid organ in the body and is located in the right upper quadrant of the abdomen. The liver receives approximately one-third of the cardiac output. This organ serves to synthesize plasma proteins such as globulins and albumin, which are important to the function of maintaining osmotic balance of the blood. Additionally, many of the coagulation factors, including fibrinogen, prothrombin, and factors (II, V, VII, IX, and X), are synthesized in the liver. The production of these factors is significantly dependent on the presence of vitamin K. Kupffer's cells in the liver assist in the removal of worn red blood cells, while hepatocytes conjugate bilirubin, a by-product of this cell destruction, so that it can be excreted.

FUNCTIONS OF THE HEMATOLOGIC SYSTEM

Formation of RBCs and Hemoglobin

One of the most important functions of the hematologic system is the formation of blood cells. During fetal development, red blood cells are produced in the yolk sac, and toward the third trimester of gestation, the liver becomes the main organ for production of RBCs. Finally, in the few weeks before birth, RBCs are produced primarily in the bone marrow; this production continues until we die. As age increases, the production of RBCs decreases. Earlier in this chapter, the process for development of erythrocytes, leukocytes, and lymphocytes from precursor and intermediate cells was discussed. All blood cells originate from the pluripotential hematopoietic stem cell.

Hemostasis

Hemostasis is the ability of the body to stop bleeding. Typically, the first stage of this process is vasoconstriction of the smooth muscle of the vascular wall to reduce blood flow to the area of injury and preserve blood volume. The endothelium releases biochemical mediators, which promote vasoconstriction upon injury. The two primary agents are endothelin and thromboxane A2. Platelets are then mobilized to the site of injury, where they adhere to the damaged vascular surface. Platelets are activated by many conditions or substances, such as shear stress, collagen, serotonin, thrombin, epinephrine, or ADP (adenosine diphosphate). The platelets morph, swell, and become sticky, so that they adhere to each other and allow for attachment of many factors, thus forming a platelet plug. Platelets degranulate and release serotonin, von Willebrand factor, adenosine diphosphate (ADP), fibrinogen, and thromboxane A2 from cell vesicles. These substances serve to recruit more platelets and clotting factors to the site of injury. If the site of injury is small, this will usually be successful in blocking further blood loss. A stronger plug is generated when fibrin threads attach to the platelets. The coagulation cascade is initiated based on phospholipids in the platelet membrane.

Oxygenation

Each hemoglobin molecule can transport four molecules of oxygen, which bind with the iron on the molecule chain. The types of hemoglobin chains in the molecule determine how readily the molecule binds oxygen. Oxygen, which is combined with hemoglobin in the lungs, is released in the peripheral capillary tissues where the oxygen tension is lower. Approximately 97 percent of the oxygen is transported in this manner; the other 3 percent is dissolved in plasma. PaO_2 measures the oxygen carried in the arterial plasma.

The propensity for the release of oxygen is determined by the oxyhemoglobin dissociation curve. The dissociation is based on several factors, but primarily hemoglobin saturation and PaO_2. Other factors influencing or causing shifts on the curve are pH, temperature, levels of 2,3-DPG, PCO_2, and carbon monoxide poisoning.

Coagulation

Another critical function of the hematology system is *hemostasis*. Hemostasis is the ability to control bleeding. The coagulation cascade is the process that is initiated when there is insult or injury causing bleeding. There are two pathways within the coagulation cascade: the extrinsic and intrinsic pathways.

FIGURE 8.1 *Coagulation Cascade*

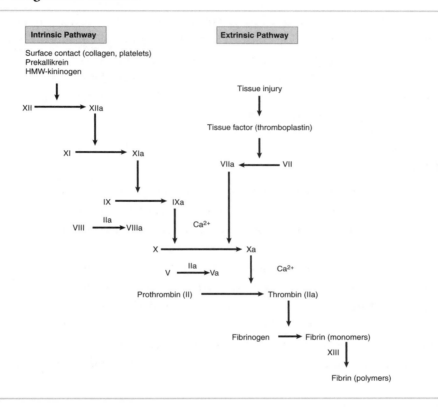

Many of the factors described in table 8.1 above function in some capacity in the cascade. In the **extrinsic pathway** (common pathway), the insult as a result of trauma or damaged tissues initiates the release of factor III. Factor VII then combines with factor X and converts factor III to factor Xa. With assistance of factor V, prothrombin (factor II) is converted to thrombin (factor IIa). Thrombin then converts fibrinogen (factor I) to fibrin (factor Ia), which is what helps bind with the initial platelet plug to strengthen the bond at the site of the injury and form a stable fibrin clot.

The **intrinsic pathway** (alternative pathway) starts slightly differently, but the end result is the production of fibrin. The intrinsic pathway starts with endothelial damage or venous stasis. One of the differences in this pathway is that it is a *slower pathway*. The intrinsic pathway begins with the endothelial damage and collagen exposure to factor XII. This exposure converts factor XII to XIIa. At each stage in the cascade, the inactive proenzyme is converted to the active enzyme by a process whereby the bond between amino acids in the protein is broken down by substances called peptidases, proteases, or proteolytic cleavage enzymes. Additional substances such as calcium, coenzymes, or phospolipids may be required to participate in the process. The cascade continues with factor XIIa combining with factor XI to convert it to factor XIa. Factor XIa converts to factor IX. At this point, with the assistance of factor VIII and platelets, the intrinsic pathway continues in the same manner as the extrinsic pathway by converting factor XIa to factor X. Vitamin K is required for this conversion.

Eventually the fibrin clot is removed by plasmin, which is a proteolytic enzyme. The body is constantly forming and dissolving clots. Activated protein C and antithrombin II are endogenous anticoagulants that play a big role in clotting. Thrombin is broken down by various factors into plasminogen, plasmin, and stable fibrin. One of the tests that can determine if the clot is beginning to break down is a blood test called serum fibrin split products, which are the final products in this process.

Iron Metabolism

Iron is a critical element in the body that is required for synthesis of hemoglobin and for other substances such as myoglobin or cytochromes. Approximately 65 percent of the total amount of iron in the body is in the hemoglobin, and 4 percent is in myoglobin. A person obtains iron through dietary intake, which is then absorbed through the intestine. There it combines with the plasma and binds loosely with apotransferrin to become *transferrin*. The transferrin is transported by the plasma to cell cytoplasm, where it also combines with apoferritin to form *ferritin*. This iron is stored for future use. When iron is needed within the body at any point, it is converted back to transferrin to be transported. This includes being transported to the cell membrane of erythroblasts. A syndrome that can develop due to the inability of the body to transport transferrin to the erythroblast cell membrane is called *hypochromic anemia*.

Reticuloendothelial System

Macrophages function as a mobile unit that serve as a phagocyte. However, another, more long-term function of the macrophages is to aid the body in phagocytosis of bacteria, viruses, necrotic tissue, and other foreign particles. They do this by becoming attached more long-term to the tissues. The body has this capability in nearly all tissues. These cells can become detached at any time and function in their original role as macrophages.

The reticuloendothelial system is the combination of the following: monocytes; mobile macrophages; fixed tissue macrophages (as described above); and specialized endothelial cells in the bone marrow, spleen, and lymph nodes. The Kuppfer cells in the liver and the Langerhaus cells in the skin are examples of these specialized cells.

TRANSFUSION OF BLOOD AND BLOOD COMPONENTS

In this section, the indications for *the primary types of blood* and *blood product transfusion* will be discussed. Additionally, a brief discussion will be done regarding *transfusion reactions* and potential *complications of blood transfusion*. Commonly in the critical care unit many of these products are administered in emergent situations. Patients who are susceptible to transfusion reactions or who have known antibodies may be premedicated with diphenhydramine and acetaminophen to prevent febrile reactions.

TABLE 8.2 *Blood Products*

BLOOD PRODUCT	INDICATIONS	NURSING CONSIDERATION
1. Fresh Frozen Plasma (FFP) Liquid portion of whole blood, separated from cells and kept frozen until ready for use	Bleeding due to lack of clotting factors V and VII, such as in disseminated intravascular coagulation (DIC), hemophilia, massive transfusion, Coumadin toxicity, **elevated PT and INR**	• Donor and patient need not have the same blood type. • Given over 30 to 60 minutes • Monitor for CHF, diuretics posttransfusion; check INR levels posttransfusion
2. Platelets Prepared from whole blood within 4 hours after collection. One 4-unit bag needs at least 4 donors.	**Usually** thrombocytopenia with platelets less than 20,000; in some cases, lower than 10,000; check hospital/treatment protocol.	• ABO matching not essential • Given in 4-unit bags (pooled) • Infuse in 30 to 60 minutes • Improves platelet levels by 5,000 to 10,000 posttransfusion • Check platelet levels posttransfusion
3. Cryoprecipitate Prepared from FFP, thawed at 4 degrees C. White precipitate is collected. Requires several donors.	Replacement of clotting factors VIII, XIII and Fibrinogen, such as in DIC, sepsis, hemophilia, elevated PT and INR	• Infuse in 30 to 60 minutes • Better in controlling bleeding than FFP because it contains more clotting factors in less volume
4. Albumin Prepared from plasma. Available in 5% or 25% grams solution. 25 gm = 500 mL plasma	Hypovolemic shock, hypotension during hemodialysis and **very** low albumin levels, sometimes given in severe third-space edema	• Infuse in 30 to 60 minutes • Diuretics sometimes given after transfusion
5. Packed Red Blood Cells (PRBC) Prepared by sedimentation or centrifugation 1 unit = approx. 250 mL	Anemia, blood loss, active bleeding, Hemoglobin <7 gm and Hematocrit <21% (check with hospital/unit protocol) **Note:** Patients who have cardiopulmonary risks may have a higher transfusion threshold.	• Watch for transfusion reactions • Follow protocols (vital signs) • Diuretics may be given after 1 unit = 4% increase in HCT

Probably one of the most common components administered in the critical care unit is **packed red blood cells** (PRBCs). The first indication for PRBCs is anemia, particularly anemia associated with symptoms of hypoxia such as shortness of breath, tachycardia, hypotension, chest pain, hypovolemia, etc. Another indication for administration of PRBCs is a decreased ability to oxygenate a patient due to diminished oxygen-carrying capacity. In the latter case, care must be taken to ensure that the patient does not show evidence of fluid overload in the event multiple units are required. In most institutions, the Hgb must be significantly decreased, < 8.0 g/dL, to indicate the need for transfusion due to the risks. Care must be taken during the transfusion of PRBCs to prevent complications if multiple units are given. If multiple units are required in a short period of time, fresh frozen plasma should be administered to prevent dilutional coagulopathies. Another consideration is that PRBCs are preserved in citrate; therefore, multiple transfusions of PRBCs may cause a reduction in serum calcium due to the binding of the patient's calcium with the citrate.

Fresh frozen plasma (FFP) is another common component administered. Fresh frozen plasma contains the clotting factors needed to maintain hemostasis. Patients with clotting factor deficiencies such as hemophilia or those who have elevated bleeding times due to warfarin will benefit from transfusion of this component. Patients may also have coagulopathy from liver disease (e.g., cirrhosis) since a majority of the clotting factors are synthesized in the liver. In these patients, as well as those on warfarin (brand name: coumadin), the administration of vitamin K will help synthesize clotting factors. This does not cause an immediate reversal of the anticoagulation, but it can be followed with the PT/INR over days. In contrast, administration of FFP will immediately reverse the anticoagulation, which may be necessary for invasive procedures. Another blood component that may be administered to the hemophiliac is cryoprecipitate. There are two clotting factors in this preparation that are not present in FFP in appreciable quantities: factor I (fibrinogen) and factor VIII.

Thrombocytopenia is the condition of decreased platelet count and is the primary indication for transfusion of platelets. Typically the platelet count must be less than 50,000 and there must be evidence of bleeding to require transfusion. Platelets may be administered rapidly and often can be pooled in a multipack for more efficient transfusion.

Albumin is a plasma protein that is synthesized in the liver. When levels of albumin drop, the most common causes are a failure to produce adequate levels of plasma proteins (liver disease) or a conditions that causes leakage of protein from plasma (renal disease, such as nephrotic syndrome). Edema may be present in these patients due to this leakage of fluid into the extracellular spaces. Administration of albumin may increase osmotic pressure and assist in shifting the fluids from the extracellular spaces to the intracellular spaces. Albumin is also indicated for patients in shock, those who have serious burns, or those with cerebral edema. Unfortunately, the half-life of albumin in the bloodstream is short due the body's enzymatic digestion of exogenously administered albumin. Further, if a person is suffering from nephrotic syndrome, the exogenously administered albumin will be subject to capillary loss as was the original albumin. The end result is that the administration of albumin is a transient solution that is quickly reversed within a few days.

Finally, the last product to be discussed is **intravenous immunoglobulin (IVIG)**. There are a few differences with this component with regard to set up and administration. IVIG does not have to be typed with the patient's blood. Additionally, it is administered with D_5W rather than normal saline, as are all other blood products. IVIG is indicated in patients with idiopathic thrombocytopenic purpura (ITP), acquired immunodeficiency syndrome (AIDS), bone marrow transplant, severe combined immunodeficiency disease (SCID), as well as a host of autoimmune disorders that are beyond the scope of this book and the CCRN.

During initiation of all blood components, the infusion should be started slowly for the first 15–30 minutes while the patient's vital signs are monitored for transfusion reaction. If there are incompatibilities with the component administered and the patient's own blood, there is a chance that the patient will develop a blood transfusion complication.

TABLE 8.3 *Blood Transfusion Complications*

COMPLICATION	CAUSE	SIGNS/SYMPTOMS	INTERVENTIONS
Acute Hemolytic Reaction: usually manifests within 5–15 minutes	ABO incompatibility or blood products containing more than 10 mL RBC; antibody in the recipient attaches to antigen in the donor blood	Chills, fever, nausea, low back pain, flushing, tachycardia, hypotension (shock), hemoglobinuria, dark urine, renal failure, and DIC	Stop transfusion, send for CBC and UA, monitor vitals, send unused blood to BB, IVF to prevent pigment nephropathy, and O_2
Mild Allergic Reaction: urticaria 2–3 minutes after the start of transfusion	Sensitivity to foreign plasma proteins	Itching, hives, flushing and hemoglobinuria	Stop transfusion, give antihistamine; BT may be continued if reaction is mild
Non-Hemolytic Febrile Reaction: most common, usually toward the end of transfusion	Sensitivity to donor's WBC, platelets, and plasma protein; due to accumulation of cytokines in stored blood	Sudden chills and fever, headache, flushing, anxiety, and muscle pains	Stop transfusion, give antipyretics (no aspirin for patients with low platelets); patient should receive leukocyte-poor blood products with special filter

TABLE 8.3 *Blood Transfusion Complications (continued)*

Anaphylactic Reaction: manifests within 1–45 minutes of start of transfusion	Sensitivity to plasma proteins; transfusion of IgA protein to IgA-deficient recipient who has developed IgA antibody	Shock, wheezing, respiratory/cardiac arrest	Stop transfusion, RRT, follow ACLS protocol for cardiac arrest; use autologous transfusion if possible
Circulatory Overload: transfusion associated circulatory overload (TACO)	Fluid overload due to rapid transfusion particularly in high-risk patients; manifests within several hours of transfusion	CHF, SOB, crackles, pulmonary congestion, neck vein distension, JVD, and tachycardia	Infuse blood slowly, diuretics after transfusion, O_2, assess breath sounds, set the patient upright
Transfusion-Related Acute Lung Injury (TRALI): most cases manifest within 6 hours	Reaction between antileukocyte antibodies and recipient's leukocytes causing pulmonary inflammation	Fever, hypotension, SOB, tachycardia, hypoxia, frothy sputum, and ARDS	Oxygen, steroids, ACLS protocol if patient is in respiratory-cardiac arrest, CXR, provide leukocyte-reduced products

HEMATOLOGIC CONDITIONS OF THE CRITICALLY ILL PATIENT

Anemia

Anemia is simply a decreased RBC level, quantity of hemoglobin, or volume of RBCs. The causes of anemia are varied, but the manifestation of anemia is most always hypoxia, which can subsequently cause end tissue damage if severe. The body compensates for anemia by increasing heart rate, which in turn increases cardiac output, and by increasing respiratory rate to increase oxygenation. Additionally, blood supply to other key organs such as gastrointestinal organs, skin, and kidneys will decrease. This can produce symptoms such as cold, clammy skin, ileus, or decreased urine output.

Anemia can be acute or chronic. **Acute anemia** typically occurs with trauma, gastrointestinal hemorrhage, or hemolysis. Immediate, extensive blood loss can significantly alter the hemodynamic status of an individual and requires emergent intervention to decrease the potential for adverse outcomes. Rapid administration of PRBCs and FFP is required to maintain hemostasis. Stabilization of the bleeding should be undertaken as well; typically this is done surgically or endoscopically. **Chronic anemia** results from conditions such as acute renal failure, dietary deficiencies, menorrhagia, or sickle cell anemia. The treatment for these conditions is based on the etiology of the disease, but it may include transfusion, injection of erythropoietin, or surgical interventions.

During history taking, it is important to question the patient regarding subjective symptoms of hypoxia. The physical examination should include observation for signs and symptoms of anemia including *pallor, shortness of breath, tachycardia,* and *hypotension. Orthostatic blood pressures* should be taken. Examination of laboratory test results is done to ascertain the degree of anemia and to determine the potential cause of the bleeding and/or hemolysis.

Thrombocytopenia

Thrombocytopenia is a decreased level of platelets in the blood. As a result, the patient is at an increased risk of bleeding when the platelet count drops below 50,000. Conditions that cause thrombocytopenia are categorized into two categories: conditions that result in *decreased production of platelets* and conditions that result in the *increased destruction of platelets.*

Malignancies such as leukemia and lymphoma are examples of conditions that cause decreased production, because the increase in cancerous cells limits the production of healthy platelets in the blood. Two of the most common conditions that result in destruction of platelets are *disseminated intravascular coagulation (DIC)* and *immune thrombocytopenic purpura (ITP).* Both of these will be discussed in more detail in this section. Many medications can also cause thrombocytopenia.

Administration of platelets is the treatment for thrombocytopenia. The patient most likely receive transfusion of platelets is one who has a platelet count less than 50,000 *and* evidence of bleeding. Other manifestations of thrombocytopenia include a skin rash called petichiae, conjunctival bleeding, and oozing from peripheral IV sticks.

Idiopathic thrombocytopenia (ITP) is also a condition of low platelet count for which the causes are not clearly known—hence, the derivation of the name. ITP is commonly a diagnosis made by exclusion of other conditions. A form of ITP is thought to be an autoimmune disease due the development of antibodies to platelet membrane glycoproteins. In addition, specific drugs may elicit this response. Examples of these drugs include sulfanamides, thiazide diuretics, chlorpropamide, quinidine, and gold. Treatment of idiopathic thromobocytopenia purpura (ITP) includes whole blood transfusion, corticosteroids, or splenectomy. Administration of platelets is not generally done except in emergencies such as uncontrolled bleeding, as the effect is generally short-lived. In severe cases of autoimmune ITP refractive to traditional therapy, the patient may be treated with chemotherapeutic agents such as vinblastine or other medications such as intravenous IGG or inferon.

Hypercoagulable Disorders

In this condition, there is evidence of a disruption of the normal coagulation processes, and the patient clots more readily. On occasion as a result of a hypercoagulable disorder, the patient may also develop a secondary bleeding disorder when platelets and clotting factors are exhausted; this is referred to as consumptive coagulopathy.

In acute conditions such as ischemia, infarction, or venous stasis, where there is decreased blood flow to specific locations, the coagulation cascade will be initiated, and a hypercoagulable state may occur. Additionally, any condition that increases the activity of platelets such as atherosclerosis, hypertension, diabetes, or smoking may cause hypercoagulopathy. Venous thromboses may occur as a result of this state. In the event the thrombus breaks loose, arterial emboli occur, and pulmonary embolus or CVA may result. Other conditions that can initiate a hypercoagulable disorder include vessel wall injury and thrombotic thrombocytopenic purpura (TTP). TTP results when there is a vessel wall injury with a resultant exaggerated immunologic response. The symptoms vary slightly in this type of response and include *fever, thrombocytopenia, acute kidney injury, altered mental status, and/or hemolytic anemia.* Additionally, the treatment is different and primarily consists of plasmapheresis and infusion of FFP.

The treatment for hypercoagulable disorders is anticoagulation, which in and of itself has a certain degree of risk in these patients. Careful monitoring of prothrombin times (PTT) while the patient is on heparin, and INRs while on warfarin, is important to ensure a patient does not hemorrhage from supratherapeutic anticoagulation. The treatment that one would anticipate with TTP (i.e., administration of platelets) is contraindicated because of its potential to worsen the hypercoagulable and thrombotic state.

Hemophilia

Approximately 85 percent of all cases of hemophilia are in males, because these are X-linked recessive disorders. There are three types of hemophilia: **hemophilia A** (classic hemophilia), **hemophilia B**, and **hemophilia C** (factor XI deficiency—Ashkenazic Jews). Hemophilia A is an abnormality or deficiency in factor VIII, while hemophilia B patients have a deficiency in factor IX. Even though the male is the individual who suffers from hemophilia in the majority of cases, it is actually the mother who carries the chromosome that has the deficiency. When the mother is a carrier and the father is normal, then the male children will have a 50 percent chance of manifesting the disease, and the female children will have a 50 percent chance of becoming a carrier.

Hemophilia causes the individual to have a propensity to bleed. There are various levels of this disease and symptoms. Most often the individual is taught how to prevent trauma that may cause bleeding. The treatment for excessive bleeding is administration of factor VIII. Factor VIII is limited in supply and is used primarily when severe bleeding occurs.

Iron Deficiency Anemia

Iron deficiency anemia is the most common form of anemia and is most often caused by *chronic blood loss* such as menorrhagia, renal failure, or gastrointestinal bleeding from chronic use of NSAIDs. One of the most interesting symptoms of iron deficiency anemia is a craving for unusual foods/substances, known as pica. These cravings include ice, dirt, chalk, or plaster. Pica frequently occurs in pregnant women with iron deficiency anemia. Ironically, the items often craved do not contain iron, and it is unknown why pica occurs.

The treatment for iron deficiency anemia is supplemental iron in an oral form. Patients who are known to have chronic blood loss conditions can be given supplemental iron to prevent anemic states.

Disseminated Intravascular Coagulopathy (DIC)

DIC occurs frequently in critically ill patients and is extremely hard to manage due to the combination of both hypercoagulable states and hemorrhage. DIC does not occur in isolation but rather as the result of other serious precipitating factors: sepsis/septic shock, major trauma/crash injuries, shock states, obstetrical emergencies such as abruptio placentae or fetal death, and malignancies including acute tumor lysis syndrome.

The precipitating factor causes *stimulation or initiation of the coagulation cascade,* as discussed earlier in the chapter. This often results from large amounts of traumatized or damaged/dying tissues. The clotting factor that is initially released to initiate the cascade is the tissue factor/tissue thromboplastin/factor III. Small clots begin to form and clog the smaller peripheral blood vessels. One example, which is common in the critical care unit, is the septic patient with circulating endotoxin from the infecting bacterial organism due to overwhelming infection. The release of endotoxins initiates the clotting cascade. Subsequently, as the peripheral vessels become obstructed with clots, the oxygen-carrying capacity of the vessels diminishes, and nourishment to the cells is limited. This causes shock and circulatory collapse.

In addition to the clotting cascade initiation, the patient also demonstrates evidence of bleeding. It is felt that the precipitating factor for the bleeding is the widespread consumption of the clotting factors. Hence, the supply (synthesis) of the clotting factors does not match the rate of consumption.

FIGURE 8.2 *Pathophysiology of Disseminated Intravascular Coagulation (DIC)*

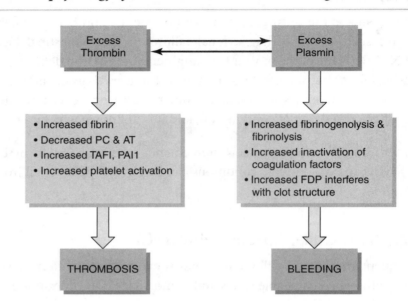

In sepsis-induced DIC, the thrombotic pathway predominates in the initial stages leading to microvascular thrombosis. Bleeding results secondary to continued thrombin generation and the ensuing loss of the coagulation factors, platelets and fibrinogen, and plasmin-mediated functions. In trauma-induced DIC, the fibrinolytic pathway is the initial major player leading to bleeding as the early manifestation, with thrombosis resulting from further continued thrombin generation and inhibition of antifibrinolytic pathways. It needs to be clarified that this concept is arbitrary, and complex interactions between several components including thrombin and plasmin exist in DIC.

The patient must be provided with supportive care to ensure that hemodynamic stability is maintained. Treatment of the cause of the coagulopathy should be a primary focus. Support with platelet transfusion may also be required if the platelet count is below 50,000 *and* there is evidence of bleeding. In the situation where the cause of bleeding is not known, FFP should also be given. Platelet transfusion should be avoided unless there is evidence of bleeding. Cryoprecipitate should also be avoided unless fibrinogen levels are low and there is active bleeding. (This does not interrupt the clotting cascade, and the patient will continue to clot.) Oxygenation must be maintained, including by intubation if required, to ensure an adequate airway and exchange of blood gases.

The use of heparin in chronic DIC patients is well established. It is contraindicated in conditions that may require surgical intervention and when platelets cannot be maintained at a level of at least 50,000. Administration of recombinant activated protein C, drotrecogin alfa (trade name: Xigris), deactivates factor V and VII, in turn, stopping the coagulation cascade.

This drug showed benefit in a subgroup of patients with sepsis and DIC. However, it was withdrawn from the market in 2011 after research data failed to demonstrate significant survival benefit for patients with severe sepsis and septic shock.

Leukemia

Leukemia is a complex malignant disease of the white blood cells. There are several kinds of leukemia based on the speed of the progression of the cloning of the white blood cell into the malignant white blood cell. The two most common types of leukemia are **acute myelogenous leukemia** (AML) and **acute lymphocytic leukemia** (ALL). There are chronic forms of the disease; however, most often these are not managed in the critical care unit. Additionally, most acute leukemias can be managed on the oncology unit. However, when serious complications arise such as sepsis and acute tumor lysis syndrome, admission to the critical care unit is required. The cloned white cells are not functional, healthy cells but rather multiply in quantity and overtake the space that normal healthy white blood cells occupy.

The cloned white blood cells in leukemia do not have the ability to function as normal white blood cells; therefore, patients have an increased likelihood of infection. They have no ability to initiate an immunologic response even to simple bacterial exposures that otherwise healthy individuals could ward off fairly easily. Patients with leukemia, WBC counts less than 4,000, and an absolute neutrophil count of less than 500 are placed in neutropenic precautions to limit exposure to infectious agents. Further, as mentioned earlier, neutropenic fever is a clinical emergency, and the patient should be hospitalized, an infectious workup undertaken, and the patient started empirically on broad spectrum antibiotics.

Tumor lysis syndrome occurs when a patient with malignancies is administered chemotherapy. In the case of both leukemia and lymphoma, the malignant cells are being produced quickly, and patients develop a large tumor burden even before the diseases are diagnosed. Chemotherapy is typically effective on these cells and causes significant lysis. Upon lysis, the cell contents are released into the bloodstream, and the by-products (uric acid, potassium, phosphorous, and calcium) can cause renal failure if they obstruct the distal tubules or collecting ducts in the kidneys.

Lymphoma

Lymphoma is another malignancy condition of tissues of the lymphatic system. The two primary types of lymphoma are **Hodgkin's disease** and **non-Hodgkin's lymphoma**. In lymphoma, the T and B lymphocytes are abnormal. The production of these abnormal cells increases dramatically because they are carried by the lymphatic system and are distributed throughout the body. Recalling from earlier discussion, the T and B lymphocytes protect the body against infection from viruses, fungi, and some bacteria. Therefore, without healthy cells of this type, the patient is less likely to develop an immune response to these organisms.

The patient is often treated with chemotherapy to eradicate the abnormal cells. Most patients admitted to the critical care unit with lymphoma have a complication such as an overwhelming infection or sepsis.

Other Conditions of the Hematologic System

Deep Vein Thrombosis

The precipitating factors that cause deep vein thrombosis (DVT) are called Virchow's triad, named after the German professor Rudolf Virchow. The three factors are 1) alterations in blood flow, specifically stasis; 2) injuries to the vascular endothelium; and 3) alterations in the coagulopathy of blood. One of the most common sites of DVT is the iliofemoral vascular system, although DVT can occur in any vessel. Immobility due to postoperative recovery on bedrest, long air flights, obesity, and advanced age are some of the most common causes of DVT.

At the site of the DVT, the extremity may become swollen, painful, and hot to touch. Diagnostic testing includes Doppler studies, D-dimer, CBC, and coagulation studies. Treatment is low molecular weight heparin or unfractionated heparin for renal patients. The risk for patients with DVT is that the thrombus will break loose and travel to the lungs, causing pulmonary embolus.

Heparin-Induced Thrombocytopenia (HIT)

Heparin-induced thrombocytopenia is platelet deficiency that develops after the initiation of heparin therapy. There are two types of HIT: *Type I*, where mild thrombocytopenia develops within a few days after initiation of heparin therapy, and *Type II*, where an immune syndrome develops and IgG attaches to the platelet, causing clumping and subsequently thrombosis. The second type develops approximately 5–14 days after exposure to heparin.

In **Type I HIT**, the heparin may continue, and the patient should be observed for symptoms for bleeding due to low platelets. In **Type II HIT**, the heparin must be stopped and symptomatic treatment begun. Type II HIT occurs in only about 3–5 percent of the patients on unfractionated heparin and 0.5 percent of patients on low molecular weight heparin.

The critical care nurse must be aware of this syndrome and of the potential for formation of thrombus. Venous or arterial clots may form, although venous clots are more likely. The patient should be treated with *direct thrombin inhibitors* (e.g., argatroban and lepirudin).

SPECIAL SITUATIONS

Bone Marrow and Stem Cell Transplantation

Patients with malignancies who have received chemotherapy and radiation in doses high enough to destroy their bone marrow will often benefit from bone marrow and peripheral stem cell transplantation. These processes reconstitute the patient's hematologic and immunological systems with healthy cells that can reproduce. The donor marrow or stem cells are harvested and infused intravenously into the recipient and travel via a natural homing mechanism to the patient's bone marrow.

There are *three types of transplantation* in this category. The first is what is referred to as an **allogenic** bone marrow transplant. A donor is identified via HLA matching (human leukocyte antigen) to ensure compatibility with recipient. A relative is the most likely donor in this type of transplantation. A sibling has a 25 percent chance of a match. There is only a small chance that an unrelated donor will match. The second type of bone marrow transplant is the **autologous** donation. Prior to treatment with chemotherapy or radiation, the patient's own marrow is harvested, then later infused back into the patient. With this type of transplantation, the risk of rejection is eliminated; however, there is always the potential that the transplanted marrow contains the malignant cells the patient was being treated for. Therefore, this option is more successful in patients with solid tumors and unaffected bone marrow. The final type of transplantation is done by **stimulation of the patient's own marrow to produce colony-stimulating factors**. The stem cells produced from this process are then harvested through pheresis. After the chemotherapy or radiation, the stem cells are reinfused to the patient. Similarly to the autologous donation, the risk of rejection is absent. There is a slight benefit with this type of transplant in that the ability for the stem cells to re-engraft is quicker than for marrow, thus lessening the time the patient is unable to illicit an immune response.

One of the most significant complications of transplantation of bone marrow or stem cells is potential for infection due to the absence of a cellular immune function while the patient is being prepared for the transplantation. This compromise can last up to a year. A complication of chemotherapy and radiation is thrombocytopenia, which can place the patient at risk for bleeding. There is also a risk of renal insufficiency from many of the medications required to either address infection or rejection. Damage can also occur to the venous system of the liver from high-dose chemotherapy or radiation. Graft versus host disease (GVHD) can occur as long as 100 days after transplantation due to grafted T lymphocytes attacking the recipient. This can occur in up to 40–50 percent of recipients.

PRIMARY ORGANS OF THE IMMUNOLOGICAL SYSTEM

Bone Marrow

Bone marrow has been discussed in the earlier section on organs of the hematologic system.

Thymus

The thymus is a gland that is located in the upper chest under the sternum. Early in an individual's life, lymphocytes are produced in the bone marrow and released and travel to the thymus, where they mature into T cells prior to being released into the blood circulation. The thymus gland actually changes size over the life of a human. In fetal development and infancy, it grows very quickly as the T cell maturation process is active, and the gland slowly degenerates as the person matures into adulthood.

Spleen

The spleen is also considered a lymphoid organ and functions to filter RBCs from the circulation, but it also filters antigens to be evaluated by the lymphocytes. The spleen is a very vascular organ. It provides lymphocytes and a source of plasma cells and, therefore, antibodies for cellular and humoral-specific immune responses.

Lymph Vessels/Lymph System

The lymph system is a series of vessels and nodes that serves to collect plasma and leukocytes from the tissues that are not returned to the circulatory system. The combined substances are called *lymph* and play a role to balance fluid levels in the tissues and prevent edema from retained fluids in the tissues. Propulsion of the lymph is done by skeletal muscles. Because lymph does not contain any of the clotting factors, it coagulates slowly. The lymph fluid returns to the circulation via the right subclavian vein and thoracic duct and eventually to the left subclavian vein. On occasion, the lymph nodes swell due either to WBCs or leukocytes responding to an infectious process or to malignant cells that have migrated away from the primary site.

Tonsils and Adenoids

There is a mixed debate about the effectiveness of the role of the tonsils and adenoids in immunity. It is felt that in the first year of life, these glands do provide some protection against infection by trapping bacteria and viruses. Years ago, it was fairly common to have the tonsils and adenoids removed; however, today surgical removal is done only in the case of repeated, frequent infections.

Skin

The skin is one of the largest organs in the body, and it serves as the first line of defense to protect the body against infections. The outermost layer of epidermis serves as a tough protective barrier against environmental hazards. Additionally, the dermis contains mast cells, which are in the connective tissue and function to perform the functions of secretion, phagocytosis, and production of fibroblasts.

FUNCTIONS OF THE IMMUNOLOGICAL SYSTEM

The immunological system is a very sophisticated set of organs and processes that protects the human body against nearly all types of invasive organisms. The capability to resist infection with these organisms is called *immunity*. In this section, we will discuss the two types of immunity: *acquired/adaptive immunity* and *innate immunity*. As stated above, the first line of defense to protect the body against the invasion of infectious microorganisms is the skin. It is a *mechanical barrier*. The second line of defense is *inflammatory*. Inflammatory responses are considered more rapid responses than the immune response.

Innate Immunity

Initial Primary Barriers

Innate immunity is considered to be a set of processes that is directed to respond as a first line of defense and is nonspecific with regard to the organism being targeted. These responses include the anatomic and physiological barriers to infectious agents. As mentioned above, the skin is the first line of defense against microorganisms and is part of the innate immune response. Another simple barrier is the pH of the skin and stomach, which is slightly negative. Some body functions serve as a means of a mechanical defense through flushing or mechanical removal of the organism. Examples of these include the emptying of the bladder, coughing and sneezing to remove respiratory pathogens, or gastrointestinal motility. All of these are examples of the innate immune response. Immune cells that react nonspecifically to foreign particles and organisms such as macrophages, neutrophils, eosinophils, basophils, and natural killer cells are also part of the innate immune system.

Inflammation

When inflammation occurs, the innate immune response brings about a hallmark set of events. This begins with vasodilation of the capillary bed of the site of inflammation. The capillary membrane becomes more permeable, allowing fluid and immune cells to move into the area. Mediators of inflammation called eicosanoids, specifically thromboxane and leukotriene, help to increase the movement of additional inflammatory cells to the area. The physical symptoms include *erythema* (redness at the site), *edema, warmth at the site of inflammation,* and *pain.*

Phagocytosis

The next stage of the response is phagocytosis. Neutrophils and macrophages are phagocytes, as described earlier, and function to ingest and digest antigens such as microorganisms, dead cells, and cellular debris. During this process, the cell is able to recycle useable products and allow evaluation of the protein pieces by T cells.

Along with the above processes, a complement system is initiated. This is a group of proteins that, when activated or triggered by an immune response, transform specific proteins into cytokines. These products stimulate further transformations, which ultimately result in massive cell destruction of the invading organisms.

Acquired (Adaptive) Immune Response

The human body also has the ability to develop a more specific response to individual antigens, which include bacteria, viruses, toxins, and foreign tissue. Acquired immunity is more focused on extracellular organisms or hypersensitive reactions to allergens. Immunizations are a type of acquired immunity and provide a level of protection that is significantly stronger (as much as 100,000 times). There are two types of acquired immunity: humoral immunity and cell-mediated immunity. Both of these types of immunity are initiated by antigens. An antigen is described as a substance that, when introduced into the body, stimulates the production of an antibody.

Development of Antibodies

Antibodies are essentially proteins that sit on the surface of a B lymphocyte that is secreted into the blood at the time of exposure to an antigen. Immunoglobulins on the B cell bind the antigen on the cell surface. Antibodies are normally not present at birth but are transferred passively from the mother to the baby via the placenta or colostrum in breast milk. Antibodies are also introduced into the body by immunizations or following natural infections.

Humoral Immunity

Humoral immunity is named after the term *humours* or body fluids where the immune response is stimulated by substances known as antigens. In response to the antigen, the body stimulates the B cells to produce antibodies that bind with the antigen on the surface of the cell. Prior to stimulation, the clones of the B lymphocytes stay dormant in the lymphatic tissue. Upon presentation of the antigen, macrophages phagocytize the antigen and "present" it to the B lymphocyte and the T lymphocyte. The T cell assists as a helper cell, while the B cells specific for the antigen enlarge and transform eventually into gamma globulin antibodies (immunoglobulins). These immunoglobulins then perform specific functions to protect the body, including agglutination, precipitation, neutralization, and lysis.

Formation of the T Lymphocyte

Refer to the earlier section on formation of leukocytes, including T lymphocytes.

Cell-Mediated Immunity

Cell-mediated immunity is focused primarily on the intracellular microorganisms, viruses, and cancer cells, and it is responsible for delayed hypersensitivity or allergic reactions and tissue rejection. This type of immunity does not involve antibodies or the complement pathway but rather involves cytotoxic T lymphocytes. With repeated exposure to allergens, activated helper and cytotoxic T cells are formed. Within a day of a subsequent exposure, the activated T cells diffuse from the circulating blood into the skin (or other areas such as the lungs) to respond to the toxins from the allergen. This produces a local response where tissue damage can occur.

Cytokines

Cytokines are secreted by cells and are considered vasoactive and biologically active mediators. There are many types of cytokines that have various activities, including proliferation of B and T cells and antiviral and thrombopoietic actions. Some of the most commonly known cytokines include interleukin-1, interleukin-2, tumor necrosis factor alpha (TNF-α), interleukin-6, interleukin-8, and interleukin-10. Interferons are another category of cytokines that play a larger role in viral infections. Most cytokines play a role in the initial inflammatory response and are triggered by the innate immune system. The presence of these cytokines then plays a differential role in the orchestration of other lymphocytes.

Eicosanoids

Eicosanoids are fatty acids that regulate processes within the body. Examples of these substances are prostaglandins, thromboxanes, and leukotrienes. These are short-lived compounds that signal cells in specific areas. For example, thromboxanes have both cardiovascular and hematologic effects. The hematologic effect of this eicosanoid is platelet aggregation. Medications can inhibit eicosanoid production and can, in fact, affect other physiological processes. NSAIDs (nonsteroidal anti-inflammatory drugs) block the enzyme cyclooxygenase, which converts arachidonic acid to prostaglandins and thromboxanes.

CONDITIONS OF THE IMMUNOLOGICAL SYSTEM

Allergic/Hypersensitive Reactions

An allergy is sensitivity to a substance most commonly known as an *allergen*. There are various levels of allergic reaction to these allergens, ranging from a simple, mild sensitivity to a severe, anaphylactic, life-threatening reaction.

In hypersensitive reactions, it is the frequency and degree of exposure that can cause subsequent, more severe reactions over time. At the time of the first exposure to an allergen, abnormally large amounts of IgE antibodies are formed. When the individual has a repeated exposure, IgE triggers the release of histamine, heparin, and other cytokines, which can cause more systemic symptoms such as bronchiole constriction, peripheral vasoconstriction, airway obstruction, pulmonary edema, hypovolemia, shock, and circulatory collapse.

The treatment of these types of reactions includes medications such as epinephrine, diphenhydramine, bronchodilators, and steroids. Hemodynamic support may be required if the reaction causes serious hypotension or compromising arrhythmias such as supraventricular tachycardias.

Anaphylactic Shock

Anaphylactic shock is a type of distributive shock that is the result of a severe hypersensitivity reaction. This is a life-threatening event that requires immediate intervention to prevent complications and poor outcome. The ultimate effect of anaphylactic shock can be altered tissue perfusion and hypoxia and subsequent initiation of the general shock state.

Allergens that are ingested, inhaled, or absorbed through the skin cause an antibody-antigen response, which precipitates the immune response. The first time the individual is exposed to the antigen, the antigen-specific IgE (immunoglobulin) is stored as an attachment to the mast cells and basophils. The more frequently the individual is exposed to the allergen, the more the secondary immune response is initiated, which triggers the release of chemical mediators. On occasion, the individual who is not sensitized can have an anaphylactic response to the allergen.

During these severe reactions, eosinophils phagocytize the antibody-antigen complex and other debris. These antigens release enzymes that inhibit vasoactive mediators—secondary mediators that can increase capillary permeability and favor vasodilation. This initiates the cascade whereby peripheral vasodilation results in decreased venous return, loss of intravascular volume, and hypovolemia. Altered tissue perfusion occurs as a result of the loss of cardiac output, and if left untreated or treated ineffectively, it can result in airway obstruction or cardiovascular collapse.

The treatment for anaphylactic shock is to treat the patient symptomatically and immediately respond with hemodynamic support: securing of the airway, mechanical ventilation, vasopressors, fluids, administration of epinephrine, and removal of the allergen.

Human Immunodeficiency Virus (HIV) and Autoimmune Deficiency Syndrome (AIDS)

The treatment for HIV and AIDS has dramatically changed over the years due to extensive research in an attempt to find a cure for these diseases. Individuals who may have succumbed to these diseases in the past are living many years beyond initial expectations. The first known diagnosed case of AIDS occurred in 1981. AIDS is the disease that is caused by HIV, which progressively destroys the immune system, exposing the individual to infections.

Exposure to HIV occurs through unprotected sexual contact or intravenous needles that are shared by individuals who have HIV. It is considered a blood-borne pathogen disease. The scientific name for the virus is human T lymphocyte virus-3 (HTLV-3). Once HIV has attached to the cell membrane of a CD4 T-lymphocyte, RNA from the virus enters the cell and undergoes enzymatic transformation to DNA, and this DNA is inserted into the genome of the CD4 T-lymphocyte. The CD4 T-lymphocyte then produces virion when it is activated to respond to another infection or inflammatory response. The above description is a gross oversimplification of the replication cycle of HIV, but a more detailed discussion is beyond the scope of the CCRN. Once the immune system has been compromised significantly (as determined by the CD4 count), the patient is susceptible to a number of opportunistic infections, such as fungal, parasitic, and viral infections.

Typically, treatment is at first a combination of drugs targeted toward HIV, as well as empiric antibiotics. The HIV medications typically include those that inhibit the replication of the RNA protein and new drugs that prevent the virus from entering the cell. If patients also have evidence of infection, they are treated appropriately with antibiotics, antifungals, or antivirals as appropriate. At this time there is still no cure for the disease, though patients may have a much longer life span than they would have years ago.

Immunosuppression

Immunosuppression is simply a deficit in the immunological system that prevents an individual from launching a defense against infection. There are physiological conditions that cause immunosuppression, as well as medications that stimulate immunosuppression. Patients are often admitted to the critical care unit due to a condition that has caused immunosuppression as an adverse effect.

During organ transplantation, patients are purposefully immunosuppressed to prevent the likelihood of rejection. Antirejection medications work primarily on B cells and T cells in an attempt to suppress not only the donor allograft but also the individual's own immune system. The challenge with this process is that the patient is then exposed to the potential for opportunistic infections and therefore must be protected, for example with neutropenic precautions.

NURSING CONSIDERATIONS IN PATIENTS WITH HEMATOLOGIC OR IMMUNOLOGICAL CONDITIONS

The critical care nurse plays an important part in the care and management of the patient with these two types of conditions. As mentioned earlier, hematologic and immunological conditions are not often the primary reason a patient presents to the critical care unit; however, they do become conditions that dramatically impact the care of the patient throughout his stay.

History and Physical

During the course of taking the patient's history, it is imperative that the critical care nurse focus her questions to determine if the patient has evidence or symptoms of hematologic or immunological conditions. The following are areas in the history which may be indicative of these conditions:

- Current, past, or recurrent infections, including HIV

- Malignancies

- Liver abnormalities

- Renal abnormalities

- Any problems with prolonged bleeding or clotting disorders, including splenectomy

- Past history of blood or blood component transfusion

- Replacement of heart valves

- Recent surgeries, including dental surgery

A review of systems should also be done with the patient or, if the patient is unable to respond to the questions, including those about the following signs and symptoms, the family.

- Any evidence of fever, chills, weakness, malaise, night sweats, pain, altered mental status

- Conditions of the skin, including petechiae, changes in color, rashes, bruising

- HEENT: Headaches, vision changes, bleeding from nose or gums, problems or pain with swallowing

- Cough, hemoptysis, dypnea, orthopnea

- Feelings of palpitations, dizziness when standing, chest pain

- Nausea, vomiting, passing blood in stool, weight changes, anorexia, or bloating

- Hematuria, menorrhagia, enlarged nodes at any location (groin, axillary, neck)

- Changes in musculoskeletal system, pain, swelling

Along with these observations and questions, a family history, a social history, and a list of current and recent past medications should be taken. A complete head-to-toe physical assessment should be done, including observations that relate to evidence of bleeding or clotting disorders, infectious processes such as skin breakdown, abnormal lung sounds, etc. and any evidence of hemodynamic instability.

Diagnostic Testing

A chart of normal laboratory data relating to these systems is shown in table 8.4. Recognizing that this is not a complete listing of all laboratory tests is important. Additionally, each laboratory has a custom set of normal values (based on the calibration of instrumets used), and therefore these should be verified by the critical care nurse.

Cultures will be done if there is suspicion of an infection so that the site can be determined and treated appropriately. If transfusion of blood products is required, the patient will need to be typed and cross-matched. If the patient has unusual antibodies, more extensive testing will be required to get a safe blood match.

Radiological testing should include chest films if a respiratory infection is suspected. Ultrasound testing is helpful if there needs to be an assessment of the spleen or liver, particularly if there is suspicion of malignancy.

TABLE 8.4 *Normal Lab Values*

Test	Expected Normal Value
WBC	4,000–10,000/mcL
Neutrophils	50–65%
Bands	3–6%
Monocytes	3–7%
Basophils	0–1%
Eosinophils	0–3%
Lymphocytes	25–40%
RBC	Men 4.5–5.5 × 10^6/L
	Women 4.0–5.0 × 10^6/L
Hgb	Men 14–17.4 g/dL
	Women 12–16 g/dL
Hct	Men 42–52%
	Women 36–48%
Platelets	140,000–440,000/mm^3
Bleeding time	3–10 min
INR	0.9–1.2
PT	11–13 sec
PTT	30–45 sec
FSP	Negative at 1:4 dilution
Iron	Men 75–175 mcg/dL
	Women 65–165 mcg/dL
TIBC	240–450 mcg/dL
Fibrinogen	200–400 mg/dL

Another common test for patients with suspected leukemia or lymphoma is bone marrow aspiration and biopsy. Surgical biopsy of lymph nodes may also be required.

Skin tests will be helpful to determine if the patient has sensitivity to allergens or antigens. Skin tests can also be helpful for diagnosing some infections such as tuberculosis and coccidiomycosis.

Appropriate Nursing Diagnoses

Critical care nurses have the ability to identify the highest priority in patient care needs and devise a plan of care that will address the goals and interventions for those priorities. It is helpful also to have a multidisciplinary team that evaluates these priorities on a daily basis and engages in the recovery of the patient.

Key nursing diagnoses for patients with hematologic and immunological conditions include the following:

- Risk for infection related to disease or treatment (e.g., neutropenia)

- Risk for hemorrhage related to disease or treatment (e.g., thrombocytopenia)

- Altered gas exchange related to anemia, abnormal loss of RBCs

- Alterations in hemodynamic stability relating to shock states (e.g., septic shock, anaphylactic shock, hemorrhagic shock)

- Coping difficulties related to new diagnosis of malignancy or abnormality in blood components

With the information the critical care nurse has gained via the physical assessment and the above nursing diagnoses, specific interventions can be determined and put into place. Many times due to the nature of the conditions, these are emergent interventions that should be implemented immediately to prevent complications. Most often with conscientious and meticulous care, these patients can recover with good outcomes.

Review Questions

Questions 1–3 pertain to the following scenario:

Shortly after a blood transfusion is initiated, the patient begins complaining of shortness of breath and chest pain. Vital signs are blood pressure 100/56, pulse rate 110, respirations 22, and temperature 101.8 °F. Later, the patient developed hemoglobinuria and tea-colored urine.

1. What should be the nurse's next immediate action?

   A. Administer sublingual nitroglycerin.

   B. Notify the attending physician.

   C. Stop the transfusion immediately.

   D. Continue to monitor the patient's vitals and provide supportive care.

2. What type of blood reaction is described in the above scenario?

   A. hemolytic reaction

   B. anaphylactic reaction

   C. febrile reaction

   D. circulatory overload

3. This reaction was most likely caused by

   A. an allergic reaction to the plasma proteins in the transfused blood.

   B. reaction of the patient's antibodies with the donor's leukocytes.

   C. an incompatible blood type having been given to the patient.

   D. the transfusion having been administered too quickly.

4. A 32-year-old female presents with the unusual urge to eat inedible objects, such as dirt and plaster. Which of these is the most likely cause of this behavior?

   A. disseminated intravascular coagulopathy (DIC)

   B. thrombocytopenia

   C. iron deficiency anemia

   D. sickle cell disease

5. Which of these findings in a client diagnosed with disseminated intravascular coagulation (DIC) will require immediate attention?

   A. The patient is difficult to arouse.

   B. The urine has a dark tea color.

   C. The temperature is 102.2 °F.

   D. The patient wants to get out of bed.

6. To assess the extent of fibrinolytic activity in a client with disseminated intravascular coagulation (DIC), which of these lab values will the nurse closely monitor?

   A. hemoglobin and hematocrit

   B. platelets

   C. prothrombin time and INR

   D. fibrin degradation products

7. Which of these statements about an individual with type AB blood is **incorrect**?

   A. The blood possesses both A and B antigens.

   B. The blood possesses both A and B antibodies.

   C. The individual can donate to type AB only.

   D. The individual can receive blood from all blood types.

8. Patients with clotting factor deficiencies such as hemophilia will benefit from the transfusion of which blood component?

   A. packed red blood cells (PRBC)

   B. whole blood

   C. fresh frozen plasma (FFP)

   D. platelets

9. Shortly after administration of an IV antibiotic, your patient begins complaining of shortness of breath with expiratory wheezes, hives, and hypotension. Which of these life-saving interventions should be performed immediately?

   A. oxygen via non-rebreather mask

   B. epinephrine subcutaneously

   C. crystalloid fluid bolus

   D. removal of the allergen

10. Which cells release histamine, stimulating an inflammatory response?

    A. mast cells

    B. T cells

    C. B cells

    D. monocytes

Review Answers and Explanations

1. C

Patients who develop a new onset of fever, chills, shortness of breath, chest pain, restlessness, joint pain, back pain, abdominal pain, nausea/vomiting, tachycardia, tachypnea, urticaria, or hypotension during a blood transfusion are at high risk for having a transfusion reaction. The nurse should immediately stop the transfusion and notify the physician.

2. A

Hemolytic blood reactions typically occur within the first 10 minutes after starting the blood but can occur at any time during the transfusion. These reactions can be associated with fever, chills, nausea, chest tightness, restlessness, apprehension, joint pain, back pain, tachycardia, tachypnea, and hypotension.

3. B

Hemolytic reaction usually occurs as a result of the antibodies in the patient's plasma attacking the antigens on the donor's leukocytes, specifically the erythrocytes. This causes hemolysis of the red blood cells. The most common reason for this is an incompatibility issue. Hemoglobinuria and tea-colored urine indicates hemolysis of RBCs.

4. C

Patients with iron deficiency anemia can experience a craving to eat unusual nonfood substances, which can include ice, dirt, or clay, along with other items. This often will disappear rapidly with iron replacement even before there is a rise in hemoglobin.

5. A

Change in mental status signals a potential cerebral hypoxia or intracranial bleeding. This requires prompt evaluation. (B) A dark tea-colored urine is most likely due to concentrated urine and/or hematuria. Although it is a cause for a concern, the client's lethargy requires more immediate attention. (C) A temperature of 102.2 °F is a cause for concern; however, the priority is evaluating the neurological changes. (D) A client's expressed interest to get out of bed does not require an emergency response.

6. D

Fibrin degradation products are a byproduct of fibrinolytic activity (breakdown of clots). FDP reflects primary fibrinolysis. (A) Hemoglobin and hematocrit are indicators of blood loss, not fibrinolytic activity. (B) Platelets are monitored to assess thrombocytopenia and ability to clot, not fibrinolytic activity. (C) In DIC, prothrombin time and INR are monitored to track ability to clot, not fibrinolytic activity.

7. B

Patients with AB blood have A and B antigens on the surface of the cells, not antibodies.

8. C

Fresh frozen plasma contains many of the clotting factors that are deficient in many of the clotting deficiencies. FFP is efficacious for treatment of deficiencies of factors II, V, VII, IX, X, and XI when specific factors are not available or are inappropriate.

9. B

A patient with systemic manifestations of an anaphylactic reaction should receive epinephrine as part of the treatment. Epinephrine is the drug of choice for life-threatening reactions.

10. A

Mast cells release histamine when an allergen is encountered and cause an inflammatory response in the area.

The Neurologic System

9

Approximately 12 percent of the questions on the CCRN exam cover the neurologic system.

The nervous system is a complex network of cells, tissues, and specialized organs. It is the center of thinking, judgment, memory, cognition, communication, behavior, emotion, sensation, and movement. It exerts both direct and indirect control of the body systems. For example, a traumatic brain injury affecting the motor strip of the temporal lobe may result in seizures and/or loss of limb movement.

ANATOMY REVIEW

The entire nervous system is made up of two types of cells: **neurons**, which transmit or conduct nerve impulses, and **neuroglial cells**, which support the neurons. Each neuron consists of a **cell body**, an **axon**, and **dendrites** (see figure 9.1). Myelinated axons are called **white matter**. Nonmyelinated axons are called **gray matter**. The myelin sheath is interrupted at intervals by the **nodes of Ranvier**. The nodes of Ranvier allow movement of ions across the cellular membrane.

FIGURE 9.1 *Neuron*

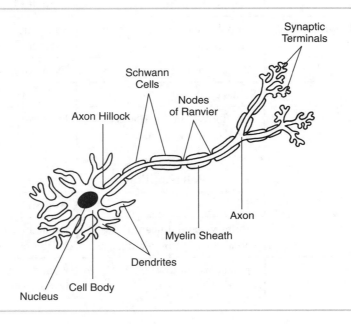

Neurotransmitters

In the central nervous system, **neurotransmitters** are chemical substances that inhibit, excite, or modify the responses of another cell. In general, each neuron releases the same transmitter at all of its terminals. Table 9.1 lists the neurotransmitters.

TABLE 9.1 *Neurotransmitters: Site and Action*

Amines		
Classes	**Site**	**Action**
Acetylcholine	Brain, brain stem, basal ganglia, and autonomic nervous system	Usually excitatory; some inhibitory effects of parasympathetic nervous system (e.g., heart by vagus)
Serotonin	Medial brain stem, hypothalamus, dorsal horn of spinal cord	Inhibits spinal pain pathway; helps control mood and sleep

Catecholamines		
Classes	**Site**	**Action**
Dopamine	Substantia nigra to basal ganglia	Usually inhibitory
Norepinephrine	Brain stem, hypothalamus	Usually excitatory, sometimes inhibitory
Amino acids	Sympathetic nervous system	Sometimes excitatory, sometimes inhibitory
Aspartate	Brain, spinal cord	Excitatory
Gamma-amino-butyric acid (GABA)	Brain, basal ganglia, cerebellum, spinal cord	Sometimes excitatory, sometimes inhibitory
Glutamic acid	Sensory pathways	Excitatory
Glycine	Spinal cord	Inhibitory
Substance P	Pain fibers of dorsal horns of spinal cord, hypothalamus	Excitatory

Polypeptides		
Classes	**Site**	**Action**
Endorphins	Pituitary gland, thalamus, spinal cord, hypothalamus	Excitatory to systems that inhibit pain
Enkephalins	Spinal cord, brain stem	Excitatory to systems that inhibit pain

Neuroglial Cells

The second types of cells in the nervous system are **neuroglia (glia)**. They support the neurons by providing protection, structural support, and nutrition. In the central nervous system, there are four types of neuroglia: **astrocytes**, **ependymal cells**, **oligodendroglia**, and **microglia**. The neuroglia are very important for their support of the neurons but also for their capability of division and replication throughout adulthood. This ability makes glial cells susceptible to abnormal cell division (cancer).

The central nervous system (CNS) has two major divisions: the **brain** and **spinal cord**. The brain is composed of the cerebrum, the brain stem, and the cerebellum. The spinal cord is the conduit for the ascending sensory and descending motor neurons. This is the pathway for two-way communication between the brain and the periphery.

Bones

The bones of the skull and the vertebral column prevent injury to the brain and the spinal cord. The skull is the bony, rigid framework of the head. It is composed of the 14 bones of the face and the 8 bones of the cranium. The four major suture lines are **sagittal**, **coronal**, **lambdoidal**, and **basilar**.

Meninges

The brain and spinal cord are covered with a series of membranes called the **meninges**. These include the **dura mater**, the **arachnoid**, and the **pia mater**.

Brain

The **cerebrum** is the largest part of the brain. Each hemisphere has an outer layer of neurons called the white matter and an inner layer of gray matter. These two hemispheres are connected by a thick band of white fibers called the **corpus callosum**. The corpus callosum allows the two hemispheres to communicate. Each hemisphere receives sensory and motor impulses from the opposite side of the body. The majority of people are left-brain dominant. The left side controls language, while the right side controls perception.

Ventricles

There are **four ventricles** (or chambers) within the brain. The chambers are filled with cerebrospinal fluid and are linked by ducts (also called foramen) that permit circulation. **Cerebrospinal fluid** (CSF) is a clear, colorless fluid produced by the **choroid plexus**, located in the ventricles. Reabsorption occurs via the **arachnoid villi**.

FIGURE 9.2 *Cross Section of Spinal Cord and Components of a Spinal Nerve*

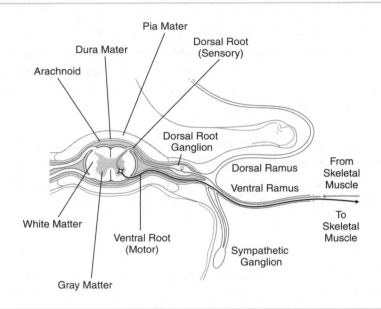

FIGURE 9.3 *Brain*

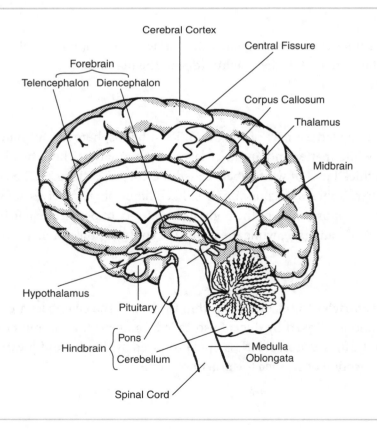

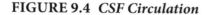

FIGURE 9.4 *CSF Circulation*

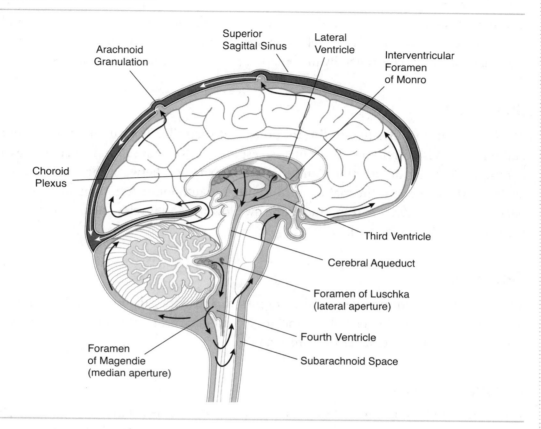

Basal Ganglia

The **basal ganglia** are found deep within the cerebral hemispheres. They consist of several collections of nuclei: the **lenticular nucleus**, the **caudate nucleus**, the **amygdaloid body**, and the **claustrum**. The basal ganglia coordinate communication between the cerebral cortex and the cerebellum that controls motor activity. Lesions of the basal ganglia produce abnormal movements, including chorea, althetosis, hemiballismus, and dystonic posturing.

Lobes

The lobes of the cerebral hemispheres are **frontal**, **parietal**, **temporal**, and **occipital**.

Diencephalon

The diencephalon is composed of the **thalamus**, **epithalamus**, and **hypothalamus**. The thalamus is the initial processing area for sensory input. The epithalamus forms the roof of the third ventricle and the pineal gland. The hypothalamus regulates temperature, appetite, water metabolism, emotional expression, thirst, and a portion of the sleep-wake cycle.

Hypophysis

The **hypophysis** (pituitary gland) is connected to the hypothalamus by the hypophyseal stalk. There are two lobes, each releasing specific hormones into the systemic circulation (see chapter 7). It is controlled by information processed in the hypothalamus.

Brain Stem

The brain stem includes the **midbrain**, **pons**, and **medulla**. The midbrain is the center for auditory and visual reflexes. The pons is responsible for arousal and sleep and assists in controlling autonomic functions, and it relays information between the cerebrum and cerebellum. The medulla is the main control center for autonomic functions such as control of heart rate, blood pressure, respiration, and swallowing, and it relays neural signals between the brain and the spinal cord.

Cerebellum

The **cerebellum** is located behind the brain stem and under the occipital lobe of the cerebrum. Functions of the cerebellum include coordination of voluntary muscle movement, equilibrium, and maintenance of trunk stability.

Cerebral Circulation

The source of blood to the brain occurs via the **internal carotid arteries** (anterior circulation) and the **vertebral and basilar arteries** (posterior circulation). These arteries join at the base of the brain to form the **circle of Willis** (cerebral arterial circle). The two anterior cerebral arteries (ACA) supply the medial portion of the frontal lobes. Two middle cerebral arteries (MCA) supply the outer portions of the frontal, parietal, and superior temporal lobes. The two posterior inferior cerebral arteries (PICA) supply the medial portions of the occipital and inferior temporal lobes.

Venous blood drains from the brain via the dural sinuses, which drain into the two jugular veins. Knowledge of the major arteries of the brain and the areas supplied is necessary for understanding and evaluating the signs and symptoms of brain tumors, cerebral vascular disease, and trauma.

Blood-brain Barrier

The **blood-brain barrier** maintains a functionally stable environment for the central nervous system. It does this by selectively allowing a restricted number of molecules and cells across the barrier. For example, white blood cells (WBCs) generally do not have access to the brain, making the brain an immunoprivileged site. While protecting the brain, this feature impairs the effectiveness of many drugs used to treat nervous system problems.

Spine

The **spine** is a flexible column formed by series of bones called **vertebrae**. There are 33 vertebrae: 7 **cervical**, 12 **thoracic**, 5 **lumbar**, 5 **sacral** (fused into one), and 4 **coccygeal** (fused into one). The vertebrae serve multiple functions: protection of the **spinal cord**, support of the head, and assistance with spinal flexibility. Also part of the spinal column, **discs** function as shock absorbers between vertebrae and act like ligaments, allowing flexibility.

Spinal Cord

The **spinal cord** extends from the medulla to the level of the first lumbar vertebrae. It exits the cranial cavity through the **foramen magnum**. A cross section of the spinal cord reveals **gray matter** in an **H** pattern in the central portion. It is surrounded by **white matter**. The **ascending tracts** carry specific sensory information to the higher levels of the CNS. The information comes from specialized sensory receptors in the skin, muscles, joints, viscera, and blood vessels. **Descending tracts** carry impulses from the higher levels to the lower motor neurons. The **lower motor neurons** are the final step of the nerve impulse before stimulation of skeletal muscle. **Upper motor neurons** are located in the brain stem and cerebral cores and also influence skeletal muscle movement. Damage to the upper motor neurons, sometimes seen in multiple sclerosis, may cause weakness, atrophy, hyperreflexia, or spasticity. Circulation to the spinal cord comes from three sources: **anterior spinal**, two **posterior spinal**, and branches of the descending aorta.

Peripheral Nervous System

The **peripheral nervous system** (PNS) is composed of the spinal nerves, cranial nerves, and the autonomic nervous system. The **spinal nerves** consist of 31 pairs exiting from the spinal cord. They include 8 cervical, 12 thoracic, 5 lumbar, 5 sacral, and 1 coccygeal. Each spinal nerve has both a sensory and a motor component for a specific area of the body or dermatome. The spinal nerves are composed of a dorsal root and ventral root as they enter and exit the spinal column. The dorsal root is responsible for carrying sensory information into the spinal cord, while the ventral root is composed of motor neurons carrying signals from the upper motor neurons to the muscles.

Sensory Receptors

Sensory input is collected throughout the body by receptors of pain, temperature, touch, vibration, pressure, visceral sensation, and proprioception. This information is transmitted to the cortex along with input from the special senses: vision, taste, smell, and hearing.

FIGURE 9.5 *Cranial Nerves and Brain Stem*

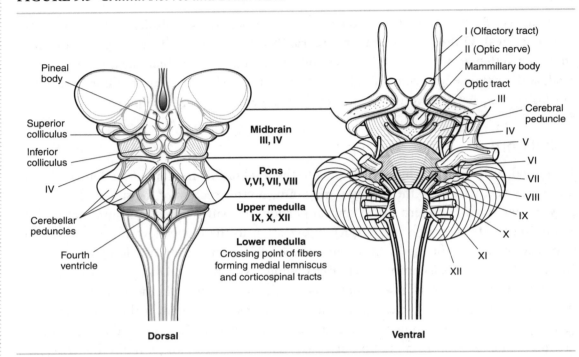

Cranial Nerves

The **cranial nerves** provide both motor and sensory innervation for the head, neck, and viscera. There are 12 cranial nerves. Anatomically they begin in and emerge from the cranium. See figure 9.5 and tables 9.2 and 9.4 for more detail.

Autonomic Nervous System

The **autonomic nervous system** (ANS) has two components: **sympathetic** and **parasympathetic** (see table 9.3). The two systems function together to maintain homeostasis of the body's internal environment. The sympathetic nervous system is responsible for the flight-fight response, such as increased heart rate, dilation of the pupils, constriction of the visceral vasculature and dilation of the vasculature, increase in the blood supply to the skeletal muscles, and decreased intestinal motility. The sympathetic and parasympathetic nervous systems act in opposition to each other.

Reflexes

A **reflex** is a response to a stimulus that occurs without conscious control. One way to classify reflexes is as stretch, cutaneous, and pathologic. Muscle stretch reflexes are also called **deep tendon reflexes** (DTRs). Cutaneous reflexes are termed **superficial reflexes**. Superficial reflexes occur when noxious stimulation is applied to the skin. The response is withdrawal from the irritant. An example is contraction of the abdominal muscles when the skin is

TABLE 9.2 *Cranial Nerve Function*

Nerve	Function
I. Olfactory	*Sensory:* Smell
II. Optic	*Sensory:* Sight
III. Oculomotor	*Motor:* Eye movements; contraction of iris
	Parasympathetic: Smooth muscles of eye socket
IV. Trochlear	*Motor:* Eye movement
V. Trigeminal (3 branches)	
Ophthalmic	*Sensory:* Forehead, eye, and superior nasal cavity
Maxillary	*Sensory:* Inferior nasal cavity, face, upper teeth, and superior mucosa of mouth
Mandibular	*Sensory:* Jaw surfaces, lower teeth, anterior tongue, and inferior mucosa of mouth
	Motor: Muscles for chewing
VI. Abducens	*Sensory:* Eye movement
VII. Facial	*Motor:* Muscles of expression, cheek muscle
	Sensory: Taste of anterior two-thirds of tongue
VIII. Vestibulocochlear (2 components)	
Vestibular	*Sensory:* Balance
Cochlear	*Sensory:* Hearing
IX. Glossopharyngeal	*Sensory:* Pharynx and posterior tongue (including taste)
	Motor: Superior pharyngeal muscles, swallowing
X. Vagus	*Sensory:* Viscera of chest and abdomen
	Motor: Larynx, middle and inferior pharyngeal muscles
	Parasympathetic: Heart, lungs, most of GI tract
XI. Accessory	*Motor:* Movement of neck muscles
XII. Hypoglossal	*Motor:* Movement of tongue

stroked. **Primitive or pathologic reflexes** are normal in infants and toddlers but should not be present in healthy adults. Presence of a pathologic reflex in an adult indicates interference with the normal CNS function. The upward movement of the great toe with flaring of the pedal digits (Babinski's reflex) is an example of a pathologic reflex, indicative of upper motor neuron disease. Sensory information from the specific peripheral location is responsible for the motor impulses that return to the same peripheral location. This is called a reflex arc.

TABLE 9.3 *Sympathetic versus Parasympathetic Response*

System	Sympathetic Response	Parasympathetic Response
Neurological	Pupils dilated Heightened awareness	Pupils normal size
Cardiovascular	Increased heart rate Increased myocardial contractility Increased blood pressure	Decreased heart rate Decreased myocardial contractility
Respiratory	Increased respiratory rate Increased respiratory depth Bronchial dilation	Bronchial constriction
Gastrointestinal	Decreased gastric motility Decreased gastric secretions Increased glycogenolysis Decreased insulin production Sphincter contraction	Increased gastric motility Increased gastric secretions Sphincter dilation
Genitourinary	Decreased urine output Decreased renal blood flow	Normal urine output

Age-Related Changes

As the human body ages, patients begin to experience both motor and sensory changes. Chronic diseases of the bones, muscles, or joints can have a detrimental effect on the nerves' motor function. With aging there is a decrease in both muscle bulk and nerve electrical activity. This causes diminished muscle strength and a decrease in reaction and movement time. Sensory function is diminished due to a decrease in total sensory receptors, decrease in electrical activity, and atrophy or degeneration of the taste buds, olfactory bulb, and vestibular system of the inner ear. Reflexes may diminish due to degeneration of the myelin sheath. Cognitive function continues at the same level as in younger years, unless disease impairs the brain. For example, arteriosclerosis and hypertension may lead to a cerebrovascular accident (CVA) that causes brain damage.

PHYSICAL ASSESSMENT

Assessment of the neurologic system begins with the history. The health history interview collects subjective data. The second portion is the physical examination of the neurologic system, which collects objective data. A complete neurological health history assists the nurse to identify strengths and weaknesses and determine the extent of any problems involving the nervous system. If the patient is alert, able to state his name, where he is, and what day it is, proceed with the health history. When the patient is comatose or too lethargic to cooperate, the nurse must access secondary sources, such as family or significant others.

Mental Assessment

When assessing patients with altered levels of consciousness, use the Glasgow Coma Scale (GCS). The Glasgow Coma Scale is the most widely recognized, standardized level of consciousness (LOC) assessment tool. The score is based on three categories: eye opening, verbal response, and best motor response. The best possible score is 15 and the lowest score is 3, but a score of 8 or less generally indicates a significant alteration in level of consciousness. Mental assessment should always be conducted off any sedation or with a sedation break.

TABLE 9.4 *Glasgow Coma Scale (GCS)*

Eye(s) Opening	
Spontaneous	4
To speech	3
To pain	2
No response	1
Verbal Response	
Oriented to time, place, person	5
Confused/disoriented	4
Inappropriate words	3
Incomprehensible sounds	2
No response	1
Best Motor Response	
Obeys commands	6
Moves to localized pain	5
Flexion withdraws from pain	4
Abnormal flexion	3
Abnormal extension	2
No response	1
Best response	*15*
Comatose patient	*8 or less*
Totally unresponsive	*3*

TABLE 9.5 *Cranial Nerve Assessment*

Nerve	Function	Assessment
I. Olfactory	Smell	Identify common, nonirritating substances. Not usually done; unreliable in infant/child.
II. Optic	Vision	Use Snellen or Rosenbaum Pocket Vision Screener. Randomly read from a newspaper or magazine. Assess visual fields using confrontation test.
III. Oculomotor	Tested together	Eyelid elevation and extraocular movement
IV. Trochlear	Control eye	Pupil constriction and extraocular movement
V. Trigeminal nerve	Ophthalmic	Corneal reflexes with puff of air/cotton wisp
	Maxillary	Clench jaw
	Mandibular	Pin prick
VI. Abducens	Muscles	Movement through six cardinal directions
VII. Facial nerve	Taste	Usually deferred
	Facial movement	Raise eyebrows, close eyelids, puff out cheeks, smile, and frown.
VIII. Acoustic nerve	Cochlear (hearing)	Have patient listen to sounds.
	Vestibular (balance)	Walk heel to toe; walk on tip-toes; walk on heels.
IX. Glossopharyngeal	Swallowing	Have patient swallow water.
X. Vagus	Gag reflex	Touch back of throat with tongue blade.
XI. Spinal accessory	Neck muscles	Have patient shrug shoulders and turn head against resistance.
XII. Hypoglossal	Tongue muscles	Have patient open mouth, stick out tongue, and wiggle it side to side.

Motor Assessment

The nerves of the motor system originate from the spinal cord and control muscle movement. The motor examination begins with the neck and proceeds from proximal (upper) to distal (lower) extremities. Major muscle groups are assessed for specific functions (see table 9.6).

TABLE 9.6 *Major Muscle Groups of the Upper and Lower Extremities*

Level	Muscle	Action
C5, C6, C7	Serratus anterior	Movement of shoulder
C5, C6	Deltoid; supraspinatus	Abduction of shoulder
C5, C6	Biceps brachii	Flexion of elbow
C5, C6	Brachioradialis	Flexion of elbow
C7, C8	Triceps brachii	Extension of elbow
C6, C7	Extensor carpi radialis; extensor carpi ulnaris	Extension of wrist
C7, C8	Flexor carpi radialis; flexor carpi ulnaris	Flexion of wrist
C7	Extensor digitorum; extensor indicis proprius; extensor digiti minimi	Extension of fingers
C8, T1	Flexor digitorum superficialis, profundus, and lumbricalis	Flexion of fingers
T1	Dorsal interossei; abductor digiti quinti	Abduction of fingers
C8, T1	Palmar interossei	Adduction of fingers
C8, T1	Opponens pollicis	Opposition of thumb
T12, L1, L2, L3	Iliopsoas	Hip flexion
L2, L3, L4	Adductor brevis, longus, and magnus	Hip adduction
L4, L5, S1	Gluteus medius	Hip abduction
L5, S1, S2	Gluteus maximus	Hip extension
L2, L3, L4	Quadriceps	Knee extension
L5, S1, S2	Hamstrings	Knee flexion
L4, L5	Tibialis anterior; peroneus tertius; extensor digitorum longus; extensor hallucis longus	Ankle dorsiflexion
S1, S2	Gastrocnemius; soleus	Ankle plantar flexion
L4, L5	Tibialis posterior	Foot inversion
L4, S1	Peroneus longus; peroneus brevis	Foot eversion

Sensory Assessment

Evaluation of the sensory system tests the patient's ability to perceive various types of sensations. The *body areas usually assessed* are face, neck, deltoid regions, forearms, hands (top), chest, abdomen, thighs, lower legs, and feet (top). Superficial sensation is tested using various modalities: light touch, pin prick, pain, and temperature.

Deep sensation evaluates vibration, deep pressure pain, position, and discriminate fine touch.

Normally, the patient should be able to sense vibration over the bony prominences.

Instruct the patient to close his eyes when testing position sense (**proprioception**). Lightly grasp the patient's finger or great toe and gently move it up or down. Instruct the patient to indicate verbally which direction the digit is in. Vary the direction to prevent the patient from anticipating the digit location.

When testing for **stereognosis**, ask the patient to close his eyes and place an object (coin, paper clip, key) into the patient's hand. Instruct the patient to feel the object. Ask the patient to name the object.

To test **graphesthesia**, ask the patient to close his eyes; then draw a letter, number, or shape in the patient's open hand.

Reflex Assessment

Evaluation of reflexes provides important information on the status of the central nervous system in both conscious and unconscious patients. Altered reflexes may be the earliest signs of a pathological condition. There are three categories of reflexes: deep tendon, cutaneous, and pathologic. **Deep tendon reflexes** (muscle-stretch reflexes) occur in response to a sudden stimulus (e.g., tapping with a reflex hammer). It is important to use the correct technique to elicit the specific reflex. With the muscle relaxed and the joint in neutral position and supported by the examiner, the tendon is tapped directly with the reflex hammer. Normally the muscle contracts with a quick movement of the limb or structure. Cutaneous reflexes occur in response to cutaneous sensation, such as the cremasteric reflex, where brushing on the inner upper thigh results in contraction of the cremaster muscle.

Pathological reflexes are also called primitive reflexes because they are normally seen in infants and then disappear (see table 9.7). If these reflexes reappear, they are found in patients suffering from dementia syndromes or Parkinson's disease. Grading of pathological reflexes is documented as presence (+) is abnormal and absence (−) is normal. Examples of primitive reflexes are the Moro (startle response), stepping, rooting, sucking, tonic neck flex, plantar, palmar grasp, upgoing Babinski, and Galant reflexes.

TABLE 9.7 *Pathological (Primitive) Reflexes*

Reflex	Technique
Grasp	Stimulation of palm results in a grasp.
Snout	Stimulation of circumoral region results in puckering of lips.
Sucking	Stimulation of lips, tongue, or palate results in sucking movement.
Rooting	Stimulation of lips results in head moving toward stimulus.
Palmomental	Stimulation of palm results in contraction of the chin muscles.
Glabellar	Eyes blink each time the glabellar area (between eyes) is tapped. Normal: Blinking stops after first few taps.

TABLE 9.8 *Neurodiagnostic Studies*

Study	Purpose	Nursing Care
Lumbar puncture	Obtain CSF for analysis. Measure CSF opening pressure.	Have patient empty bladder. Position in lateral decubitis position, with back arched, knees flexed on chest, chin touching knees. Keep flat in bed for 6 to 8 hours to prevent headache. Monitor neurological status and vital signs. Encourage fluids and administer IV fluids; give analgesics PRN. Complications: headache; abscess; low back pain; meningitis; CSF leak; spinal cord puncture
Skull x-rays	Identify skull/facial fractures, tumor, cranial anomalies, bone erosion, air/fluid levels in sinuses, calcification, foreign bodies.	Linear/basal fractures often missed by routine x-rays
Spine x-rays	Identify vertebral dislocation or fracture; degenerative disease; bone erosion; tumor; calcification; structural defects; injury.	Prevent fracture displacement by maintaining spinal precautions.
Computed axial tomography (CT)	Identify acute vs. chronic bleeding; hydrocephalus; abscess; tumors.	Sedation may be given. If contrast given, check for allergies and renal function. Encourage fluids post-test.

TABLE 9.8 *Neurodiagnostic Studies (continued)*

Study	Purpose	Nursing Care
Magnetic resonance imaging (MRI)	Identify strokes, tumors, trauma, seizures, edema, and herniation. Gadolinium (non-iodine contrast media) may be used.	Contraindicated in patients with iron-based (ferrous) implanted objects (artificial joints, pacemakers, bullets or metal fragments, clips/wires). Sedation may be required. Patient must lie still during test.
Magnetic resonance angiography (MRA)	Visualizes blood flow in extracranial and intracranial blood vessels. Identifies vascular lesions (stenosis, aneurysms, arteriovenous malformations).	Similar to MRI. Assess bony prominences for pressure areas.
Magnetic resonance spectroscopy (MRS)	Differentiate tumor vs. abscess or infection vs. autoimmune destruction.	Similar to MRI.
Functional magnetic resonance imaging (fMRI)	Conduct functional mapping of the brain using chemical changes in response to specific tasks.	Similar to MRI.
Cerebral angiography (angiogram)	Visualize cerebral vasculature. Identify aneurysms, AVM, vasospasm, tumors.	Sedation may be given. Check for allergies and renal function. Post-test: Maintain bed rest 6–12 hours. Maintain hydration. Monitor vital signs; assess puncture site for hematoma or bleeding; conduct frequent neuro checks; check pedal pulses, color, sensation, and temperature of affected extremity. Complications: Anaphylaxis; seizures; stroke; thrombosis; PE; shock; aphasia; vision changes.
Digital subtraction angiography (DSA)	Same as angiogram.	May be done arterially or via IV. If done arterially, nursing care is the same as for angiogram. When done via IV, there are fewer complications since it is less invasive.
Positron emission tomography (PET)	Provides 3-D structure and functional view of the brain. Evaluates oxygen and glucose metabolism. Measures cerebral blood flow.	Sedation may be given. Check for allergies and renal function. Maintain hydration. Monitor vital signs; conduct frequent neuro checks.

TABLE 9.8 *Neurodiagnostic Studies (continued)*

Study	Purpose	Nursing Care
Single-photon emission CT (SPECT)	Same as for PET scan. Uses contrast that emits gamma rays.	Same as for PET scan.
Myelogram	Visualizes spinal subarachnoid space. Detects spinal cord lesions (obstructions, compression, herniated intervertebral discs).	If done with oil-based contrast, maintain bed rest for 4–8 hours. With water-soluble contrast, elevate head of bed. Maintain hydration. Complications: Anaphylaxis, headache, nausea, vomiting, backache, neck ache, chest pain, seizures, dysrhythmias.
Electroencephalography (EEG)	Identifies areas of abnormal electrical discharge in the brain or encephalopathy.	Withhold caffeine, tobacco, alcohol, anticonvulsants, stimulants, tranquilizers, and antidepressants 24–48 hours prior to test. Shampoo hair before and after test.
Magnetoencephalography (MEG)	Similar to EEG with addition of biomagnetometer, which detects magnetic fields generated by neural activity. Identifies location of seizure, stroke, or injury.	Similar to EEG.
Electromyography (EMG)	Nerve conduction studies. Identifies muscle disease, peripheral, neuropathies, nerve compression, nerve regeneration, muscle recovery.	May be uncomfortable. Contraindicated in patients taking anticoagulants, with bleeding disorders, or with skin infections.
Evoked potentials (EPs)	Evaluate electrical responses of brain to external stimuli. Identify spinal cord injury, tumors, neuromuscular or cerebrovascular disease, traumatic brain injury, peripheral nerve disease.	Similar to EEG.

TABLE 9.9 *Cerebrospinal Fluid Analysis*

Parameter	Normal Value	Analysis
Opening pressure	60–200 mm H_2O	<60—dehydration; blocked CSF >200—brain tumor, abscess, or cyst; subdural hematoma; hydrocephalus; cerebral edema
Appearance	Clear, colorless	*Xanthochromia* is often due to the breakdown of blood products. *Turbidity or cloudiness* is often due to increased WBCs, elevated protein levels, or infection.
RBCs (red blood cells)	None	Cell count of RBCs indicates bleeding; serial reductions in tubes sent from LP may indicate a traumatic tap.
WBCs (white blood cells)	0–8/L	Elevations may indicate meningitis, tumors, or multiple sclerosis.
Protein	15–45 mg/dL	Elevations with infection, tumor, hemorrhage, tumors, and multiple sclerosis.
Glucose	45–75 mg/dL	Elevations are not significant; decrease indicates infection.
Microorganisms	None	
pH	7.35	
Specific gravity	1.007	

TABLE 9.10 *Types of Evoked Potentials*

Type	Stimulus	Purpose
Visual Visual evoked potential (VEP) Pattern reversal electrical potential (PREP) Visual electrical response (VER)	Rapidly changing geometric designs or flashing lights	Locate lesion in visual pathway or visual cortex.
Auditory Auditory evoked potential (AEP) Auditory brain stem evoked potential (ABEP)	Multiple clicks to each ear via earphones	Locate lesion; evaluate the central auditory pathways of the brain stem; follow the course of recovery.

TABLE 9.10 *Types of Evoked Potentials (continued)*

Type	Stimulus	Purpose
Somatosensory Somatosensory brain stem evoked potential (SBEP) Somatosensory evoked potential (SEP)	Electrical stimulation of selected peripheral nerves	Differentiate lesions of the peripheral nerve from those of subcortical or cortical central sensory pathways.
Carotid Doppler scan	Detects atherosclerotic carotid artery disease.	No specific follow-up care is required.
Transcranial Doppler (TCD)	Measures blood flow velocity of the cerebral arteries; identifies vasospasm, emboli, vascular stenosis, and brain death.	When vasospasm is identified, patient may require treatment via angiography.

PATHOLOGIES

Vascular Hemorrhage (Bleeding)

Subarachnoid hemorrhage (SAH) is bleeding into the subarachnoid space. There are multiple causes of SAH, including cerebral aneurysms, arteriovenous malformations, traumatic injury to an artery, hypertensive intracranial bleeding, and hemorrhage from a brain tumor. A cerebral aneurysm is a dilation of the artery due to weakness of the middle and inner layers of the vessel wall. Most cerebral aneurysms occur at bifurcations of the large arteries at the base of the brain (circle of Willis; see figure 9.6). Aneurysms are classified as saccular or berry (ballooning of the wall with a stemlike attachment to the vessel), fusiform (usually a large atherosclerotic bulge), dissecting (bleeding into the inner layers of the arterial wall), or mycotic (infected lesion of the vessel wall).

SAH from aneurysm rupture affects approximately 30,000 Americans each year. The incidence of SAH is greater in women and increases with age. Mortality from ruptured aneurysms is 25 percent, with the majority of these patients dying within 24 hours of the initial bleeding. Significant morbidity is seen in approximately 50 percent of SAH survivors.

Presenting signs and symptoms of SAH include severe headache, brief loss or altered level of consciousness, nausea, vomiting, photophobia, focal neurologic deficits, and a stiff neck. The headache is often referred to as a "thunder clap" headache or the "worst headache of my life" by patients. Kernig's (reflex contraction and pain in the hamstring muscles when attempting to extend the leg after flexion) or Brudzinski's (flexion of the hips when the neck is flexed from a supine position) sign is sometimes present. These signs are seen in patients with meningeal irritation. SAHs are graded using several scales (Botterell, Hunt/Hess, or World Federation of Neurologic Surgeons).

FIGURE 9.6 *Circle of Willis*

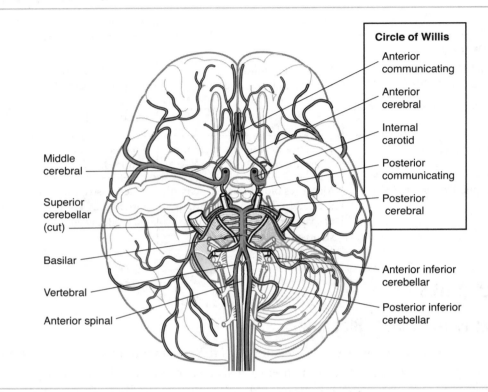

Hunt/Hess Classification of SAH

Grade I: Asymptomatic or minimal headache and slight nuchal rigidity

Grade II: Moderate to severe headache, nuchal rigidity, no neurologic deficit other than cranial nerve palsy

Grade III: Drowsiness, confusion, or mild focal deficit

Grade IV: Stupor, moderate-to-severe hemiparesis, possible early decerebrate rigidity, and vegetative disturbances

Grade V: Deep coma, decerebrate rigidity, moribund appearance

Diagnostic Studies

Diagnostic studies used for assessment of SAH include presenting signs and symptoms, computed tomography (CT) scan, lumbar puncture, and angiography. Noncontrast CT scan is the "gold standard" for definitive SAH diagnosis. In over 90 percent of patients, CT scan demonstrates blood in the subarachnoid space when performed within 24 hours of the onset of symptoms. When the CT is negative, lumbar puncture (LP) is performed to obtain cerebral spinal fluid for color, a pressure reading, protein, and cell counts. If the LP is performed more than five days after the SAH, the CSF is xanthochromic (dark amber) due to breakdown of the blood products. If the CSF is cloudy, an infectious process such as bacterial meningitis is the diagnosis, not SAH. Transcranial Doppler (TCD) studies are used to assess for vasospasm. After the diagnosis is made, a cerebral angiogram is performed to show the size, shape, and location of the aneurysm and any vasospasm.

Fischer Grade Scale of Radiological Appearance of SAH

Grade I: None evident

Grade II: Less than 1 mm thick

Grade III: More than 1 mm thick

Grade IV: Any thickness with interventricular hemorrhage or parenchymal extension

Management

Aneurysm treatment includes symptom management and either surgical or endovascular methods. Before definitive repair is attempted, symptom control may include airway management, blood pressure control, seizure control, and electrocardiogram (ECG) changes. Patients with a GCS score less than 8 or patients without airway protective reflexes should be electively intubated and mechanically ventilated. Hypertension is a common symptom prior to surgery. SAH patients should be hemodynamically monitored in the ICU. Since there is loss of cerebral autoregulation after an intracranial hemorrhage, maintaining diastolic blood pressure at 120–150 mm Hg is recommended before definitive treatment. Blood pressure should not be lowered too rapidly, as this can cause cerebral ischemia. Management of hypertension may require IV sodium nitroprusside or labetalol. Seizure control should start with fosphenytoin. The most common dysrhythmias that occur after SAH are prolonged QT interval, and torsade de pointes. All of these sequelae of SAH require close monitoring of the patient's neurological status, reduction of environmental stimuli, and analgesia for pain.

Complications

Common complications of SAH are rebleeding, hydrocephalus, and vasospasm. Rebleeding of the aneurysm occurs most often 2–10 days after the initial rupture. As the clot that initially sealed the rupture site undergoes fibrinolysis, there is a risk of rebleeding. This may be accompanied by a sudden worsening of headache, severe nausea and vomiting, decrease in level of consciousness (LOC), and new focal neurological deficits. **Hydrocephalus** is the progressive dilatation of the ventricular system when the production of CSF exceeds the absorption rate. In obstructive hydrocephalus, the arachnoid villi become plugged with blood, preventing reabsorption of the CSF. The patient will have a change in LOC, such as excessive drowsiness, stupor, or coma. CT scan will demonstrate enlarged ventricles. Management involves insertion of a ventriculostomy to drain CSF periodically, especially when the intracranial pressure (ICP) is above the predetermined level, often 20 mm Hg. If the obstruction does not resolve, a ventriculoperitoneal shunt may be required long-term.

Cerebral vasospasm is a narrowing of a cerebral blood vessel that causes reduced blood flow distally and may cause ischemic deficits or cerebral infarction. Approximately 30 percent to 50 percent of SAH patients experience cerebral vasospasm. The patient may have a decrease in LOC, such as excessive drowsiness, focal neurological deficits (paresis/paralysis of a limb, cranial nerve deficits, and aphasia), or coma. CT scan should be done to rule out rebleeding or hydrocephalus. Management of vasospasm includes the use of nimodipine and triple H therapy (hypervolemia, hypertension, and hemodilution). Vasospasm can easily be determined by transcranial Doppler sonography (TCD), utilized often with SAHs.

The goal of hypervolemia is to maintain a PAOP (wedge pressure) of 14 to 20 mm Hg and/or CVP of 10 to 12 mm Hg. The goal of hypertension is to maintain systolic blood pressure of 120 to 150 mm Hg before definitive treatment and 160 to 200 mm Hg after treatment. The goal of hemodilution is to maintain a hematocrit of 30 percent to 33 percent. Nimodipine (brand name: Nimotop) is a calcium channel blocker that is lipid soluble and therefore able to cross the blood-brain barrier. It is believed to work at the cellular level as a neuronal protector. Serial TCD studies monitor flow velocities in the cerebral vessels. When intracranial blood flow velocities are greater than 100 to 120 cm/sec, this suggests vasospasm; if they are greater than 200 cm/sec, it suggests severe vasospasm.

Definitive Treatment

Surgery is indicated within 48 hours for grade I, II, or III SAHs. Surgery is usually delayed for grades IV and V. Several surgical methods can be used: clipping, wrapping, or ligation. Clipping involves occlusion of the aneurysm neck with a ligature or metal clip. This is the most common surgical method when there is a well-defined arterial neck. Wrapping the aneurysm with muscle or fibrin foam reinforces the sac. Proximal ligation of a feeding vessel is rarely done. Endovascular procedures include coiling and intravascular balloon placement. Coiling involves placing multiple platinum coils inside the aneurysm. A clot forms around the coils, and eventually the base of the aneurysm scars over and is cut off. Intravascular balloon placement involves placing a silicone microballoon into the aneurysm.

Arteriovenous Malformation

Arteriovenous malformation (AVM) is a congenital miscommunication or "tangling" of high-pressure arterial flow with low-pressure venous flow without the intervening capillary network. This shunting of blood causes ischemia and atrophy to the adjacent tissues. Arterial blood flow creates venous engorgement, causing higher than normal pressure. Since there is no muscle layer in veins, rupture of the engorged veins occurs. AVM has three morphologic components: feeding arteries, nidus, and draining veins. The feeding arteries supply blood flow to the AVM. The nidus is the central tangle of vessels. Drainage of blood occurs via the dilated veins.

Clinical Presentation

Presenting signs and symptoms of AVM include intracranial hemorrhage, seizures, headache, and progressive focal neurologic deficits. Intracranial hemorrhage is the most common initial presenting manifestation of AVM, occuring in 50 percent to 60 percent of patients. Symptoms include sudden onset of headache, nausea/vomiting, paresis or plegia, and decreased level of consciousness. Seizures are the second most common presentation of AVM, occurring in 20 percent to 25 percent of patients. Recurrent headache that is unresponsive to the usual drug therapy, new onset of migraine-like headache, or worsening of migraine symptoms (in patients with history of migraine) may be the only manifestation seen with AVM in 15 percent of patients. Progressive focal neurological deficits symptoms depend on the specific area of the brain deprived of adequate blood supply. They may also be related to repeated small hemorrhages from the AVM.

Diagnostic Studies

Diagnostic studies for AVM include CT scan, magnetic resonance imaging (MRI), magnetic resonance angiography (MRA), and four-vessel angiography. CT scan without and with contrast may reveal the bleeding site and any tissue abnormalities. MRI gives a more comprehensive analysis of the AVM, and MRA examines the blood vessels instead of the brain tissue. The "gold standard" is four-vessel angiography, allowing for AVM analysis and grading of the blood flow into and out of the vessels.

Management

Before definitive repair is attempted, symptom control may include airway management, blood pressure control, headache management, and seizure control. When the patient is unable to protect her airway, she should be electively intubated and mechanically ventilated. AVM patients should be hemodynamically monitored in the ICU. Hypertension may cause rebleeding, and hypotension may cause ischemia. Blood pressure should be maintained within 10 percent of prehemorrhage levels. Hypertension can be treated with labetalol (brand name: Normodyne) or hydralazine (brand name: Apresoline). Hypotension may require vasopressors such as phenylephrine (brand name: Neo-Synephrine). Antiseizure medications such as fosphenytoin should be given when seizures are present.

TABLE 9.11 *Surgical Grading Scale for Cerebral Arteriovenous Malformations (AVM)*

Category	Criteria	Point Value
Size (maximum dimension)	< 3 cm	1
	3–6 cm	2
	> 6 cm	3
Location	Noneloquent brain	0
	Eloquent brain	1
Venous drainage	Superficial only	0
	Deep	1

Definitive Treatment

Treatment of arteriovenous malformation includes symptom management and either surgical, radiation, or endovascular methods or conservative management. Surgery for AVM is elective and if possible is delayed as much as three weeks to stabilize the patient and allow time for the body to recover from the effects of the hemorrhage. The goals of surgery are the complete removal of the AVM (prevent further hemorrhage) and excision of the lesion without causing injury to adjacent brain tissue (see table 9.11). If the AVM is very large (> 6 cm), embolization of large feeding vessels may be required prior to excision. Radiosurgery involves focusing radiation beams into selected tissue with the goal of inducing an inflammatory response in the AVM walls, resulting in thrombosis and obliteration of the lesion. Several types of ionizing radiation have been used to treat AVMs, including x-rays, gamma rays, and proton/helium beam radiation. Pretreatment embolization may also be utilized. Endovascular methods (embolization) may be curative, palliative, or adjunctive to surgical excision or radiosurgery. The goal of embolization is permanent occlusion of the AVM, especially when it is deep in the brain cortex or not surgically accessible. Conservative management involves lifestyle changes to decrease the chance of hemorrhage, including activity restrictions, smoking cessation, and control of seizures (if present).

Traumatic Brain Injury

Trauma happens when external forces impact the body causing structural and/or physiological alterations or injuries. The external forces can be chemical, electrical, mechanical, radiation, or thermal forms of energy. Knowledge of the mechanism of injury helps caregivers to anticipate and predict the extent of injury. Brain injury is the leading cause of trauma-related deaths in people younger than 45 years of age and occurs twice as often in males. It is estimated that over 2 million traumatic brain injuries occur each year in the United States. There are approximately 75,000 deaths, and significant disability is seen in 70,000–90,000 people per year. Some 200,000 brain injuries are sports-related (Center for Head Injury Statistics).

Etiology

Traumatic brain injury (TBI) occurs when mechanical forces are transmitted to brain tissue. These mechanisms are kinetic energy (KE) and force (F). The formula for kinetic energy is

$$KE = \frac{M}{2} \text{ (mass divided by 2)} \times V^2 \text{ (square of the velocity)}$$

The formula for force is

$$F = M \times A \text{ (deceleration)}$$

The impact force is determined by the force, duration, direction, and rate. In an automobile accident, there are three separate collisions that occur: vehicle hits object, victim strikes internal parts of vehicle, and soft tissue strikes the hard body surfaces. For example, an unbelted occupant in a 30 mph collision slams into the interior surfaces with the same impact as though he fell from a three-story building (Bader & Littlejohns, 2004).

Blunt trauma is seen in motor vehicle crashes, motorcycle crashes, pedestrian–motor vehicle crashes, bicycle injuries, falls, sports, and assaults. Blunt head trauma is caused by contact, acceleration-deceleration, and rotational forces. Contact injuries occur when an object strikes the head. The velocity of the impact determines whether the injury is restricted to the scalp or skull (low velocity) or includes the brain (high velocity). Acceleration-deceleration injuries occur when the skull strikes (or is struck by) an object. The brain is carried by force until it strikes the inside of the skull (coup injury). When the impact is strong enough, the undissipated force pitches the brain in the reverse direction, striking the opposite side of the skull (contrecoup injury). Rotational injury, often occurring with acceleration-deceleration injuries, results in tearing or shearing of tissues. This includes injuries to the spinal cord and neck.

Penetrating trauma injuries are caused by objects that penetrate the skull, producing significant focal damage but little acceleration-deceleration or rotational injury. The most common instruments used in penetrating trauma are guns (low/high velocity), knives, and sharp objects (knives, metal rods). With these injuries, there is deep penetration into the brain tissue and the possibility of damage to the ventricular system. A low-velocity (stabbing) injury is limited to the entry tract, and the greatest concern is bleeding and infection. Gunshot (high-velocity) injuries cause extensive damage related to entry of bone fragments; the bullets spin irregularly, creating multiple paths and shock waves that cause extensive brain damage.

Trauma to the head may result in both primary and secondary injuries to the brain. Primary brain injury is the result of direct trauma to the brain. Secondary injury occurs as a result of injury to the brain and includes hypoxia, cerebral edema, hypertension, hypercapnia, and elevated intracranial pressure. Secondary injuries occur hours or days after the initial trauma and are a result of the body's response to the primary injury. The goal when caring for a TBI patient is to support maximum recovery from the primary brain injury and at the same time prevent, minimize, and reverse the occurrence of secondary injuries.

Skull Fractures

Direct contact is the mechanism of skull injury. The extent of injury depends on several factors, including the skull's thickness at the point of impact and the weight, velocity, and angle of impact of the intruding object. Upon impact, several actions are set in motion. The object velocity at the point of impact causes an indentation, which may be temporary or permanent. Stress waves are set in motion and radiate throughout the entire skull. When there is a high-velocity impact, a depressed skull fracture with or without a dural tear and cerebral laceration may occur. With a low-velocity impact, the area of indentation rebounds outward and may result in no fracture, a linear fracture, or a comminuted fracture. The fracture line extends from the point of impact toward the base of the skull.

Skull fractures are classified as linear, comminuted, depressed, open depressed, or basilar skull. **Linear** fractures are a single fracture line in the bone. In a **comminuted** fracture, the bone is splintered or shattered into pieces. **Depressed** fractures occur when one or more sections of bone fragment become embedded in the brain tissue. The scalp and/or the dura may or may not be torn. The patient may require surgery to debride the wound and elevate the bone fragments. An **open depressed (compound) fracture** has openings in the scalp and dura and bone fragments in the tissue. The patient is at greater risk for infection because the blood-brain barrier is violated. A **basilar skull fracture** is a linear fracture at the base of the skull that is associated with a dural tear. Signs and symptoms include spinal fluid and/or blood leaking from the ears or nose, raccoon's eyes (periorbital ecchymosis), and Battle's sign (bruising of the mastoid bone). The patient should be monitored for meningitis, encephalitis, and epidural hematoma.

Brain Injuries

Concussion is the mildest form of brain injury and is characterized by brief loss of consciousness (LOC). The patient complains of headache, dizziness, and possibly nausea/vomiting. Focal neurologic deficits and altered LOC usually clear in 6–12 hours. Post-concussion syndrome is common and may include short-term memory deficits, headache, cognitive difficulties, visual disturbances, lack of coordination, and lethargy. These "minor" injuries can have devastating long-term effects.

Contusions are bleeding of small vessels and necrotic brain tissue caused by acceleration-deceleration movement of the brain within the skull. Neurologic deficits may include changes in LOC, cranial nerve dysfunction, hemiparesis or hemiplegia, seizures, and intracranial hypertension. The clinical effect depends on the size, location, and related cerebral edema.

Diffuse axonal injury results from white matter shearing associated with rotational and acceleration-deceleration forces. There is disruption of the axons and neuronal pathways in the brain hemispheres, diencephalon, and brain stem. Neurologic deficits include coma, confusion, posttraumatic amnesia, and prolonged recovery. Treatment is support of vital functions and maintenance of intracranial pressure within normal parameters. Mortality rates vary between 33 and 50 percent depending on the severity of the initial injury. Many patients may survive in a vegetative state characterized by periods of wakefulness and sleep but without observable signs of cognition.

Diagnostic studies include CT scan, MRI, and MRA. These may show brain edema, areas of small hemorrhage (severe contusion), and detection of associated injuries (carotid or vertebral dissection). EEG may show brain wave abnormalities, and evoked potentials may show slowing of impulse transmission through the brain stem.

Intracranial Hemorrhage

Traumatic intracranial bleeding is a common complication of brain injury. Bleeding may begin immediately after the injury, but its presence may not become clinically apparent until enough blood accumulates to cause signs and symptoms. The time between bleeding and the appearance of clinical symptoms may be minutes to weeks, depending on the site and rate of bleeding. Hemorrhage can be a late development in a patient with a "minor" traumatic brain injury (TBI) when there is minimal loss of consciousness. Other patients with hemorrhage may remain unconscious from the moment of injury. The types of bleeding associated with TBI are epidural hematoma, subdural hematoma, and intracerebral hemorrhage.

Epidural hematoma (extradural hematoma) is bleeding into the potential space between the lining of the skull (periosteum) and the dura mater. Epidural hematoma (EDH) is seen in 4 percent to 8 percent of all head traumas and 20 percent to 30 percent of all hematomas. Most EDHs are arterial in origin (85 percent) and are often associated with linear skull fractures that cross major blood vessels. The most frequent site is the **middle meningeal artery** located under the temporal bone. Occasionally, EDHs may be due to tearing of the dural venous sinuses. As the hematoma enlarges, the dura is gradually torn away from the skull, creating pressure on the underlying brain and causing a mass effect.

The classic description of an epidural hematoma is "talk and die." Patients have a brief loss of consciousness, followed be a lucid ("honeymoon") period lasting from minutes to several hours. The lucid period is followed by rapid deterioration in LOC from drowsiness to lethargy and then to coma, as mass effect and herniation develop. The most common clinical presentation is headache, vomiting, seizures, unilateral hyperreflexia, positive Babinski sign, ipsilateral occulomotor paralysis, contralateral hemiparesis/hemiplegia, and elevated ICP. Once LOC begins to deteriorate, coma occurs rapidly. Bradycardia and respiratory distress are late signs.

Diagnostic Studies

Diagnostic studies include skull and spine radiographs, CT scan of the head, and MRI. Radiographs (x-rays) may reveal associated skull or spine fractures. CT scan will show an area of increased density and may show midline shift. Lumbar puncture is contraindicated due to elevated ICP.

Epidural hematomas require immediate surgical intervention to remove the clot. Postoperative infection is usually not a concern since meninges and blood-brain barrier are intact. Prompt diagnosis and treatment prevents mortality (5 to 10 percent) from EDH.

Subdural hematoma (SDH) is bleeding between the dura mater and arachnoid layer. This is usually caused by **shearing of the cortical veins** that bridge the dura and arachnoid membrane as a result of acceleration-deceleration and rotational forces. Subdural hematoma is seen in 15 percent to 30 percent of patients with head trauma and 50 percent to 70 percent of all hematomas. It may occur with minimal trauma when patients have a coagulation disorder or are taking anticoagulants. The majority of SDHs are seen in older patients with brain atrophy or a history of alcohol abuse. Subdural hematomas are classified based on the time interval and appearance of blood/fluid composition (see table 9.12).

TABLE 9.12 *Subdural Hematoma Classification*

Time Interval	Blood/Fluid Composition
Acute SDH: 0 to 48 hours	Clotted blood that is hypodense is seen on CT scan.
Subacute SDH: 3 to 20 days	Clot lysis has begun, and blood products and fluids are present.
Chronic SDH: 3 weeks to months	Hemolysis of the clot draws fluid into the area, causing swelling. The SDH is hypodense on CT scan.

Clinical Presentation

Clinical presentation of SDHs varies based on classification. Acute SDHs may present gradually or with rapid deterioration of the LOC from drowsiness, slow cerebration, and confusion to coma. Patients may also have pupillary changes and hemiparesis/hemiplegia.

Subacute SDH symptoms are similar to those of acute SDH but occur at a slower rate. Chronic SDH symptoms include headache, slow cerebration, confusion, papilledema, slowed pupillary responses, and possibly seizures. The symptoms develop gradually and may be misdiagnosed as Alzheimer's disease, "old age," or cerebral atrophy.

Diagnostic Studies

Diagnostic studies include skull and spine radiographs, CT scan of the head, and MRI. Radiographs (x-rays) may reveal associated skull or spine fractures. CT scan will show an area of increased density and may show midline shift.

Management

Treatment of large hematomas requires immediate surgical intervention (craniectomy, craniotomy, or burr holes) to remove the clot. Postoperative infection is a concern since meninges and blood-brain barrier are entered to remove the clot. Patients with small SDH and minimal symptoms may be followed with close observation with serial CT scans. Once the clot liquefies, burr holes are made in the skull, and the fluid is drained. A drain is placed to prevent reaccumulation of fluid in the subdural space. Elderly patients and those with a history of alcohol abuse tend to rebleed after surgical evacuation and require careful monitoring. Prompt diagnosis and treatment prevents mortality (20 percent) from SDH.

Intracerebral hemorrhage (ICH) is bleeding into the cerebral parenchyma and may be caused by caused by trauma, tumors, bleeding disorders, anticoagulant therapy, or hypertension. When the ICH is from trauma, the injury may be due to a penetrating missile or from severe acceleration-deceleration forces that cause laceration of the deep cerebral tissues. ICH occurs in 2 to 20 percent of patients with head trauma.

Clinical Presentation

Clinical presentation of ICH varies with the area of brain involved, size of the hematoma, and rate of blood accumulation. These patients may or may not show symptoms of intracranial hypertension. Symptoms may include headache, decreasing LOC progressing to deep coma, contralateral hemiplegia, ipsilateral dilated pupil, and, as ICP increases, the development of transtentorial herniation.

Diagnostic Studies

Diagnostic studies include skull and spine radiographs, CT scan of the head, and MRI. Radiographs (x-rays) may reveal associated skull or spine fractures. CT scan will show an area of increased density and may show midline shift. MRI will show the hematoma and any associated edema.

Treatment is based on the location and extent of bleeding. Surgery rarely improves neurological outcome. Most patients are managed medically with supportive care and management of increased ICP.

Secondary Brain Injury

Secondary injury is any complicating injury occurring as a result of physiologic events related to the primary brain insult, such as ischemia, inflammation, excitotoxicity, and metabolic insults. Severe head trauma begins a cascade of ischemic and cellular-level biochemical changes that can lead to neuronal injury and cell death. Some changes occur almost immediately after injury, some later. Any systemic (extracerebral) or neurological (intracerebral) complication can compromise adequate oxygen and nutrient delivery to the brain's cells, causing hypoxia or ischemia. The ischemia can begin or worsen the pathological cascade of events that leads to secondary brain injury.

Ischemia is a mismatch between oxygen supply and oxygen demand. Cerebral ischemia is defined as cerebral blood flow (CBF) of less than 20 mL/100 g per minute. If oxygen demand is not matched by oxygen delivery, irreversible cellular injury begins, and toxic metabolites build up in the blood. When blood flow is reduced, neurons increase their extraction of oxygen from the surrounding tissues. Inadequate blood flow to the brain and/or reduced oxygen content of the blood causes clinical manifestations. These manifestations include alterations in LOC, motor impairments, and ultimately coma. Multiple physiological stressors impact cerebral blood flow and cerebral perfusion; these include hypotension (due to blood loss), shock, underlying cardiovascular disease, and increased intracranial pressure. Other complications of CBF and cerebral perfusion alterations include alterations of neurotransmitter activity, glucose transport and utilization, protein synthesis, and cellular membrane stability. Prevention and management of cerebral ischemia require maintenance of adequate blood flow and cerebral perfusion of brain tissues.

Cerebral edema is the intra- or extracellular swelling in response to injury and ischemia, which is associated with increased brain tissue volume. The edema usually peaks two to four days after a TBI and is associated with increased ICP. Cerebral edema is a serious complication and can be life threatening since the edema puts pressure on the brain tissue, causing neurologic deficits. Severe cerebral edema can produce transtentorial herniation and progress to brain stem compression, herniation, and death. There are three types of cerebral edema: vasogenic, cytotoxic, and interstitial.

Vasogenic edema is extracellular edema of the white matter in the brain. It results from increased capillary permeability and an increase in pinocytotic vesicles in the blood-brain barrier. These alterations allow plasma-like filtrate, including large protein molecules, to leak into the extracellular space. This increases the distance that oxygen, substrates, and waste products must travel to and from cells and exerts pressure on the cells and blood vessels, compressing them and contributing to increased ICP. Vasogenic edema may be caused by trauma, infection, abscess, hypoxia, or tumor. The use of corticosteroids (dexamethasone) is effective only with brain tumors. Mannitol, an osmotic diuretic, may be helpful in the acute phase. The extent of cerebral edema can be minimized in the acute phase by controlling oxygenation, ventilation, and blood pressure.

Cytotoxic edema is an increase of fluid in the neurons, glial, and endothelial cells as a result of ATP-dependent sodium-potassium pump failure. Fluid and sodium accumulate within the cells, leading to diffuse brain swelling involving both gray and white matter of the brain. Cytotoxic edema is associated with hypoxic or anoxic episodes (cardiac arrest, asphyxiation), water intoxication, hyponatremia, and syndrome of inappropriate antidiuretic hormone (SIADH) secretion. Corticosteroids (dexamethasone) are not effective in treating cytotoxic edema. Osmotic diuretics may be beneficial in the acute stage when hypoosmolarity is present.

Hydrocephalus is caused by a buildup of CSF pressure within the ventricular system that forces CSF into the periventricular white matter. It is associated with acute or subacute hydrocephalus and benign intracranial hypertension (pseudotumor cerebri). Hydrocephalus may be communicating (nonobstructive) or noncommunicating (obstructive). Communicating hydrocephalus is due to a defect in the absorption of CSF at the arachnoid villi or sagittal sinus. Noncommunicating is caused by a blockage of CSF at or above the fourth ventricle. Corticosteroids and osmotic diuretics are not effective. A decrease in CSF production occurs with the administration of acetazolamide (Diamox). Treatment includes temporary drainage of CSF via a ventriculostomy until the condition is corrected by surgical placement of a shunt.

Cellular excitotoxicity occurs when the traumatic brain injury causes a massive depolarization of the brain cells. There is a rapid increase in excitatory neurotransmitter release (glutamate, aspartate) that changes the normal ionic gradients of the neuronal membranes, glial cells, and cerebral vascular endothelial cells. This change begins a chain of disruption of crucial cellular processes. Aerobic metabolism and production of adenosine triphosphate (ATP) stops quickly, reducing the energy stores of the affected cells. Potassium leaves the cells, allowing calcium, sodium, and water to enter the damaged cells and resulting in edema.

Intracranial pressure is the force normally exerted by the CSF that circulates around the brain, spinal cord, and cerebral ventricles. The normal range of ICP for adults is 0 to 10 mm Hg (15 mm Hg is considered the upper limit of normal).

When patients have cerebral trauma or other neurological disorders, the normal homeostatic mechanisms may be disrupted, causing a sustained elevated ICP that may result in death. The intracranial space has three components: brain (80 percent), CSF (10 percent), and blood (10 percent). Essential to the understanding of the pathophysiology of ICP is the Monro-Kellie hypothesis. The hypothesis is based on these principles:

1. The brain is in an enclosed space.

2. Cerebral blood volume is constant.

3. Outflow of venous blood equals the incoming arterial blood flow.

The **Monro-Kellie hypothesis** states that if the volume of one component increases, a reciprocal decrease in the volume of one or both of the others must occur or an increase in ICP will result.

Autoregulation of cerebral blood flow (CBF) includes multiple compensatory mechanisms that maintain the intracranial volume in homeostasis, including CSF displacement from the subarachnoid space and ventricles via the foramen magnum to the spinal subarachnoid space and via the optic foramen to the basal subarachnoid cisterns; compression of the low pressure dural sinuses; decreased production of CSF; and vasoconstriction of the cerebral blood vessels. However, the amount of displacement is limited. Once the compensatory mechanisms are exceeded, the ICP increases, and intracranial hypertension is the result. Mean arterial pressure (MAP) of 50 to 150 mm Hg does not change CBF when autoregulation is present. With intracranial hypertension, CBF becomes dependent on the perfusion pressure. **Intracranial hypertension** is a sustained elevated intracranial pressure (ICP) of 20 mm Hg or higher.

Cerebral blood flow varies with changes in cerebral perfusion and constriction or dilatation of the cerebrovascular vessels. Normal cerebral blood flow in adults is 50 mL per 100 g per minute.

The brain comprises 2 percent of body weight, but it requires 15 percent to 20 percent of the total cardiac output and 15 percent to 20 percent of oxygen consumed at rest.

Systemic Factors That Alter CBF

Increase	Decrease
Hypercapnia	Hypocapnia
Hypoxemia	Hyperoxemia
Decreased blood viscosity	Increased blood viscosity
Hyperthermia	Hypothermia
Vasodilators	Vasopressors
	Intracranial hypertension

Intracranial Pressure Monitoring

Intracranial pressure monitoring is the standard of care in the ICU and is the most significant factor in determining the morbidity and mortality of neurosurgical patients. There are four sites used for monitoring ICP: the intraventricular space, the epidural space, the subarachnoid space, and the parenchyma. When the **intraventricular** space is used, a catheter is inserted into the anterior or occipital horns of the lateral ventricle. The use of a three-way stopcock allows both ICP monitoring by a pressure transducer and drainage of CSF as needed. This method is also called ventriculostomy. Advantages of this method are that it allows direct measurement of ICP and instillation of medications or contrast media for diagnostic studies. Disadvantages include increased risk of infection (2 to 5 percent), hemorrhage, CSF loss, midline shifting, and increased cerebral edema.

The **epidural** sensor method uses a fiberoptic sensing device inserted via a burr hole into the epidural space between the skull and the dura mater. Advantages are that the sensor is easier to insert, is less invasive, and generates a lower infection rate (less than 1 percent). Disadvantages are that it is unable to drain excess CSF and that pressure readings are higher than measured by other methods.

When a **subarachnoid** screw or bolt is used, the device is inserted into the subarachnoid space through a burr hole and connected to an external transducer. Advantages include easier insertion method than with a ventriculostomy, direct measurement of ICP, low no penetration into the brain, and low risk for infection (1 to 2 percent). Disadvantages are that CSF drainage is not possible, the device requires frequent recalibration, it may become occluded with debris (clots, tissue) causing inaccurate measurements, and it is more easily dislodged than a catheter.

In the **intraparenchymal** method, a fiberoptic-tipped probe is inserted through a burr hole and placed 1 cm into the brain tissue. It is then connected to an external monitor, providing waveforms for evaluation. Advantages are that it is easy to insert, head position has no effect on readings, and placement is not dependent on ventricular size or position. Disadvantages include CSF drainage is not possible; it cannot be re-zeroed once it is in place; the probe is fragile and easily bent, broken, or kinked; and there is an increased risk of intracerebral bleeding and infection.

ICP Waveform Monitoring

Monitoring systems allow the ICU nurse to observe the ICP waveform pattern. The ICP waveform is similar to an arterial hemodynamic waveform. A normal ICP waveform has three defined peaks of decreasing height, identified as P_1, P_2, and P_3. P_1 is an upward spike called a systolic or percussion wave, which represents the blood being ejected from the heart. Extreme alterations in blood pressure produce changes in P_1. P_2 is a second upward spike called the tidal wave; it is more variable, ends on the dicrotic notch, and is indicative of brain compliance. When P_2 is equal to or higher than P_1, decreased compliance exists and can be helpful in predicting the risk for increases in ICP. P_3 follows the dicrotic notch and represents closure of the aortic valve.

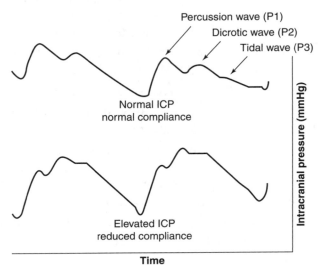

External Ventricular Drain (EVD)

External ventricular drain, also known as an extraventricular drain or ventriculostomy, is a device used in neurosurgery that relieves elevated intracranial pressure and hydrocephalus when the normal flow of cerebrospinal fluid around the brain is obstructed. This is a plastic tube placed by neurosurgeons and managed by ICU nurses and critical care paramedics to drain fluid from the ventricles of the brain and thus keep them decompressed, as well as to monitor intracranial pressure.

TABLE 9.13 *External Ventricular Drain*

Assessment:	Key Points:
• HOB 30° unless otherwise ordered	• Clamp (hold drainage) whenever the HOB changes in relation to the height of the cylinder
• Neuro assessment **Q1hr**	• Label EVD tubing to prevent inadvertent access
• Verify order for drain height (mm HG or cmH2O) and drainage parameters (mL/hour) **Q-Shift/PRN**	• NO pressure bag required
• Maintain cylinder in an upright position	• RN may NOT flush or obtain CSF sample
• Document CSF outputs **Q1hr**	• Prime system with normal saline
• Color and clarity of CSF drainage	• Integra EVD is MRI safe
• Tubing for kinking	• Zero: level EVD transducer to the **Tragus** (ear)
• Dressing **Q1hr**	
• Note the presence of tidaling of the CSF in the tubing (fluctuations of the meniscus)	

TABLE 9.13 *External Ventricular Drain (EVD) (continued)*

Notify the Provider If:	Complications:.
• Dressing has CSF fluid	• CSF leakage
• ICP >20 for more than 5 min	• Aneurysmal rebleeding
• Outpouring of bright red blood and/or CSF	• Drain blockage
• No drainage for 2 hr	• Infection
• Absence of CSF tidaling	
• Dressing is damp, loose, or solid	

Herniation Syndromes

Herniation is defined as the displacement of brain structures due to increased ICP. It causes a sequence of neurologic signs and symptoms related to compression of brain structures and compromised cerebral blood flow. There are four types of brain herniation syndromes caused by expanding mass lesions: cingulate, central, uncal, and tonsillar (infratentorial). In cingulate herniation the brain squeezes under the falx cerebri. The brain stem herniates caudally in central herniation. In uncal herniation, the uncus and the hippocampal gyrus herniate into the tentorial notch. The cerebellar tonsils herniate through the foramen magnum in tonsillar herniation.

Cingulate Herniation

In cingulate herniation (most common), the innermost part of the frontal lobe is forced under part of the falx cerebri (the dura mater at the top of the head between the two hemispheres of the brain). Cingulate herniation can be caused when one hemisphere swells and pushes the cingulate gyrus by the falx cerebri. This does not put as much pressure on the brain stem as the other types of herniation, but it may interfere with blood vessels in the frontal lobes that are close to the site of injury (anterior cerebral artery), or it may progress to central herniation. Interference with the blood supply can cause dangerous increases in ICP, which can lead to more dangerous forms of herniation. Symptoms for cingulate herniation are not well defined. Usually occurring in addition to uncal herniation, cingulate herniation may present with abnormal posturing and coma. Cingulate herniation is believed to be a precursor to other types of herniation.

Central Herniation

In central herniation (transtentorial herniation), the diencephalon and parts of the temporal lobes of both of the cerebral hemispheres are squeezed through a notch in the tentorium. Downward herniation can stretch branches of the basilar artery, causing it to tear and bleed. The result is usually fatal.

Uncal Herniation

In uncal herniation, the innermost part of the temporal lobe, the uncus, can be squeezed so much that it goes by the tentorium and puts pressure on the brain stem. The *tentorium* is a structure within the skull formed by the dura mater. Tissue may be stripped from the cerebral cortex in a process called *decortication*. The uncus can squeeze the third cranial nerve, which controls parasympathetic input to the eye on the side of the affected nerve. This interrupts the parasympathetic neural transmission, causing the pupil of the affected eye to dilate and fail to constrict in response to light as it should. A dilated, unresponsive pupil is an important sign of increased intracranial pressure. The progression of pupil constriction/dilation in uncal herniation is dependent upon the level of involvement, and the pupil can be constricted but reactive at the point of upper brain involvement, fixed and either nonreactive or sluggishly reactive at the point of brain stem involvement, and "blown" or fixed and dilated either unilaterally or bilaterally in lower brain stem compression. Commonly, a blown pupil is considered a late sign of increased intracranial pressure. Cranial arteries may be compressed during the herniation. Compression of the posterior cerebral artery may result in loss of the contralateral visual field. This type of herniation can also damage the brain stem, causing lethargy, slow heart rate, respiratory abnormalities, and pupil dilation. Uncal herniation may advance to central herniation.

Tonsillar Herniation

In tonsillar herniation (downward cerebellar herniation), the cerebellar tonsils move downward through the foramen magnum, possibly causing compression of the lower brain stem and upper cervical spinal cord as they pass through the foramen magnum. Increased pressure on the brain stem can result in dysfunction of the centers in the brain responsible for controlling respiratory and cardiac function.

Complications

The patient may become paralyzed on the same side as the lesion causing the pressure or on the side opposite the lesion. Increased pressure on the midbrain, which contains the reticular-activating network that regulates consciousness, will result in coma. Damage to the cardio-respiratory centers in the medulla will cause respiratory and cardiac arrest.

Infections

Infections of the central nervous system include meningitis, encephalitis, and intracranial abscess. **Meningitis** (bacterial, fungal, viral) is an inflammatory process of the meninges and CSF within the subarachnoid space. The infecting organism multiplies rapidly, stimulating-inflammatory cytokine (interleukin-1[IL-1], tumor necrosis factor [TNF]) release. Blood-brain barrier permeability is altered, allowing PMNs into the brain. These events cause formation of purulent exudate that obstructs CSF flow, vasogenic edema, and increased ICP. Early and aggressive diagnosis and treatment help to prevent the development of complications. Presenting signs and symptoms may include progressively worsening headache, fever, nausea, vomiting, photophobia, nuchal rigidity, positive Kernig's and Brudzinski's sign, altered LOC, and seizures. Diagnosis is usually determined by clinical examination and lumbar puncture.

The CSF is cloudy or xanthochromic and shows elevated pressure, elevated protein, decreased glucose, and the presence of WBCs. CT scan of the head may show hydrocephalus or diffuse enhancement in severe cases. Management includes symptom control, patient isolation (meningococcal), and administration of appropriate anti-infectious agents. Nursing care includes monitoring for LOC changes, maintenance of low-stimulation environment, and medication administration.

Encephalitis is inflammation of brain tissue usually caused by a virus (most common), fungus, bacteria, or parasite. Incidence is highest in children younger than 10 years of age; then it decreases and is constant until about 40 years of age, when it decreases further. It is most common in the immunosuppressed. Acute encephalitis is usually caused by a viruses such as herpes simplex, Epstein-Barr, equine, and arbovirus. Arbovirus and equine viruses (transmitted by ticks and mosquitoes) include West Nile, malaria, Eastern equine, Western equine, and St. Louis varieties. Presenting signs and symptoms may include progressively worsening headache, fever, nausea, vomiting, photophobia, nuchal rigidity, positive Kernig's and Brudzinski's sign, altered LOC, and seizures. Diagnosis and management is the same as for meningitis.

Encephalopathy is structural or functional abnormality of the brain. It can result from any disease that changes brain structure or function, including liver or renal failure, infection, brain tumors, increasing hydrocephalus, and environmental hazard exposure. Hypoxic-ischemic (anoxic) encephalopathy is brain injury arising from lack of oxygen; this can result from cardiac arrest, exsanguination, or drop in pO_2. Metabolic encephalopathy occurs when an organ other than the brain fails; for instance, hepatic/renal failure, hypo/hyperglycemia, or sepsis. Infectious encephalopathy is caused by viruses. Initial treatment for encephalopathy depends on the cause. Nursing care includes monitoring for LOC changes, maintenance of low-stimulation environment, oxygen therapy, and medication administration.

Intracranial abscesses are localized infections in the brain tissue caused by bacteria outside the cranium that are carried intracranially by the bloodstream. The most common abscess sites are the cerebrum, epidural, and subdural spaces. Presenting signs and symptoms may include fever, lethargy, focal neurologic deficits, speech and motor deficits, pain, and seizures. Diagnosis is made using CT scanning and lumbar puncture. Medical management includes both intravenous and intrathecal antibiotics, after the infecting agent is identified. Surgical excision and drainage may be required to remove as much purulent drainage as possible. Nursing care includes monitoring for LOC changes, maintenance of low-stimulation environment, and medication administration. If the patient requires surgery, the head of the bed should be elevated 30 degrees to facilitate venous drainage.

Neuromuscular Disorders

Neuromuscular disorders, such as Guillain-Barré syndrome, myasthenia gravis, and muscular dystrophy, affect the nerve impulses that control voluntary muscle groups and generally cause muscle weakness and/or pain. In some neuromuscular disorders, the nerves themselves are damaged; in others, the receptor sites are compromised. Many neuromuscular disorders are genetic, but some are caused by autoimmune disorders. Though cures do not exist for many neuromuscular disorders, they can be treated with medications and other therapies to improve symptoms and prolong life.

Guillain-Barré syndrome is an inflammatory process of the nervous system characterized by demyelination of the peripheral nerves. Incidence of Guillain-Barré syndrome (GBS) is 1 to 2 per 100,000 people in the United States. It affects all ages, races, and genders equally. A flu-like illness, one to three weeks prior to symptoms, has been implicated in 60 to 70 percent of GBS cases. The syndrome is thought to be autoimmune, triggered by the infectious event. Macrophages attack normal myelin, producing demyelination of the axons. Presenting signs and symptoms include acute onset of bilateral lower extremity muscle weakness that ascends rapidly upward; tingling; hypoactive or absent deep tendon reflexes (DTRs), cranial nerve deficits; impaired respiratory muscle function, which can progress to respiratory failure; and autonomic nervous system dysfunction. One of the most common differentiating symptoms of Guillain-Barré is that paralysis initiates in the peripheral nerves and moves more centrally. Therefore, frequent assessments measuring negative inspiratory force (NIF) and vital capacity (VC) should be done minimally every hour during the early identification phase. Intubation may be required to maintain airway protection and adequate ventiliation.

Diagnosed in as many as 20 people in a population of 100,000, **myasthenia gravis (MG)** is a chronic disorder characterized by muscle weakness and rapid fatigue of the voluntary muscles, including muscles of the face, throat, mouth, eyes, arms, and legs. MG is usually caused by an acquired immunological abnormality, where antibodies attack or block up to 80 percent of muscle receptor sites. In some cases, MG is not caused by an autoimmune disorder; rather, it is caused by a genetic abnormality of the neuromuscular junctions. MG is neither directly inherited, nor is it contagious. Although onset typically appears in women in their 20s or 30s and in men in their 70s or 80s, MG affects both genders and all races and can occur at any age. Symptoms of MG include drooping eyelid(s), double or blurred vision, slurred speech, difficulty chewing or swallowing, weakness in arms and/or legs, chronic muscle fatigue, and difficulty breathing.

Although there is no cure for MG, symptoms are generally treated with medications (such as cholinesterase inhibitors, corticosteroids, and immunosuppressant drugs), thymectomy (removal of the thymus gland), plasmapheresis (plasma exchange), and, in some cases, intravenous immunoglobulin.

Muscular dystrophy (MD) is a general term referring to over 30 different progressive and degenerative diseases—all of which result in muscle weakness and loss—usually caused by an absence of or insufficient dystrophin. Depending on the type of MD, onset of symptoms in individuals can appear anywhere from infancy to middle age or later. The most common forms of MD include *Duchenne, Becker, facioscapulohumeral*, and *myotonic*. Duchenne is a rapidly progressive form of MD with onset between three and five years of age that generally affects boys. Most individuals with Duchenne MD are unable to walk by the time they reach age 12, and they may require a respirator. Duchenne MD is hereditary, and girls can be carriers of the disease. Becker MD is similar to Duchenne MD, although it is less severe. Onset of facioscapulohumeral MD is generally seen in teenagers, affecting muscles around the face, shoulders and chest, arms, and legs. Progression of facioscapulohumeral MD is often slow, and symptoms range from mild to debilitating. Myotonic MD has onset in adults. Symptoms of this form of MD include prolonged muscle spasms, cataracts, cardiac abnormalities, and endocrine complications.

There is no cure for any form of MD; treatments to ease symptoms include therapies, such as physical, occupational, respiratory, and speech; corrective surgery; orthopedic devices; and medications, such as corticosteroids, anticonvulsants, and immunosuppressants.

Surgical Procedures

Neurosurgical procedures include craniotomy, craniectomy, cranioplasty, and burr holes.

Craniotomy is surgical opening of the skull to allow for access to brain tissue. There are three types of craniotomies: supratentorial, infratentorial, and transsphenoidal. Supratentorial approach is just above the tentorium and is used to access the cerebral hemispheres (frontal, parietal, temporal, occipital). This approach is used to

- remove intracranial tumors, hematomas, abscesses, or seizure foci.
- clip or ligate aneurysm or AVMs in the anterior circulation.
- secure placement of ventricular draining shunts (venous, pleural, peritoneal).
- ensure debridement of fragments or necrotic tissue and/or elevate and realign bone fragments.

Infratentorial approach is below tentorium in the posterior fossa and is used to access the brain stem (midbrain, pons, medulla) and cerebellum. This approach is used for removal of cerebellar tumors and hemorrhages, acoustic neuromas, brain stem tumors, cranial nerve tumors, and abscesses. The transsphenoidal approach is frequently used to remove pituitary tumors or to control pain associated with metastatic cancer.

Craniectomy is excision of a portion of the skull without replacement and may be used for decompression after cerebral debulking or removal of bone fragments from a skull fracture.

Cranioplasty is the repair of skull using synthetic material. **Burr holes** are small holes drilled through the skull allowing access to the underlying structures. They are frequently used for evacuation of epidural or subdural hematomas, insertion of an intraventricular catheter for CSF drainage, or insertion of ICP-monitoring device.

Complications of cranial surgery may include intracranial hypertension, brain ischemia or infarction, hemorrhage, CSF leak, CNS infection, seizures, fluid and electrolyte imbalance, hydrocephalus, deep vein thrombosis, or stress ulcers. Most neurosurgery patients are admitted to an ICU for close observation and extensive physiological monitoring. Patients will have a turban-style head dressing covering the incision and require frequent monitoring for bleeding or CSF drainage. After the dressing is removed, the incision is monitored for redness, drainage, or signs of wound infection. Frequent neurologic assessments are needed to identify and prevent possible complications. Medication administration is needed to control conditions that may increase the cerebral metabolic rate, including anticonvulsants, analgesics, antipyretics, sedation, and muscle paralytics or barbiturates if indicated. Maintain capillary perfusion pressure (CPP) of 60 to 100 mm Hg by preventing and treating hypertension or hypotension. DVT and stress ulcer prophylaxis should be ordered by physicians as per ICU protocols.

Seizures

A **seizure** is a sudden, uncontrolled discharge of electrical impulses in the brain. Seizures are frequently a symptom of an underlying pathology. Seizures secondary to systemic or metabolic pathology are not considered epilepsy if the seizures stop when the pathology is resolved. A **convulsion** is the abnormal motor response or jerking movements that occur during a seizure. About 3 million people in the United States have epilepsy, and there is an increase of approximately 200,000 new patients each year.

Etiology

Seizure generation has two components: a seizure focus and the neuronal connections to that focus. The seizure focus is a group of hyperexcitable neurons. The area of the brain that is connected to the focus will determine the seizure manifestations. For example, a slow-growing brain tumor near the frontal lobe will eventually cause a seizure to occur. The seizure focus is near the motor cortex, adjacent to the increasing tumor mass. When the hyperexcitable focus discharges, it is transmitted to the motor strip, and a clonic seizure is the result.

Causes of seizures include CNS infections, inborn errors of metabolism, congenital malformations, acquired metabolic disorders, and structural lesions. Acquired metabolic disorders such as hypoglycemia, uremia, and electrolyte and acid-base disturbances may complicate care and cause seizures in TBI, SCI, stroke, and cranial surgery patients.

Clinical Manifestations

The clinical manifestations of a seizure are determined by the site of the disturbance (focus). Phases of a seizure include **prodromal phase**, **aural phase**, **ictal phase**, and **postictal phase**. The prodromal phase is the signs or activity before the seizure (e.g., headache or feeling depressed). The aural phase is a sensation or warning that the patient remembers. An aura can be visual, auditory, gustatory, or visceral in nature (e.g., an odor or flashing lights). The ictal phase is the actual seizure, when the individual is frequently unresponsive. The postictal phase is the period immediately following the seizure. During this phase the patient is usually confused, disoriented, and drowsy and does not remember the seizure. If left alone, the patient may sleep deeply for several hours. A seizure may include some or all of the phases.

Additional clinical manifestations may include **automatisms**, **clonus**, **autonomic symptoms**, or **Todd's paralysis**. Automatisms are coordinated, involuntary motor activities that occur during the seizure. Examples include lip smacking, chewing, fidgeting, and pacing. Clonus is the descriptive term for the pattern of spasm with muscle rigidity followed by muscle relaxation. Autonomic symptoms occur in response to stimulation of the autonomic nervous system. These symptoms include pallor, sweating and increased secretions, epigastric discomfort, flushing, piloerection, or dilation of pupils. Todd's paralysis is a temporary, focal weakness or paralysis following a seizure that can last up to 24 hours.

Types of Seizures

Seizures are divided into two major classes: generalized and partial. Generalized seizures originate in all of the regions of the brain cortex. There is no aura or warning, but there is loss of consciousness. The seizure may last for a few seconds or several minutes.

- *Absence seizures* usually occur during childhood and last 5–10 seconds. If the seizure lasts for more than 10 seconds, there may be automatisms such as eye blinking or lip smacking. They frequently occur in clusters and can occur dozens or even hundreds of times per day. The electroencephalogram (EEG) will show a 3 Hz (cycles per minute) spike and wave pattern unique to this type of seizure.

- *Atypical absence seizures* usually begin before age five and are associated with mental retardation and a tendency for multiple seizure types. They last longer and are associated with muscle spasms.

- *Myoclonic seizures* are characterized by sudden, brief arm muscle contractions. Consciousness is usually not impaired.

- *Clonic seizures* demonstrate rhythmic, repetitive clonic movements of the arms, neck, and face. These movements are bilateral and symmetric.

- *Tonic-clonic* (formerly called grand mal) *seizures* are the most common type of generalized seizure. The seizure will progress through all of the seizure phases and last two to three minutes. Because of the suddenness of this type of seizure, injuries such as limb fractures, tongue biting, and head trauma can occur. These seizures can occur any time of the day or night, whether the patient is awake or not. Seizure frequency is highly variable.

- *Atonic seizures* (drop attacks) involve a sudden loss of muscle control, usually in the legs, that results in falling to the floor, increasing the possibility of injury.

- *Partial seizures* begin in a specific brain region, and consciousness is usually not impaired. The clinical manifestations depend on the region of the brain where the seizure focus starts. There may be an aura or warning signs.

- *Simple partial seizures* do not involve a loss of consciousness. Depending on the seizure focus, there may be motor, sensory, autonomic, or higher-level cognitive clinical manifestations.

- *Complex partial seizures* are the most common type of epileptic seizure in adults. Consciousness and awareness of surroundings is lost. Automatisms may occur. The seizure typically lasts one to three minutes.

Status Epilepticus

Status epilepticus is defined as either continuous seizures lasting more than five minutes or two or more different seizures with incomplete recovery of consciousness between them. The most common cause of status epilepticus is an abrupt stopping of antiepileptic drugs (AEDs). Clinically, status epilepticus can present with tonic, clonic, or tonic-clinic movements. It is a medical emergency since it is often accompanied by respiratory distress brought on by hypoxia or anoxia. Morbidity and mortality for status epilepticus is 20 percent. Subclinical status epilepticus is seen with partial seizures but can only be verified by EEG. It is estimated that between 50,000 and 100,000 patients experience status epilepticus each year in the United States.

During status epilepticus, cerebral metabolism is increased. Initially, compensatory mechanisms increase CBF and metabolism, increase autonomic activity with catecholamine release, and cause cardiovascular changes. These changes can lead to hyperglycemia, hypertension, increased cardiac output, increased central venous pressure, tachycardia, increased salivation, sweating, hyperpyrexia, vomiting, and incontinence. Hyperglycemia is due to the increased release of epinephrine and activation of hepatic gluconeogenesis. Hypertension is caused by the increased CBF in response to the increased metabolic demands for oxygen and glucose. Tachycardia is the result of the increased cardiac output. Hyperpyrexia is due to the excessive muscle activity and increased catecholamine release. Anaerobic muscle metabolism causes lactic acidosis. The elevated catecholamines and lactic acidosis promote cardiac dysrhythmias, and autonomic dysfunction causes excessive sweating and vomiting, leading to dehydration and electrolyte disturbances.

When metabolic demands can no longer be met, decompensation occurs. This causes decreased CBF, systemic hypotension, increased ICP, and failure of cerebral autoregulation. The patient develops both metabolic and respiratory acidosis due to the hypoxia, hypoglycemia from depleted energy stores, hyponatremia, and hyper- or hypokalemia. Lack of oxygen and glucose stimulates the production and release of glutamate, changing the electrical balance and causing calcium influx and the development of oxygen free-radicals. These changes make the brain cells electrically unstable and cause cellular injury. As the seizure activity continues, the patient may develop pulmonary edema, cardiac dysrhythmias, rhabdomyolysis, damage to striated muscle fibers, and acute intravascular coagulation. Prompt diagnosis and treatment are imperative since the duration of the seizure is a good predictor of outcomes.

Management

Status epilepticus (SE) is a medical emergency associated with significant morbidity and mortality (20 percent). Initial management includes providing the standard ABCs of life support, administering medications, finding and treating the underlying cause, and preventing and treating any complications. Establishing a patent airway with adequate ventilation is the first priority of treatment. This may require insertion of an artificial airway or intubation if the mouth cannot be opened. Oxygen supplementation or mechanical ventilation may be required. Protection from injury is the next priority. Loosening of constrictive clothing, turning the patient on his side, padding of immediate area, and not restraining the patient's movements will minimize or prevent injury. Medications need to be given to stop the seizure activity, if possible. For adults, the first choice is lorazepam (brand name: Ativan) or diazepam (brand name: Valium) for stopping the seizure. Then, medications to prevent seizure recurrence include phenytoin (brand name: Dilantin), fosphenytoin (brand name: Cerebyx), or phenobarbital (brand name: Luminal). Other agents used for refractory SE are pentobarbital (brand name: Nembutal), midazolam (brand name: Versed), and propofol (brand name: Diprivan). Close monitoring for hypotension and respiratory distress is necessary until seizure activity has ended. Once SE is terminated, diagnostic studies will be ordered to determine the underlying cause of the seizure activity.

Seizure Diagnostic Studies

- CT scan or MRI of the brain (to rule out tumors, hemorrhage)

- Routine laboratory studies (CBC, electrolytes, LFTs, toxicology screen)

- Skull x-rays (to rule out fractures, bone erosion, or separated sutures)

- EEG (if no seizure activity on standard test, may require 24-hour continuous test)

- Other: PET scan; SPECT scan

Note: CBC = complete blood count; CT = computed tomography; LFTs = liver function tests EEG = electroencephalography; MRI = magnetic resonance imaging; PET = positron emission tomography; SPECT = single proton emission computerized tomography.

Stroke

Cerebrovascular accident (CVA) is commonly known as stroke or "brain attack." Stroke is the fifth leading cause of death (130,000 per year) and the leading cause of adult disability in the United States. There are 795,000 new or recurrent strokes each year (CDC, 2015). There are two major types of stroke: hemorrhagic and ischemic. **Hemorrhagic stroke** is caused by a blood vessel that breaks and bleeds into the brain. Fifteen percent of strokes are hemorrhagic, but these account for more than 30 percent of all stroke deaths. **Ischemic stroke** is caused by a blood clot that blocks or plugs a blood vessel in the brain. About 85 percent of all strokes are ischemic. Transient ischemic attacks (TIAs) occur when the blood supply to the brain is briefly interrupted.

Etiology

Stroke is characterized by the onset of neurological deficits due to decreased oxygen supply that causes cellular changes, leading to the destruction of neural tissue and brain damage. Ischemic strokes are caused by either a thrombus or an embolus. A thrombus (blood clot) may develop secondary to atherosclerotic plaque blocking blood flow and stimulating platelet aggregation or hypercoagulable states (cancer, polycythemia). Emboli are small clot or plaque particles that travel distally and lodge in small blood vessels. Risk factors for emboli include atrial fibrillation, coronary artery disease, bacterial endocarditis, valvular heart disease, deep vein thrombosis, and air/fat embolism. A hemorrhagic stroke occurs when a cerebral blood vessel ruptures and blood leaks into the brain tissue. The major risk factor for hemorrhagic stroke is poorly controlled, long-standing hypertension. The most common sites of hemorrhagic stroke are basal ganglia (50 percent), thalamus (30 percent), cerebellum (10 percent), and pons (10 percent).

Pathophysiology

Stroke is the sudden development of focal neurological deficits caused by interruption of blood flow to brain tissue. Since the brain cannot store glucose or oxygen, it is dependent on a constant supply of these nutrients. Once cerebral blood flow is insufficient to maintain neuronal activity, ischemic injury occurs. The severity of neuronal injury in ischemic tissue is proportional to the reduced cerebral blood flow. In the infarction core area, brain tissue deprived of blood and oxygen dies. The area surrounding this core is known as the ischemic penumbra. The neurons of the ischemic penumbra become electrically silent but remain potentially viable for several hours. If the ischemia is not reversed, irreversible damage occurs. Severe brain tissue ischemia initiates a cascade of metabolic events, including increased lactic acid production, release of glutamate, and ATP depletion. In addition, sodium and calcium enter the cells, cytotoxic edema develops, and mitochondrial death occurs.

TABLE 9.14 *Inclusion and Exclusion Criteria for rtPA Use in Patients with Stroke*

Inclusion and Exclusion Characteristics of Patients with Ischemic Stroke Who Could Be Treated with rtPA within *3 Hours from Symptom Onset*	Inclusion and Exclusion Characteristics of Patients with Ischemic Stroke Who Could Be Treated with rtPA from *3 to 4.5 Hours from Symptom Onset*
Inclusion Criteria	**Inclusion Criteria**
• Diagnosis of ischemic stroke causing measurable neurologic deficit • Onset of symptoms <3 hours before beginning treatment • Age ≥18 years	• Diagnosis of ischemic stroke causing measurable neurologic deficit • Onset of symptoms 3 to 4.5 hours before beginning treatment

TABLE 9.14 *Inclusion and Exclusion Criteria for rtPA Use in Patients with Stroke (continued)*

Exclusion Criteria	Exclusion Criteria
• Head trauma or prior stroke in previous 3 months • Symptoms suggest subarachnoid hemorrhage • Arterial puncture at noncompressible site in previous 7 days • History of previous intracranial hemorrhage • Elevated blood pressure (systolic >185 mm Hg or diastolic >110 mm Hg) • Evidence of active bleeding on examination • Acute bleeding diathesis, including but not limited to — Platelet count <100,000/mm³ — Heparin received within 48 hours, resulting in an aPTT greater than the upper limit of normal — Current use of anticoagulant with INR >1.7 or PT >15 seconds • Blood glucose concentration <50 mg/dL (2.7 mmol/L) • CT demonstrates multilobar infarction (hypodensity >1/3 cerebral hemisphere)	• Age >80 years • Severe stroke (NIHSS >25) • Taking an oral anticoagulant regardless of INR • History of both diabetes and prior ischemic stroke
Relative Exclusion Criteria Recent experience suggests that under some circumstances—with careful consideration and weighing of risk to benefit—patients may receive fibrinolytic therapy despite 1 or more relative contraindications. Consider risk to benefit of rtPA administration carefully if any 1 of these relative contraindications is present: • Only minor or rapidly improving stroke symptoms (clearing spontaneously) • Seizure at onset with postictal residual neurologic impairments • Major surgery or serious trauma within previous 14 days	**Notes** • The checklist includes some U.S. FDA-approved indications and contraindications for administration of rtPA for acute ischemic stroke. Recent AHA/ASA guideline revisions may differ slightly from FDA criteria. A physician with expertise in acute stroke care may modify this list. • Onset time is either witnessed or last known normal. • In patients without recent use of oral anticoagulants or heparin, treatment with rtPA can be initiated before availability of coagulation study results but should be discontinued if INR is >1.7 or PT is elevated by local laboratory standards.

TABLE 9.14 *Inclusion and Exclusion Criteria for rtPA Use in Patients with Stroke* *(continued)*

• Recent gastrointestinal or urinary tract hemorrhage (within previous 21 days) • Recent acute myocardial infarction (within previous 3 months)	• In patients without a history of thrombocytopenia, treatment with rtPA can be initiated before availability of platelet count but should be discontinued if platelet count is <100,000/mm^3.
Abbreviations: aPPT, activated partial thromboplastin time; INR, international normalized ratio; PT, prothrombin time; rtPA, recombinant tissue plasminogen activator	**Abbreviations:** FDA, Food and Drug Administration; INR, international normalized ratio; NIHSS, National Institutes of Health Stroke Scale; PT, prothrombin time; rtPA, recombinant tissue plasminogen activator

Clinical Manifestations

Symptoms of stroke are sudden: numbness or weakness of the face, arm, or leg (especially on one side of the body); confusion, trouble speaking or understanding speech; trouble seeing in one or both eyes; trouble walking, dizziness, or loss of balance or coordination; or severe headache with no known cause.

Diagnostic Studies

When stroke is suspected, prompt (within three hours of symptom onset), accurate diagnosis and treatment are necessary to minimize brain tissue damage. Diagnosis includes a medical history and a physical examination, including neurological examination, to evaluate the level of consciousness, sensation, and function (visual, motor, language) and determine the cause, location, and extent of the stroke. A noncontrast CT scan is performed as soon as possible. CT scanning is widely available, requires 15 minutes or less to complete, can be evaluated quickly, and differentiates between ischemic and hemorrhagic stroke. Treatment for ischemic stroke can save brain tissue rapidly. Laboratory tests commonly ordered include complete blood count (CBC), electrolytes, renal panel, coagulation panel, liver function studies, and others depending on presenting symptoms.

Treatment

Emergency department treatment of acute ischemic stroke includes assessment for conditions that mimic stroke, thrombolytic therapy, and treatment of complications. Acute stroke therapies try to stop a stroke while it is happening by quickly dissolving the blood clot causing an ischemic stroke or by stopping the bleeding of a hemorrhagic stroke. Hemorrhagic stroke treatment and management was discussed with brain injuries. Other conditions requiring rapid evaluation are hypoglycemia, toxic or metabolic disorders, migraines, brain tumors, and seizures. Thrombolytic therapy (rtPA) is the most common treatment for ischemic stroke in selected patients. Treatment must be completed within three hours of symptom onset, and patients must meet inclusion/exclusion criteria. Before starting rtPA, two peripheral IV catheters are inserted, and all invasive procedures are completed. All anti-thrombotics are withheld for 24 hours to prevent bleeding complications.

There are two schools of thought governing administration of rtPA therapy. The first approach is to give 0.9 mg/kg (maximum of 90 mg) with 10 percent of the total dose as an initial intravenous bolus over 1 minute, followed by the remaining 90 percent over 60 minutes. The second approach is to determine rtPA dose by the patient's weight:

- More than 67 kg: 15 mg IV bolus over 1–2 minutes, then 50 mg over 30 minutes, then 35 mg over next 60 minutes = 100 mg total dose infused over 1.5 hours.

- Less than 67 kg: 15 mg IV bolus over 1–2 minutes, then 0.75 mg/kg (maximum 50 mg) over 30 minutes, then 0.5 mg/kg (maximum 35 mg) over the next 60 minutes = 100 mg total dose infused over 1.5 hours.

Post-Treatment Management

After initial treatment in the ED, the patient will be admitted to the intensive care unit (ICU) for frequent monitoring of complication from either the stroke or treatment. There is an increased risk of conversion from an ischemic stroke to a hemorrhagic stroke. Vital signs and neurologic checks are done every 15 to 30 minutes for 6 to 12 hours. Neurological deterioration needs to be communicated immediately and the patient prepared for a STAT CT scan to rule out hemorrhage. Blood pressure monitoring and management vary depending on treatment modalities, and the patient may require vasoactive medications. The cerebral edema that is a result of the ischemia may require invasive monitoring or even surgery. Blood glucose levels require close monitoring and management to prevent hyperglycemia. Secondary complications include decreased airway maintenance, risk for aspiration, decreased level of consciousness, cranial nerve deficits, and deep vein thrombus.

Space Occupying Lesions

Primary brain tumors are classified by cell type: glioma, meningioma, pituitary adenoma, acoustic neuroma, or metastatic tumor. Metastatic brain tumors are of the cell type of the primary tumor. Tumors may be invasive and cause pressure on the intracranial structures, resulting in focal deficits (paralysis, paresthesia, visual deficits) depending on location. Alternatively, tumors may cause intracranial hypertension, resulting in papilledema, vomiting, seizures, headache, and changes in LOC and behavior. Tumors are diagnosed with imaging, EEG, and biopsy. Treatment depends on the tumor's size, location, and etiology but may include administration of glucocorticoids to reduce brain edema; maintaining airway and oxygenation; preparation for surgery, radiation, or chemotherapy; and monitoring for complications such as fluid and electrolyte imbalance, brain ischemia, hydrocephalus, and seizures.

Review Questions

1. Examining a patient for cranial nerve dysfunction, the nurse is attempting to assess extraocular movement (EOM) through the six cardinal fields. Which nerve is **not** assessed by this test?

   A. II optic

   B. III oculomotor

   C. VI abducens

   D. IV trochlear

2. The nurse is assessing a new admission who is a 45-year-old female with new diagnosis of SAH. She is complaining of a headache, neck stiffness, and n/v. Her VS are 210/106; HR 92; RR 18. You anticipate that interventions for your patient would **not** include

   A. placement of an arterial line for hemodynamic monitoring.

   B. tight blood pressure control of 120–150 mm Hg.

   C. rapid reduction in BP.

   D. cardiac monitoring for ECG changes.

3. Cerebral vasospasm is a common complication of SAH causing reduced blood flow to vital brain tissue. Which of these is an appropriate management technique?

   A. hemoconcentration

   B. administration of lipid-soluble calcium channel blocker Nimodipine

   C. carotid Doppler exams

   D. CVP of 2–6 mm Hg

4. The nurse is assessing a 25-year-old male who was in a motorcycle crash and sustained a traumatic brain injury by blunt trauma from being ejected more than 15 feet from his bike. On your assessment, you notice he is becoming more lethargic and is not answering questions. Given his mechanism of injury, which of these can be excluded as a possible cause of his mental status change?

   A. subdural hematoma

   B. shear axonal injury

   C. cerebral infarction

   D. vasogenic edema

5. Your patient has been diagnosed with Fisher Grade IV SAH and has additionally developed noncommunicating hydrocephalus with increased ICP. Which of these interventions will most likely be beneficial for this patient?

   A. administration of an osmotic diuretic (mannitol)

   B. insertion of a ventriculostomy

   C. administration of corticosteroids

   D. hyponatremia

6. Symptoms of bradycardia, increased blood pressure, and respiratory abnormalities (Cushing's triad) would **not** be associated with which of these?

   A. increasing ICP

   B. uncal herniation

   C. cerebral vasospasm

   D. effects of secondary brain injury

7. The nurse cares for a 36-year-old male who fell 18 feet from a ladder and has suffered what is suspected to be a complete cord transaction at level of C5–6. The potential complications of this injury in the acute phase would **not** include

   A. orthostatic hypotension.

   B. bradycardia.

   C. respiratory insufficiency.

   D. hyperreflexia.

8. A 56-year-old male is admitted to your unit with complaints of bilateral lower-extremity weakness that started approximately 24 hours ago and has rapidly progressed in an ascending manner. He states he is having some shortness of breath, and you note that his blood pressure and HR are both elevated. Which of conditions most likely fits this symptomatology?

   A. myasthenia gravis

   B. Guillain-Barré syndrome

   C. cauda equina syndrome

   D. acute CVA

9. Priority nursing intervention in a patient who is in status epilepticus would **not** include

   A. establishing and/or maintaining a patent airway.

   B. administration of a benzodiazepine.

   C. padding of immediate area for safety.

   D. urgent CT scan.

10. A 62-year-old patient who presented with left-sided weakness and slurred speech, has just returned from stat CT scan. The reading of the CT scan is negative for any bleeding or acute process with acute CVA suspected, and the patient may be a candidate for tPA therapy. Which of these criteria would exclude him from being a candidate for tPA therapy?

    A. symptom onset of 5+ hours

    B. blood pressure of 165/88

    C. age of 62

    D. negative CT scan

Review Answers and Explanations

1. A

II optic is tested for visual acuity by a chart of numbers/letters (Snellen chart). Checking EOMs will assess oculomotor, abducens, and trochlear nerves.

2. C

Do not lower blood pressure rapidly, because it will reduce cerebral perfusion and may cause ischemia to areas already compressed by the injury. Tight control of blood pressure (B) using titratable agents that will not cause precipitous drops in blood pressure is best. Monitoring with an invasive pressure line gives the most accurate readings for titration (A). Additionally, cardiac monitoring is needed, as ECG changes and dysrhythmias are common in SAH (D).

3. B

Nimodipine is able to cross the blood-brain barrier due to its lipid solubility and prevents vessel wall spasm. It is thought to be neuroprotective and is used as part of the management in SAH patients. Hemodilution is used in SAH as part of triple H therapy with a goal Hct of approximately 30. Additionally, the CVP goal for hemodilution is 10–12 mm Hg. TCDs (C) are used regularly to assess for vasospasm, not carotid Dopplers.

4. C

Cerebral infarction is not a likely cause considering the mechanism and known complications of TBI. After a mechanism with rapid acceleration and deceleration forces, common injuries that occur include SDH (A) as well as axonal injury (B). Secondary injury also includes vasogenic edema (D).

5. B

After insertion of a ventriculostomy, temporarily drain CSF and effectively decrease ICP secondary to ventricular obstruction. Osmotic diuretics (A) and corticosteroids (C) will not be effective in this type of hydrocephalus, and urgent drainage of CSF is likely to be the only solution.

6. C

If the patient were experiencing cerebral vasospasm, you would observe more changes in the patient's mental status, secondary to tissue ischemia, due to spasm of cerebral arteries and reduction of blood flow. The other choices relate to the Monroe-Kellie doctrine of fixed space with fixed pressures, and all deal with an increase in ICP and pressure on the brain stem.

7. D

Hyperreflexia is not seen in the acute phase. You will observe flaccidity for the first one to two weeks; then the patient will begin to become spastic with hyperreflexia. During neurogenic shock, with loss of sympathetic tone and vasodilatation, the result is bradycardia (B) and hypotension (A). Respiratory insufficiency (C) must also be considered a risk with cervical injury.

8. B

When an individual has Guillain-Barré syndrome, he will experience rapidly ascending deficits that begin with the lower extremities and the peripheral nerves. Deficits then quickly move more central and may eventually affect the respiratory muscles. If this happens, the result will be respiratory depression; autonomic dysfunction may also occur as it ascends. The other syndromes listed do not present in this manner.

9. D

An urgent CT scan for this patient is not the priority and will be part of the workup after the patient has been stabilized and the seizure has broken. Initial management of a status patient includes the ABCs and rapid treatment of the seizure with benzodiazepines and antiseizure drugs (B). Padding of the patient's area (C) must be done for safety, as restricting limbs is not recommended and may potentially hurt the patient.

10. A

The tPA window in most facilities is now 4.5 hours from last known well status. It is extremely important to obtain the time of "last known well" when evaluating a patient for tPA therapy. Once beyond this window, tPA is contraindicated, and the patient may then become a candidate for interventional radiology therapies such as intra-arterial tPA.

The Gastrointestinal System

OVERVIEW OF THE GASTROINTESTINAL SYSTEM

Approximately 6 percent of the questions on the CCRN exam cover the gastrointestinal (GI) system.

The GI system is basically composed of a long tube that extends from the mouth to the anus and accessory organs of digestion (the liver, gallbladder, and pancreas). The primary purpose of the GI system is to break down ingested food and provide the body with nutrients, while eliminating waste. The gastrointestinal wall is composed of four layers: serosa, muscularis, submucosa, and mucosa. The outer connective tissue layer, called the serosa, secretes mucus to prevent friction with visceral organs of the abdomen. The muscularis is a muscular layer that provides the rhythmic contraction needed to break down food. The submucosa contains connective tissue, elastic fibers, blood vessels, lymphatic vessels, and the enteric autonomic nervous system. The innermost layer, the mucosa, absorbs nutrients and fluids and receives the majority of the blood supply. In the small intestine, this innermost layer is referred to as the microvilli. In times of critical illness, the mucosa may erode due to trauma, hypoperfusion, stress, medications, or surgery. The erosion may lead to bleeding or infection.

Components

The organs that make up the GI tract are the mouth, esophagus, stomach, small intestine, large intestine, rectum, and anus. Accessory organs assisting with digestion are the liver, gallbladder, and pancreas (see figure 10.1).

Primary Functions

The functions of the digestive system are ingestion and propulsion of food, secretion of digestive juices, mechanical and chemical digestion, absorption of digested food, and elimination of waste products through bowel movements. The accessory organs secrete substances necessary for digestion to occur. Secretions from the liver, gallbladder, and pancreas are delivered to the second portion of the duodenum through ducts. The liver produces bile, which is stored between meals in the gallbladder. The bile is released in response to ingestion of fats. The pancreas releases enzymes that assist in digestion of carbohydrates, proteins, and fats.

FIGURE 10.1 *Human Digestive Tract*

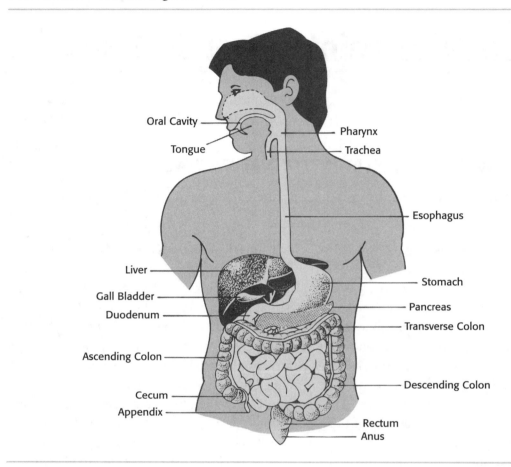

ANATOMY AND PHYSIOLOGY

Organs of the Gastrointestinal Tract

- **Mouth:** Food is chewed and mixed with saliva in the mouth. Salivary glands secrete salivary amylase, which digests carbohydrates to disaccharides. Saliva production is controlled by the sympathetic and parasympathetic nervous system but not controlled by hormones. The pH of saliva is 7.4, which helps to neutralize acids and prevent tooth decay. Saliva production is about 1,000 mL in 24 hours.

- **Esophagus:** The upper third of the esophagus has striated *voluntary* muscle, the middle third has striated and smooth muscle, and the lower third has only smooth muscle. The upper third is fully voluntary, where the contractions of the middle and lower third of the esophagus are involuntary. The vagus nerve innervates the esophagus. Swallowing occurs in the esophagus as food is propelled to the stomach. The peristaltic action of sequential contraction and relaxation is mediated by the swallowing center in the brain. Sphincters at the upper and lower end of the esophagus prevent regurgitation.

- **Stomach:** Food is stored in the stomach during eating as digestive enzymes partially digest and move the partially digested food, called chyme, into the duodenum. The upper sphincter of the stomach between the stomach and esophagus is called the cardiac sphincter, also known as the gastroesophageal (GE) junction. The lower sphincter is known as the pyloric sphincter, which relaxes to expel food into the duodenum. The stomach is divided into the fundus, body, and antrum.

The stomach is relatively sterile of bacteria due to acid secretion. The contents of the stomach are acidic secondary to the presence of hydrochloric acid (HCl). Hydrochloric acid is secreted by the parietal cells in the stomach and involves acetylcholine, gastrin, and histamine. HCl secretion can be blocked by certain medications: histamine receptors (H2-blockers) and proton pump inhibitors (PPIs) such as famotidine and omeprazole, respectively.

The main digestive enzyme in the stomach is pepsin, which is secreted by the chief cells of the stomach. Pepsin is originally secreted as a zymogen (pepsinogen), which is an inactive form of the enzyme. When the pepsinogen is exposed to the acidic lumen of the stomach, the HCl cleaves the pepsinogen into the active enzyme.

The stomach also synthesizes intrinsic factor, which is necessary for the absorption of vitamin B12 in the ileum of the small intestine. Gastric ulcers may involve a gram-negative bacteria, *Helicobacter pylori*, which damages the gastric mucosa. Some medications, like aspirin and ibuprofen, can damage the gastric mucosa and cause ulcerations.

- **Small Intestine:** The small intestine is about 20 feet long and consists of three segments: the duodenum, jejunum, and ileum. The ileocecal valve controls the flow of digested food from the ileum into the large intestine and prevents reflux into the small intestine. Major nutrients are absorbed by the small intestine villi and microvilli, which cover numerous intestinal folds, creating a mucosal surface known as the brush border. The brush border contains enzymes that break down disaccharides and dipeptides, because by the time the chyme reaches the small intestine, enzymes from other parts of the GI tract have broken down the nutrients to the level of disaccharides and dipeptides, but these cannot be absorbed. The disaccharidases (e.g., maltase and lactase) and dipeptidases need to be broken down into monosaccharides (e.g., glucose) and amino acids to be absorbed.

- **Large Intestine:** The large intestine contains mucus-secreting goblet cells and is about six feet long. It consists of the cecum, appendix, colon (ascending, transverse, descending, and sigmoid), rectum, and anus. Water reabsorption is the primary function of the large intestine. The large intestine is sterile at birth but becomes colonized with *Escherichia coli*, *Clostridium welchii*, and *Streptococcus* bacteria within a few hours. Intestinal bacteria help to metabolize bile salts and synthesize vitamins and drugs.

Accessory Organs

- **Liver:** The liver, the largest organ in the body, is located under the right diaphragm in the right upper quadrant. The liver secretes bile, excretes bilirubin, metabolizes fats, serves to detoxify drugs (e.g., Tylenol and narcotics), converts glycogen to glucose during times of fasting, stores vitamins and nutrients, synthesizes the majority of the proteins that maintain oncotic pressure (e.g., albumin), synthesizes the majority of clotting factors that are dependent on vitamin K, and metabolizes ammonia (a breakdown product of protein metabolism in the GI tract) to urea.

- **Gallbladder:** Located under the liver in the right upper quadrant, the gallbladder holds about 90 mL of bile. Within 30 minutes of an individual eating fat, bile is secreted into the duodenum from the gallbladder via the action of a hormone called cholecystokinin (CCK).

- **Pancreas:** This organ is located behind the stomach with its head in the curve of the duodenum and its tail touching the spleen in the left upper quadrant. The exocrine (secretion into ducts, external to the vascular system) pancreas secretes enzymes and alkaline fluids that assist with digestion. The endocrine (secretion into the blood) pancreas secretes insulin and glucagon.

NURSING ASSESSMENT

History

Gather information about past and present symptoms. A thorough history can assist with diagnosis and treatment. Many people with GI disturbances have a functional disorder with no anatomic abnormality. Elicit information about appetite, nausea, vomiting, bowel elimination, and pain. Ask about any previous abdominal surgeries or changes in weight. A weight gain of 2.2 pounds or 1 kg is equal to 1 liter of fluid. Include family history of colon cancer, ulcer disease, or inflammatory bowel disorders. Include social history of any tobacco, drug, or alcohol use along with work or family stress. Facilitation or open-ended questions should be used to help the patient report symptoms through spontaneous associations.

Physical Assessment

Height, weight, frame size, and body mass index (BMI) are measures to provide information about nutritional status and body mass. To determine BMI, divide the patient's weight in kilograms by the height in meters squared. Desirable BMI range is 20–25, obesity is greater than 30, and underweight is less than 17.5. Assess the mouth for symmetry, color, and hydration status. Palpate the patient's lips, gingivae, and buccal mucosa. Inspect for any loose teeth or masses. Direct physical assessment of the abdomen begins by observation of the skin and inspection. Note any asymmetry, scars, or bruising. Ask the patient to take a deep breath and hold it to determine contour and palpate organs of the abdominal cavity. A bluish periumbilical discoloration, *Cullen's sign,* suggests intraabdominal bleeding. Bruising in the lower abdomen and flank area, *Grey-Turner's sign,* indicates retroperitoneal hemorrhage. Recent striae are pink or blue, but Cushing disease striae remain purple. Scars could indicate possible abdominal adhesions.

Auscultate bowel sounds and vascular sounds for one to two minutes or more. Loud bowel sounds known as borborygmi ("growling stomach") indicate hunger. High-pitched bowel sounds may indicate intestinal fluid or air under pressure as with an intestinal obstruction. Decreased or absent bowel sounds indicate obstruction or paralytic ileus. Auscultate with the bell of the stethoscope for any bruits or venous hums.

Percussion is used to assess the size of the organs and presence of fluid (ascites) or air. Tympany is the most common sound due to air in the stomach and intestine. Dullness is heard over organs and solid masses. A distended bladder produces dullness above the symphysis pubis. Mark the liver span after percussion upward along the midclavicular line of the left upper quadrant. A span of more than 2–3 cm below the costal margin indicates an enlarged liver or downward displacement from the lungs as with emphysema. Percuss downward over the lungs on the right to determine the upper border of the liver and mark it with a pen. The upper border is usually at the 5th–7th intercostal space. A larger span indicates liver enlargement. Usual liver span is 6–12 cm, but this is dependent on the size of the patient. Percuss the spleen at the midaxillary line of the left upper quadrant.

Palpation with the palm or bimanually (one hand on the other) is used to detect muscle spasm, masses, fluid, and any tenderness. Rigidity or boardlike hardness is indicative of peritonitis or internal bleeding. Attempt to palpate the gallbladder below the liver margin. A healthy gallbladder will not be palpable. If there is gallbladder disease, the patient may halt inspiration due to pain—Murphy's sign. The spleen is usually not palpable. The right kidney is more frequently palpable than the left. Aortic pulsations may be palpated to the left of the midline and should be in the anterior direction. A prominent pulsation indicates aortic aneurym. Bladder distension can be felt as a smooth, round, tense mass above the pubic bone. Abdominal reflexes can be elicited by stroking the abdomen. Rebound tenderness (Blumberg sign) is pain with sudden removal of the hand after deep palpation and indicates peritonitis.

TABLE 10.1 *Laboratory and Diagnostic Studies*

Laboratory Studies	Description	Interpretation/ Nursing Responsibilities
Liver function tests (LFTs) Aspartate aminotranspeptidase (AST, formerly SGOT) Normal result = <40 units/L Alanine transaminase (ALT, formerly SGPT) Normal result = <40 units/L Lactate dehydrogenase enzyme (LDH) Normal result = 100–330 units/L	Elevations indicate liver disease (hepatitis) or damage to cardiac muscle.	Drugs may increase liver enzymes due to hepatocellular damage. Obtain a list of medications the patient is taking.
Total bilirubin Normal result = <1.9 mg/dL Direct bilirubin (conjugated) Normal result = <0.3 mg/dL Indirect bilirubin (unconjugated) Normal result = <1.9 mg/dL	Bilirubin is a breakdown product of hemoglobin. Used to assess hepatobiliary disease. Direct bilirubin is primarily used as a marker for hepatobiliary obstruction. These tests describe the ability of the liver to conjugate bilirubin.	Elevated in obstructive jaundice.
Urinary bilirubin Normal result = negative Urine urobilinogen Normal result = <17 mcmol/L Fecal urobilinogen Normal result = 30–220 mg/100g of stool	Colorless degradation product of bilirubin found in urine and feces. The absence of urobilinogen in urine in a jaundiced patient indicates complete biliary obstruction.	Decreased fecal urobilinogen will cause clay-colored stools.
Alkaline prosphatase Normal result = 44–147 units/L	Found in liver, biliary tract, bone, intestine, and placenta.	Elevated in gallbladder disease.
Prothrombin time (PT) Normal result = 11–13 seconds	Indicator of the liver's ability to manufacture coagulation factors.	May be altered in liver disease and biliary obstruction.
Albumin Normal result = 3.4–5.4 g/dL	Plasma-binding protein synthesized by the liver.	Low in liver disease.

TABLE 10.1 *Laboratory and Diagnostic Studies (continued)*

Laboratory Studies	Description	Interpretation/ Nursing Responsibilities
Acute hepatitis panel		Observe standard and transmission-based precautions
Hepatitis A antibody (anti-HAV) Normal result = negative	IgM antibodies detect acute hepatitis A infection within 1 week. Persist for 6 months. IgG develops 4 weeks after IgM and persists for years.	Reduce contact with blood or blood-containing secretions
Hepatitis B, antigen and antibody (HbeAg, HbeAb, HbcAb, HbsAb, HbsAg) Normal result = negative	IgM antibodies against hepatitis B virus core detected 6–8 weeks after acute hepatitis B infection. IgG antibodies usually indicate acute or previous exposure.	Dispose of used needles properly Use needleless access device if available
Hepatitis C antibody (anti-HCV) Normal result = negative	Indicates past or present infection with hepatitis C.	
Hepatitis D (delta agent)	Hepatitis B delta agent is only seen in co-infected HBsAg-positive patients.	
Pancreatic enzymes		Elevated in pancreatitis.
Amylase Normal result = 23–140 units/L	Enzyme that degrades carbohydrates.	
Lipase Normal result = <160 units/L	Enzyme that degrades fatty acids. Remains elevated 7–10 days after acute pancreatitis.	

Diagnostic Studies	Description	Interpretation
Radiology	X-rays can penetrate dense tissues. Contrast of radiopaque substance may be used to visualize upper and lower bowel.	Air appears black, bone appears white, and soft tissue appears gray. Contraindicated in pregnancy. Gather information about allergies to contrast media, iodine, or shellfish.
Angiography	X-ray of vascular beds.	
Ultrasound	Visual inspection of soft tissues by using sound waves.	Bowel cleansing or clear liquids may be ordered prior to test.
Computed tomography (CT)	Noninvasive x-ray producing cross-sectional images.	Requires patient to lie still. May require sedation.

TABLE 10.1 *Laboratory and Diagnostic Studies (continued)*

Endoscopy	Uses fiberoptic instrument to visualize internal organs and tissues.	Biopsy may be taken.
Magnetic resonance imaging (MRI)	Uses magnetic imaging sources without radiation.	Ensure patient has no metal implants or jewelry on prior to test.
Biopsy	Invasive procedure resulting in collection of tissues.	

ALTERATIONS OF THE GASTROINTESTINAL SYSTEM

Acute Abdominal Trauma

Abdominal trauma accounts for 15 percent of trauma deaths. Intra-abdominal trauma may involve more than one organ system injury. Rib fracture may result in laceration or penetration of abdominal organs. The liver is the most commonly injured organ in abdominal trauma.

Common Causes

Half of all cases of acute abdominal trauma are due to motor vehicle crashes (MVCs). Wearing seat belts properly could decrease abdominal trauma during accidents. Head and chest injuries may accompany abdominal injuries. Penetrating injuries can occur from guns or knives. Blunt trauma can occur from a fall, an assault, or contact sports. Shearing, crushing, or compressing forces may rupture the bowel or other abdominal organs. Perforation of the stomach or bowel may lead to peritonitis and sepsis.

Clinical Manifestations

- Injuries to the **diaphragm**—decreased breath sounds or acute chest pain
- Injuries to the **esophagus**—pain at the site of perforation, fever, difficulty or pain with swallowing, or cervical tenderness
- Injury to the **stomach**—epigastric pain or tenderness, signs of peritonitis, or bloody gastric drainage
- Injury to the **liver**—persistent hypotension (due to massive hemorrhage) despite adequate fluid resuscitation and guarding over the right upper quadrant
- Injury to the **spleen**—hypotension (due to massive hemorrhage), tachycardia, shortness of breath
- Injury to the **pancreas**—epigastric pain, nausea, vomiting, ileus

- Injury to **small intestine**—mild abdominal pain, peritoneal irritation, fever, jaundice, intestinal obstruction ileus

- Injury to **large intestine**—pain, muscle rigidity, blood on rectal exam

Management

Initial management of abdominal trauma follows the ABCs of resuscitation. Titrate intravenous fluids to maintain a systolic pressure of 100 mm Hg and mean arterial pressure >60 mm Hg. Life-threatening injuries require immediate treatment and stabilization. Infusion of blood products may be needed. The patient is kept NPO if surgical intervention is anticipated. Assess and provide adequate pain control. Emotional support for the patient and family are key nursing interventions. Careful assessment by the nurse is vital as the patient is prepared for surgery. More teaching will be required postoperatively. Discharge teaching may involve wound and/or ostomy care.

Acute GI Hemorrhage

Gastrointestinal bleeding is a common critical care problem. Both upper and lower GI bleeds can be arterial in origin, depending on the etiology. Upper GI bleeds may present with hematemesis, nausea, and melena. They generally will present in patients with hepatic cirrhosis because of dilation of esophageal varices. If the bleeding is brisk, then instead of melena, those with upper GI bleeds may present with bright red blood per rectum. Lower GI bleeds may be arterial in origin, particularly if there is an arterio-venous malformation (AVM). About 80 percent of GI hemorrhage stops without intervention, but recurrent bleeding can become a life-threatening emergency.

Common Causes

The most frequent cause of GI bleeding is peptic ulcers. Other common causes are ruptured esophageal or gastric varices, ruptured esophageal ulcers, malignancy, esophageal perforation, tears of the esophageal mucosa, and a long history of excessive alcohol abuse. Chronic gastritis and bulimia can erode the gastric mucosa. Certain nonsteroidal anti-inflammatory medications (NSAIDs) like ibuprofen, naproxen, and aspirin can also cause GI bleeding. Anticoagulants may predispose patients to GI bleed when patients are supratherapeutic on their dosage. Any previous history of GI bleed should be determined.

Clinical Manifestations

Suspect an upper GI bleed if the patient presents with abdominal or chest pain, nausea, bloody or coffee ground emesis, vomiting, dark tarry stools, occult blood, or change in level of consciousness.

Management

Tests that the physician will likely order may include CBC, chemistry panel, activated partial thromboplastin time, protime (with INR), hepatic enzyme panel (total bilirubin, direct bilirubin, alkaline phosphatase, gamma glutamyl transferase, AST, ALT, total protein, and albumin), amylase, lipase, blood type, and cross-match. Focus on restoring circulating volume and preventing complications of hypovolemia by inserting two large-bore intravenous access lines. Emphasis should be on rapid restoration of circulating volume with either crystalloids or packed cells based on the availability of cross-matched blood. Position the patient to prevent aspiration with the head of the bed elevated and turn the patient to his side. Give supplemental oxygen and monitor the cardiac rhythm. Anticipate further treatment of insertion of nasogastric tube and administration of vitamin K or vasoactive medication (e.g., vasopressin or norepinephrine).

Patients with esophageal varices and no previous history of variceal hemorrhage should be treated with beta-adrenergic blockers unless contraindicated. Insert an indwelling catheter and administer pain medication. Endoscopic therapy has replaced previous treatments with balloon tamponade therapy. Generally, octreotide or somatostatin will be initiated on the first confirmed evidence of a GI bleed. This medication decreases the splenic blood flow, thereby helping decrease the amount of blood lost. Patients should also be started on a proton pump inhibitor twice a day. Other medications that may be used, but are not first line, are antacids and sucralfate. Patient will require bed rest and, possibly, modification of diet. Small meals at frequent intervals help to avoid stimulation of gastric acid that occurs when the stomach is empty. Bland low-fiber foods are suggested, although there is no direct evidence to suggest that these are superior to other diets. However, avoidance of alcohol, caffeine, and tobacco may decrease discomfort. Identification and elimination of stressors are important teaching components for the nurse when a patient has peptic ulcer disease.

As with many GI disturbances, nutritional support may be needed in the form of a total enteral nutrition (TEN) by way of a gastrostomy, postpyloric feeding tube, or jejunostomy tube. When the patient cannot be fed orally or by tube, then total parenteral nutrition (TPN) or peripheral venous nutrition (PVN) may be indicated. Clinical indications for TPN or PVN are malabsorptive syndromes like short-bowel syndrome, motility disorders like ileus, intestinal obstruction, perioperative nutrition for severe malnutrition, and low-flow states. The goal of supplemental nutrition is to meet nutritional requirements.

Bowel Infarction, Obstruction, Perforation

Blockage of the GI tract can occur at any level from the esophagus to the intestine. Obstruction of the small intestine is a common surgical complication due to adhesions from scar tissue in postoperative patients.

Common Causes

Esophageal obstruction is primarily the result of neoplasm. Risk factors are heavy alcohol intake and smoking. Intestinal obstruction can occur due to tumors, adhesions, or foreign bodies. Occlusion of blood supply to the mesentery results in tissue death and cellular death of the bowel. Other causes of obstruction are Schatzki ring, achalasia, esophageal spasm, or fibrosis from Crohn's disease (less common). If not treated for a long period of time, the patient may experience weight loss and possibly even visceral perforation, as the intraluminal pressure increases beyond the capacity of the intestine. Multiple medications, like anticholinergics and opioids, can reduce gastric motility, leading to a paralytic ileus. Any handling of the bowel during surgery can result in the postoperative complication of paralytic ileus, as well.

Clinical Manifestations

Esophageal manifestations are usually asymptomatic until the malignancy is large enough to cause problems with swallowing. Signs and symptoms of malnutrition occur as a result of decreased intake. Intestinal obstruction results in increased bacterial growth due to trapped fluid. Vomiting is present if the obstruction is above the jejunum. Distention occurs with lower GI obstruction. Pain and abdominal cramping increase as peristaltic action attempts to move the obstruction. Signs and symptoms of hypovolemia may result. Electrolyte and chemistry studies reveal inflammation with elevations in BUN, creatinine, sodium, and serum amylase. Leukocytosis is common with WBC elevation from 15,000–25,000.

Management

On evidence of obstruction or GI bleed, patients should be made NPO, a nasogatric tube (NGT) should be placed to intermittent suction, laboratory tests should be ordered as indicated above, and plain abdominal films should be obtained in the supine upright and decubitus positions to look for free air. If there is evidence of free air or complete small bowel obstruction, surgical exploration and correction may be necessary. Maintenance of support with fluids and electrolyte balance may be necessary until the obstruction is resolved. A pulmonary artery catheter may be inserted to determine fluid needs. An indwelling Foley catheter is inserted to measure hourly output. Broad-spectrum antibiotics may be given if peritonitis develops. Continual nursing assessment and pain management is needed. Teaching and patient support are key nursing interventions.

GI Surgeries

Types of gastrointestinal procedures vary depending on the patient's problem. Patients with obstruction, cancer, trauma, or hemorrhage may require surgical interventions. Approximately 10 to 50 percent of patients who have undergone gastric resection experience some form of dumping syndrome postoperatively. Nutritional deficiencies may result in the inability of the GI tract to absorb needed vitamins and minerals. Total gastrectomy results in a lack of intrinsic factor absorption, thus requiring B12 injections for life to prevent pernicious anemia.

Gastric Surgeries

- **Total gastrectomy:** Complete excision of the stomach with esophageal-jejunal anastomosis
- **Subtotal or partial gastrectomy:** Removal of a portion of the stomach
  - Billroth I procedure: Gastric remnant anastomosed to the duodenum
  - Billroth II procedure: Gastric remnant anastomosed to the jejunum
- **Gastrostomy:** Rectangular stomach flap created into abdominal stoma; used for intermittent tube feedings

Hernia Surgeries

- **Herniorrhaphy:** Surgical repair of a hernia with suturing of the abdominal wall
- **Hernioplasty:** Reconstructive hernia repair with mesh for reinforcement

Bowel Surgeries

- **Appendectomy:** Excision of the vermiform appendix
- **Bowel resection:** Segmental excision of small and/or large bowel with varied approaches

Laparoscopic Surgeries

- Cholecystectomies and appendectomies are routinely done through laparoscopy.
- Advantages include reduction of postoperative pain and shorter hospital stay.
- Contraindications include obesity, internal adhesions, and bowel obstruction with distention.

Preoperative Care

Nursing care involves helping explain all diagnostic tests and procedures to the patient to promote cooperation and relaxation. Proper patient education will help ensure that the patient is prepared for the type of surgery, as well as postoperative care, including insertion of IV, patient-controlled analgesia pump, NG tube, surgical drains, incision, and ostomy care. The patient should be instructed in measures that will help prevent postoperative complications, such as pulmonary toilet and splinting incision. Strict monitoring of the inputs and outputs is routine and should be done. Preoperative laboratory studies are obtained. Bowel cleansing may be ordered or modifications in diet. Antibiotics are given preoperatively to prevent bacterial growth in the colon. An ostomy nurse may be consulted if the patient is scheduled for an ostomy. The patient, if not already NPO, will be kept NPO after midnight the night before surgery. Encourage communication with the significant other and family to promote support postoperatively.

Postoperative Management

Physical assessment is completed as indicated by patient status. Vital signs are monitored for signs of infection and shock (fever, hypotension, and tachycardia). Intake and output are strictly monitored. Output from drains is collected and analyzed for abnormal amounts or signs of infection and/or bleeding. Nursing assessment of abdominal incisions is needed often to check for abnormal bleeding, odor, or dehiscence. Unstable patients may have open incisions or wound vacuums in place.

Postoperative nursing assessment should include routine evaluation of the abdomen for increased pain, distension, rigidity, nausea, or vomiting. You should expect diminished bowel sounds immediately postoperatively, but these should return upon passing of flatus or feces. If there is a fecal odor to the vomitus, it may indicate obstruction. Laboratory values are primarily monitored for any electrolyte imbalances. If the NG tube is left in place, then the nurse should check NG tube for placement and irrigate as needed with 30 mL of normal saline every two hours as needed, but this should be approved by the treating medical team, as there may be contraindications to immediate gastric fluid administration. If there are large amounts of NG output then intravenous fluid replacement may be needed.

Antiembolism stockings and foot movement devices, such as Ted hose and sequential compression devices, may be used to prevent stasis of venous blood in legs. Turning, coughing, and deep breathing are used with incentive spirometry every two hours to serve as pulmonary toilet and help prevent atelectasis and postoperative pneumonia. Pain control is paramount in postoperative care following GI surgery and early ambulation. Dressings are changed daily or as needed using aseptic technique. The patient's diet may be advanced by the primary medical team after the NG tube is removed and the presence of bowel sounds has been verified. Progression goes from ice chips, sips of water, clear liquids, full liquids, and then soft or regular foods. Dietary education and ostomy teaching (if relevant) should be reinforced by the nursing staff. It may take three months to a year before a patient can eat normally.

Possible complications of gastric surgeries include marginal ulcers where gastric acids come in contact with the operative site or anastomosis, hemorrhage, reflux, gastric dilation, or nutritional problems. Dumping syndrome is most common after the Billroth II procedure and gastric bypass operations. Management of dumping syndrome involves decreasing the amount of food taken at one time and maintaining low-carbohydrate, high-protein, dry diet. Lying down after meals and avoidance of fluids one hour before, with, or two hours after eating helps to decrease dumping syndrome.

Hepatic Failure

Loss of function of the liver can be a slow progression or a sudden, acute problem. Every organ in the body is affected by liver failure. Damage to the liver cells occurs directly from liver disease or indirectly from obstruction of bile flow or hepatic circulation. Parenchymal cells respond to noxious agents by replacing glycogen with lipids, thereby producing fatty infiltration and cell death. Cell regeneration can occur if the disease process is not too toxic, or the liver may become fibrotic, as seen with cirrhosis. Cirrhosis leads to portal hypertension, ascites, hepatorenal syndrome, and encephalopathy. The complications of cirrhosis occur mainly due to alteration in the blood flow through the liver and portal circulation. Portal hypertension can occur from increased resistance within the venous system as with cirrhosis or rarely from other causes that may increase blood flow, like arterial-portal venous fistulas from infection or neoplasm. The spleen may become enlarged due to congestion within the portal system.

Common Causes

The most common causes of **acute liver failure** are viral hepatitis and drug-induced liver injury. Causes of **chronic liver failure** are cirrhosis, chronic cholestatic disease, chronic viral hepatitis, excessive alcohol intake, malnutrition, diabetes mellitus, alpha1-antitrypsin deficiency, Wilson's disease, hemochromatosis, repeated toxin exposure, and malignant disease such as carcinoma and cholangiocarcinoma.

Types of viral hepatitis are hepatitis A, hepatitis B, hepatitis C, hepatitis D, hepatitis E, hepatitis G, and cytomegalovirus (primarily in immunosuppressed or transplant patients). Hepatitis A and E are known as infectious hepatitis and are the result of poor sanitation; hence, they are transmitted by fecal-oral route. The difference is that hepatitis A is found in situations of unsanitary food handling, where hepatitis E is a water-borne virus affecting mostly young adults. On the other hand, hepatitis B is spread through close contact with blood and body fluids of infected individuals. Health care workers are at high risk for acquiring this form of hepatitis because of contact with the blood of carriers. Hepatitis D, if present, is found in the presence of hepatitis B, but note that hepatitis B infection can occur without hepatitis D. Hepatitis C accounts for most posttransfusion hepatitis infections and is also associated with IV drug use. Hepatitis C and G are spread by close contact with the blood or body fluids of infected individuals, similar to hepatitis B. Hepatitis B and C are often transmitted sexually through the cross-contamination of blood and body fluids.

Clinical Manifestations

Manifestations of hepatic failure, including hepatitis, are systemic and vary greatly. The early phases of hepatic failure include weight loss from nausea and vomiting that may, in some cases, proceed to acute, life-threatening liver failure. Listed below are some clinical manifestations of hepatic failure.

- **General:** Decreased weight, muscle wasting, malnourishment, malaise, and fatigue

- **Cardiovascular:** Increased cardiac output and heart rate, systolic ejection murmur, bounding pulses, decreased blood pressure, dysrhythmias, and peripheral edema

- **Immune:** Leukopenia, splenomegaly, thrombocytopenia

- **Skin:** Jaundice, palmar erythema, hair loss, pruritus and dry skin, bruising and spider angiomas

- **Endocrine:** Peripheral edema, increased weight, moon face and striae, testicular atrophy, gynecomastia, decreased libido, impotence, hypoglycemia

- **Gastrointestinal:** Anorexia, nausea, steatorrhea, hyperlipidemia, melena or clay-colored stools, epistaxis, and gingival bleeding

- **Neurologic:** Hepatic encephalopathy, sensory disturbances, foot drop, ptosis, nystagmus

- **Renal:** Decreased renal blood flow and urine output, dark foamy urine, increased urine osmolality

- **Pulmonary:** Diaphragm elevation, dyspnea, decreased oxygen saturation

Management

Management focuses on supporting liver function until the organ can regenerate while protecting the other body systems from failure. Priorities include maintaining circulating volume, stabilizing hemodynamics, providing nutritional support, and controlling ammonia levels to prevent encephalopathy. Patients with acute liver failure supported in an intensive care unit have increased survival rates. Deterioration of handwriting is an early manifestation of hepatic encephalopathy due to asterixis. Nursing assessment of a patient who is irritable or drowsy may include having the patient write her name each shift to observe for subtle early changes. Cerebral edema develops in 80 percent of the patients with encephalopathy. Patients who develop cerebral edema require intracranial pressure monitoring. The medical team

TABLE 10.2 *Stages of Hepatic Encephalopathy*

Stage 1	Fatigue, restlessness, irritability, decreased intellectual performance, decreased attention span, decreased short-term memory, personality changes, sleep pattern reversal
Stage 2	Deterioration of handwriting, asterixis, drowsiness, confusion, lethargy, fetor hepaticus
Stage 3	Severe confusion, inability to follow commands, deep somnolence but arousable
Stage 4	Coma, unresponsive to pain, decorticate or decerebrate posturing

may perform a therapeutic paracentesis to provide temporary relief from pressure on the diaphragm and/or abdominal distention. Patients with ascites are usually limited to 2 g of sodium per day and restricted to no more than 1.5 L of fluid intake per day. Lactulose reduces the pH of the intestine and helps decrease ammonia levels. Oral or enteric feedings are generally withheld during the acute phase. Patients with liver failure are often hyponatremic and hypokalemic. The nature of the hyponatremia is hypervolemic and should be treated with fluid restriction, as stated above. However, the hypokalemia should be corrected in these patients aggressively, since it is a factor of the liver failure; diuretic treatment should also administered for the ascites. Liver transplant may be indicated for patients with irreversible liver disease, if they meet certain criteria. Histamine receptor (H2) antagonists are given to decrease gastric secretions and prevent gastric ulcers. Thiamine is given to reduce neuropathies. Vitamin K is given to promote production of coagulation factors, and prothrombin is given to help prevent bleeding tendencies. Sedatives, acetaminophen, and ibuprofen are avoided because of poor metabolism and increased toxicity to the liver. Aspirin is avoided because of decreased platelet aggregation.

Pancreatitis

Pancreatitis is an inflammatory disease process resulting in autodigestion of the pancreas by its own enzymes. The pancreatic enzymes, lipase, trypsin, chymotrypsin, and amylase are activated for reasons that are unclear. The pancreas becomes necrotic, and severe pain results. The patient is at risk for shock and sepsis. Mortality can be 50 percent or higher. Chronic pancreatitis results in permanent damage. Acute pancreatitis is an attack of a previously normal pancreas where permanent damage to the pancreas does not occur. In necrotizing pancreatitis, the most severe form, necrosis of the pancreas and hemorrhage can occur with shock, multiorgan failure, and death.

Common Causes

Alcohol and biliary disease, specifically gallstones, are associated with acute pancreatitis. Biliary disease is the most common cause of acute pancreatitis in nonalcoholic patients. Another cause of pancreatitis is use of certain drugs like thiazide diuretics, furosemide, steroids, and transplant medications. Hypertriglyceridemia, hypercalcemia, infection, and trauma are other known causes of pancreatitis. As many as 20 percent of pancreatitis cases have no known cause but are thought to involve biliary sludge.

Clinical Manifestations

Patients present with a broad range of symptoms from being asymptomatic to experiencing agonizing pain. Abdominal pain is the most common symptom and may be constant. Nausea and vomiting are common, and there may be foul-smelling diarrhea due to the lack of fat digestion. If hemorrhage occurs, there will be ecchymosis in the flank region (Grey-Turner's sign) and ecchymosis in the periumbilical area (Cullen's sign). Tissue damage and inflammation lead to release of chemicals that make the capillaries more permeable, leading to fluid shifts of as much as 6 liters of fluid into the interstitial compartment. Patients with pancreatitis may develop fevers, especially if they experience the complication of an abscess or pseudocyst. Hypovolemia may result with manifestations of dry mouth, low blood pressure, tachycardia, and decreased urine. Vasodilation, myocardial depression, and hypovolemia lead to shock and tissue death. Decreased renal perfusion results in acute kidney injury, formerly known as acute renal failure. Respiratory depression is the leading cause of death in acute pancreatitis.

Laboratory levels of amylase are elevated in pancreatitis within 2–12 hours after onset of the disease. However, elevated amylase levels have a lower specificity for the diagnosis of pancreatitis, compared to elevated lipase levels. Where amylase levels may return to normal within a week, lipase levels rise and remain elevated longer. In some patients, triglyceride and blood sugar levels are elevated. Hypokalemia and hypomagnesemia contribute to the hypotension that already exists. Hypocalcemia is common, and patients may exhibit bronchospasm, tetany, cardiac dysrhythmias, positive Chvostek's sign, and positive Trousseau's sign. Acute pancreatitis precipitates calcium as a soap in the abdomen, a process called saponification, causing hypocalcemia.

CT and abdominal ultrasound are diagnostic tests used to diagnose pancreatitis. Some facilities measure C-reactive protein (CRP), but this is rather nonspecific because CRP is an acute phase reactant and may be elevated for a large number of reasons. An increase level above 150 mg/L 48 hours after symptom onset indicates severe acute pancreatitis.

Management

The management of pancreatitis revolves around the following: Make the patient NPO, administer intravenous fluids, pain control with opiods (theoretically hydromorphone carries less risks than morphine in pancreatitis), NG tube to intermittent suction. Meperidine (Demerol) is frowned upon for pain control in pancreatitis patients and is less effective than hydromorphone and morphine. Morphine is believed to be less safe than hydromorphone because it carries the potential to cause a spasm of the sphincter of Oddi, causing additional injury to the pancreas.

Comprehensive critical nursing is required for patients with severe pancreatitis. Urine output should be monitored and interventions taken to manage the volume replacement. Urine output should be at least 0.5–1 mL/kg per hour. Fluid replacement is with crystalloids like lactated Ringer's or normal saline. Daily weights help to reflect overall fluid balance. Respiratory insufficiency is the most common complication of acute pancreatitis. Mechanical ventilation with positive end-expiratory pressure (PEEP) and pleural taps may be needed to relieve respiratory depression. TPN may not be useful for patients unless they have been NPO for three to five or more days. Enteral feeding may be used when the tube is placed in the jejunum. Further, there may be added benefit to the patient if H2 blockers are administered intravenously. Antibiotics are used seldom and then only when an infection is identified or if necrotizing pancreatitis is evident on radiographic imaging. The medical team may also consider the use of antibiotics if the patient clinically appears to be infected (e.g., fevers, leukocytosis, hypotension). Blood transfusions may be needed in hemorrhagic pancreatitis. Some patients require surgical intervention to treat complications of acute pancreatitis. Anxiety and problems with alcohol are addressed by providing supportive nursing discussions with encouragement to seek support groups such as Alcoholics Anonymous. The critical care RN may also be instrumental in initiating consults to social work to help the patient identify resources for outpatient support.

Gastroesophageal Reflux

Gastroesophageal reflux is caused by a backward flow of contents from the stomach into the esophagus. Inappropriate relaxation of the lower esophageal sphincter occurs for unknown reasons, resulting in heartburn. If reflux occurs often, it results in breakdown of the esophageal lining and may lead to premalignant tissue formation (Barret's esophagus) or adenocarcinoma. The scarring of the esophagus leads to stricture/fibrosis and dysphagia (difficulty swallowing).

Common Causes

Many patients with gastroesophageal reflux disease (GERD) have hiatal hernias. Reflux esophagitis exposes the esophageal mucosa to the acidic gastric contents, which gradually erode the esophageal tissue. Some patients have delayed emptying of the stomach and obesity, which causes pressure on the lower esophageal sphincter. Certain foods and medications are associated with GERD. For example, fatty foods, peppermint, alcohol, and caffeine can increase the frequency and/or severity of GERD. Medications and drugs such as nicotine, beta-adrenergic blockers, nitrates, theophylline, and anticholinergic drugs may have similar effects because they lower tone and contractility of the lower esophageal sphincter. GERD can occur at any age but is most common in people over 50 years of age.

Clinical Manifestations

The history is almost diagnostic for GERD. Patient may complain of retrosternal aching or burning, typically after large meals and worsened by lying flat or bending over. Regurgitation of fluid or food particles may predispose the patient to recurrent pneumonia or bronchospasm. Pain or difficulty swallowing may be accompanied by chest heaviness and pressure radiating to the jaw or shoulders. Due to the association with distress on eating, patients may complain of a "burning feeling" in their chest or chest pain, as well as weight loss. Since GERD can be described as chest pain, the symptoms may overlap with those of ACS. Hence, do not simply assume heartburn history is GERD, as it may be a manifestation of ACS; the reverse is also true.

Management

Diagnostic tests are needed in atypical or severe cases. The "gold standard" is esophageal manometry with pH monitoring in the lower esophagus. Endoscopy or CT of chest may

TABLE 10.3 *Acid-Controlling Agents*

	Antacids	H2 Antagonists	Proton Pump Inhibitors	Other
Mechanism of Action	Neutralizes gastric acid.	Blocks histamine by binding on surface of parietal cells.	Blocks all gastric secretion.	Mucosal protective agent provides protective barrier over active stress ulcerations by binding to the base of the area.
Interactions	Several drug interactions occur if given at the same time as other medications due to changes in the pH of the stomach to a more alkaline enviroment.	May inhibit the action of certain drugs that require acidic GI environments for gastric absorption, like ketoconazole.	May increase levels of certain drugs, like diazepam and phenytoin.	Impairs absorption of certain drugs, like tetracycline.
Side Effects and Adverse Effects	Magnesium-containing diarrhea, aluminum- and calcium-containing constipation	Headache, confusion, diarrhea, increased liver function tests, creatinine, flushing, urticaria, thrombocytopenia	Same as H2 antagonists	Constipation, nausea, and dry mouth
Major Drugs in Category	**Aluminum-containing** • Aluminum carbonate (Amphojel) **Magnesium-containing** • Milk of Magnesia • Gaviscon **Calcium-containing** • Tums **Combination** • Maalox • Mylanta	• Cimetidine (Tagamet) • Famotidine (Pepcid) • Nizatidine (Axid) • Ranitidine (Zantac)	• Lansoprazole (Prevacid) • Omeprazole (Prilosec) • Rabeprazole (Aciphex) • Pantoprazole (Protonix) • Esomeprazole (Nexium)	• Sucralfate (Carafate) • Misoprostol (Cytotec)

also be done, but these are of limited value in the context of manometry and pH monitoring. Nursing measures involve encouraging the patient to eat multiple small meals per day of low-fat foods. If obesity is present, weight loss is helpful for symptoms. Smoking cessation is suggested. Teach patients to avoid food for three hours prior to sleep and rest with the head upright following meals and during sleep. It is also useful to teach patients to not strain when defecating and to limit fats and carbohydrates in their diets. Antacids and especially PPIs are helpful in controlling symptoms. Surgical procedures involving wrapping the esophagus with the fundus of the stomach (Nissen fundoplication) are used for patients whose GERD is not relieved with medications.

Review Questions

Questions 1–5 pertain to the following scenario:

While working in the ICU, you receive a patient from the emergency room who was recently (<6 hours) injured in an altercation involving a pool-stick assault to the abdomen and trunk of the body. Upon receiving the patient, he is intubated and has a BP of 80/42, HR 132, and temp 97.8 °F. He is displaying Cullen's and Grey Turner signs along with multiple other bruises to his body. His medical history includes alcohol abuse, diabetes, and hypertension.

1. Which of these statements accurately describes the pathogenesis of acute abdominal blunt trauma?

   A. Blunt trauma to the abdomen can occur from falls, assaults, or sports.

   B. Injuries from blunt trauma to the abdomen do not show up for 24 to 48 hours.

   C. The small intestine is the organ most likely to be affected by blunt trauma to the abdomen.

   D. Blunt trauma to the abdomen is normally not life threatening.

2. Upon assessing the patient in the ICU, you note that the abdomen has become more rigid despite the NG tube placement for stomach decompression. This may be caused by which of these?

   A. rupture of the bowel

   B. swelling of soft tissue in the abdominal wall

   C. massive hemorrhaging

   D. normal pendulous abdomen due to the alcohol abuse

3. Despite rapid fluid resuscitation performed in the emergency room prior to patient transfer to the ICU, hypotension continues. What is the nursing care priority?

   A. notifying a physician

   B. typing and cross-matching for transfusion of blood components

   C. drawing hemoglobin and hematocrit laboratory studies

   D. obtaining a rapid infuser and replacing hypertonic fluids until the patient is normotensive

4. The patient is noted to have steady dark red blood in his newly placed nasogatric tube. The patient is prepped for emergency surgery. The most likely cause of this bleeding is

   A. peritonitis.

   B. obstruction of the lower GI tract.

   C. esophageal varices.

   D. neoplasm.

5. The nurse noted that the patient has a yellow hue to his skin and conjunctiva. The most likely cause of this assessment finding is which of these?

   A. pancreatitis

   B. hepatic failure

   C. gallstones

   D. adrenal insufficiency

6. What is the main pathophysiologic feature of acute pancreatitis?

    A. total necrosis of the pancreas

    B. pancreatic enzyme deficiency

    C. autodigestion of the pancreas

    D. multiple tumors in the pancreas

7. The nurse cares for a patient admitted for chronic alcohol abuse and altered mental status. The nurse notes that the patient's handwriting abilities have changed since initial admission forms. This is indicative of which of these?

    A. dementia

    B. pancreatitis

    C. diabetes insipidus

    D. hepatic encephalopathy

8. What is the leading cause of death in patients with acute pancreatitis?

    A. acute renal insufficiency

    B. hypovolemia

    C. respiratory depression

    D. cardiac dysrhythmias

9. Patients that have undergone the Billroth II procedure may have complications with malabsorption and malnutrition, most likely caused by

    A. overproduction of stomach acid.

    B. dumping syndrome.

    C. adhesions causing strictures.

    D. decreased peristalsis.

10. The nurse cares for a client diagnosed with acute pancreatitis who has a blood pressure of 87/54. Which priority intervention would the nurse anticipate?

    A. keeping the head of the bed elevated

    B. providing oral pancreatic enzyme

    C. insertion of nasogastric tube (NGT)

    D. administration of normal saline IV

Review Answers and Explanations

1. A

Blunt trauma to the abdomen with the pool stick had great force over a small area, causing the mechanism of injury to be higher. Falls and sports are two other blunt-force trauma MOIs to the abdomen. (B) is incorrect because if the liver or spleen is injured, it may be tamponed off for a while but not likely for 24 to 48 hours. (C) is incorrect because the small intestine is protected well by the greater omentum and is a hollow organ, unlike the spleen and liver. (D) is incorrect because the abdomen can hold several liters of fluid before becoming rigid. This makes trauma to the abdomen very life threatening if internal bleeding should go undetected for a long time.

2. C

A rigid abdomen is a critical assessment finding for massive hemorrhaging in the abdomen.

3. B

By obtaining type and cross-match for transfusion of blood components, you will be able to advance the patient's care. The next step would be to contact the physician so that further investigation and testing of your assessment can be done.

4. C

Esophageal varices are normally attributed to excessive alcohol intake where the esophageal tissue becomes friable and increases the chance for bleeding with just slight trauma. The alcohol intake thins the esophageal wall and causes bleeding to occur with little or no trauma to the membranes.

5. B

Jaundice is a hallmark sign of hepatic failure or infection due to the inability to rid the body of bilirubin.

6. C

Activation of pancreatic enzymes within the pancreas causes autodigestion of the pancreas and the resulting inflammation and necrosis. (A) There is no total necrosis of the pancreas, although some necrotic areas may be noted in acute pancreatitis. (B) There is no deficiency in pancreatic enzymes; the issue is excretion of the enzymes. (D) Multiple tumors are complications of pancreatitis, not initial pathology.

7. D

Deterioration of handwriting is an early manifestation of hepatic encephalopathy. Along with deterioration of handwriting, subtle changes in mentation, confusion, and drowsiness are later signs of hepatic encephalopathy.

8. C

Respiratory depression in acute pancreatitis is caused by toxic waste accumulation when there is underlying infection due to pseudocysts, abscesses, or gallstones. This accumulation of toxins causes the body to become acidotic, further developing into septicemia and causing the patient's condition to slowly decline into septic shock or respiratory depression or compromising the respiratory system. This is a slowly progressing condition; however, if it is not assessed correctly and in a timely manner, the patient may go into cardiac arrest.

9. B

Dumping syndrome occurs when large amounts of food high in sugar content are consumed and the intestines are unable to digest complex sugars.

10. D

Isotonic solutions will expand volume and correct the hypotension. (A) Elevating the head of the bed may further lower the blood pressure. (B) Pancreatic enzyme supplementation is important in the post-acute phase; the priority is correcting the low BP. (C) Gastric decompression will allow the GI to "rest," but the priority is improving BP.

The Renal System

The renal portion of the critical care nursing certification exam is approximately 6 percent of the total number of questions.

The renal system can be described as a complex filtering system that serves a variety of functions within the human body to assist in homeostasis. The primary organs of the renal system are the kidneys. The main functions of the kidneys are the maintenance of fluid and electrolyte balance, the maintenance of acid-base balance, homeostasis, and excretion of by-product waste. In addition to these organs, there is a system serving as the collective mechanism for urine, which is the by-product of the filtration of the blood. The ureters, urinary bladder, and urethra are the components of the urinary collection system. The homeostatic functions include maintaining fluid and electrolyte balance, removal of metabolic wastes, regulation of blood pressure, acid-base balance, and synthesis of red blood vessels.

The purposes of this chapter are to review renal anatomy and physiology, normal renal function, and conditions that impact renal function such as acute and chronic renal failure, acute tubular necrosis, and electrolyte disturbances and the nursing interventions that should be implemented to improve patient outcomes in the critically ill patient. A clear understanding of the basic anatomy and physiology of the renal system is necessary to apply more advanced concepts in the critically ill patient with renal disorders.

ANATOMY OF THE RENAL SYSTEM

There are two terms to describe the anatomy within the renal system and specifically the kidneys: **macroscopic** and **microscopic**. The macroscopic anatomy is that which can be visualized by inspection with the naked eye, while microscopic is that which requires specialized equipment such as a microscope.

Macroscopic Anatomy

The kidneys are two organs that are similar in shape to a bean that is flattened on one side. The typical size of a normal kidney is 4" in length, 2 to 2½" in breadth, and 1" in thickness. The kidneys are located in the retroperitoneal cavity, and one lies on each side of the vertebral column between the 12th thoracic vertebra and the 3rd lumbar vertebra. The right kidney sits lower than the left kidney in the retroperitoneal space due to the position of the liver. The kidneys are well protected in the retroperitoneal space lying behind the lower portion of the rib cage, under the abdominal musculature, and behind the parietal peritoneum. Fibrous tissues in the renal fascia form a smooth covering to protect the organs.

Within the kidneys there are three distinct layers of anatomical structures, specifically, the **cortex**, **medulla**, and **renal pelvis**. The *cortex* is the outermost portion and contains the microscopic anatomical structures of the glomeruli, proximal tubules, cortical portions of the loops of Henle, distal tubules, and the cortical collecting ducts. The *medulla* is the innermost portion and contains the medullary portions of the loops of Henle and collecting ducts. The *renal pelvis* collects urine from the calyx and funnels it to the urethra. Visually, the appearance of the medulla of the kidneys is one of multiple pyramids (approximately 6–10), which are formed by the collecting ducts. These pyramids taper to join together and form the *minor calyx,* which in turn join together to form the *major calyx.* The renal pelvis is formed by the funneling of the major calyx and function to direct urine into the ureters. The capacity of the collecting system is only 5 to 10 mL and, therefore, functionally is primarily one of a conduit or channel to drain urine. (See figure 11.1.)

Microscopic Anatomy

The **nephron** is the functional unit of the kidney (see figure 11.2). There are more than 1 million nephrons within each kidney. Structurally, there are both cortical and juxtamedullary nephrons whose function is based on their location within the kidneys. Nephrons in the cortex make up approximately 85 percent of the total nephrons. The *nephron* is comprised of two components: the renal corpuscle and the renal tubule. The renal corpuscle encompasses

FIGURE 11.1 *Macroscopic Anatomy of the Renal System*

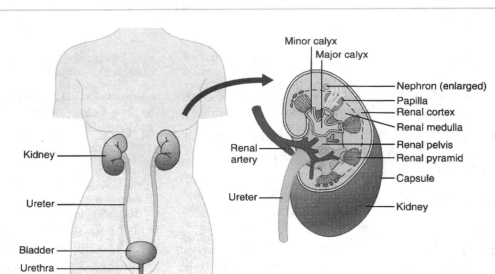

Bowman's capsule and glomerulus. The renal tubule contains the proximal convoluted tubule, *loop of Henle*, distal convoluted tube, and the collecting tubules. The kidneys will continue to function even with destruction of thousands of nephrons from diseases or other conditions.

The **glomerulus** serves as the first structure within the nephron and functions as a high-pressure capillary bed to filter the blood. The *afferent arteriole* brings blood to the glomerulus at a higher pressure than the exiting *efferent arteriole*. This variation in gradient allows for *filtration* to occur. Within the glomerulus is the basement membrane, which is semipermeable and does not allow larger particles such as albumin, protein, or red blood cells to enter the filtrate. If these are seen in the filtrate, there is likely damage to the membrane. Other factors that impact the filtration of molecules include electrical charge, protein binding, and molecular shape.

The glomerulus is surrounded by a membranous layer of epitheal cells, which is called **Bowman's capsule**. This capsule serves as a holding space for the filtrate until it moves into the proximal convoluted tubule.

The **proximal tubule** is the first section of the renal tubular system, which also includes the loop of Henle, distal tubule, and collecting tubule. The main purpose of the tubular system is reabsorption of the key solutes such as glucose, amino acids, and bicarbonate. Additionally, water and electrolytes, including potassium, sodium and calcium, are reabsorbed after being filtered by the glomerulus. Osmolality of the filtrate is adjusted by the proximal tubules through the process of reabsorption of solutes. The hyperosmolar filtrate becomes isoosmotic upon exiting the proximal tubule. The kidneys receive about 20 percent of the cardiac output with each beat and filter nearly 200 liters of fluid in a 24-hour period. This amount of filtrate, if excreted and not reabsorbed in its majority, would completely deplete the body of all water and electrolytes. The nephrons have the primary purpose of separating that which must be conserved and that which must be excreted.

The **loop of Henle** has three segments named for their position in the loop. These are the *thin descending loop,* the *thin ascending loop,* and the *thick ascending loop.* The cortical and juxtamedullary nephrons vary in the length of the loops of Henle within their structure. Shorter nephrons are located in the cortical nephrons and have excretion and regulatory functions. The longer nephrons located in the juxtamedullary nephrons serve to concentrate and dilute the urine. The permeability within these loops determines whether water or solutes, such as urea, sodium, potassium, and calcium, are reabsorbed and at what point. The thinner descending loop is more permeable to water, and therefore, urea and sodium are not reabsorbed there. This causes the iso-osmotic filtrate to become hyperosmotic as it moves into the thin ascending and thick ascending loops. Within the ascending loop, the filtrate becomes more dilute. The membrane of the thick ascending loop is impermeable to water; thus the reabsorption of electrolytes such as potassium, sodium, calcium, and bircarbonate occurs. This causes the filtrate to become hypo-osmotic.

The next entry point for the filtrate is the **distal convoluted tubule** at the cortex of the kidney. At the termination of the thick descending limbs of the loop of Henle is found the specialized cells called the **macula densa cells**. These cells are a component of the **juxtamedullary apparatus** and serve to assist in regulation of blood pressure. Sodium, potassium, and chloride are reabsorbed in the first section of the distal tubule, while this section is impermeable to water and urea. The later section regulates all these solutes based on hormonal, acid-base, and electrolyte balance. The late distal tubule reabsorbs sodium and water and excretes potassium. ADH (antidiuretic hormone) assists in the regulation of water and solutes in the late distal tubule, which changes the osmolality of the filtrate.

The final section of the nephron is the **collecting tubule**. These tubules are located initially in the cortex and extend through the medulla and empty into the papilla. Predominantly, the function of the collecting tubules is to transport sodium, potassium, hydrogen, and bicarbonate and to acidify the urine. This is done by specialized cells called *principal and intercalated cells*. ADH and aldosterone also play a critical part in water reabsorption and the dilution/concentration of urine and produce compensatory vasoconstriction in the nonessential vasculature and conservation of sodium and water within the distal convoluted tubule.

FIGURE 11.2 *Microscopic Anatomy of the Nephron*

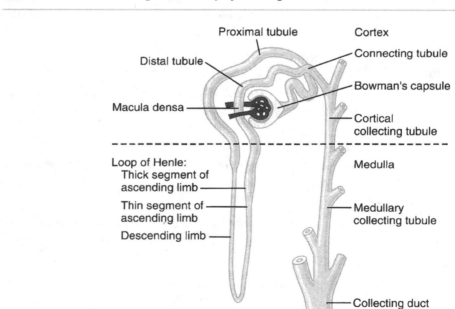

Renal Vasculature

Despite their size, the kidneys receive approximately 20 to 25 percent of the resting cardiac output. These organs are the only ones within the human body that have an arteriole-capillary-arteriole blood flow system at the microscopic level. Additionally, another distinguishing factor regarding the renal vasculature is that there are *two capillary beds,* the glomerular and the peritubular capillary beds, separated by an efferent arteriole. The capillary bed itself is more porous and creates a size and charge barrier to prevent larger molecules, such as albumin, to pass, unlike systemic capillaries.

FIGURE 11.3 *Renal Vasculature*

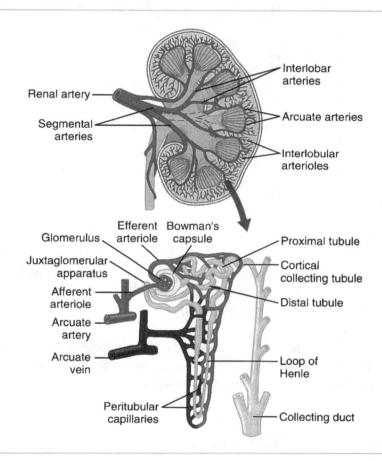

The renal vasculature (see figure 11.3) begins as the renal artery branches off the aorta and enters the kidney near the hilar region. This artery begins to branch into three smaller vessels—**interlobar, arcuate, interlobular**—which provide circulation to the renal cortex and medulla. The afferent arterioles emerge from the interlobular arteries, which extend from the renal artery to the cortex. These arterioles form the capillary bed of the glomerulus. The efferent arterioles serve as the exit system for the blood flow from the

FIGURE 11.4 *Renal Vasculature and Microcirculation*

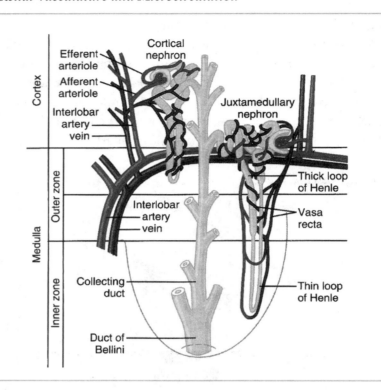

glomerular capillary bed. As above, this is different from other organs' vasculature where there is an arteriole-capillary-venule system. The arteriole-capillary-arteriole structure allows for the maintenance of intercapillary pressure regulation, which allows movement of the fluid out of the capillary bed. The efferent arterioles form the second capillary bed, which is called the peritubular capillaries (see figure 11.4).

The kidneys have the ability to regulate *hydrostatic pressure* within the capillary system by adjusting the resistance of the afferent and efferent arterioles and, in turn, changing the rates of filtration, reabsorption, or both to provide homeostasis in the body.

PHYSIOLOGY OF THE RENAL SYSTEM

Glomerular Filtration, Reabsorption, Secretion and Excretion

One of the key functions of the renal system is called glomerular filtration. This process is essentially the formation of urine. The rate of filtration of the kidneys is affected by many factors within the human body such as changes in blood pressure, tone of the arteriole system, dehydration, and obstructions of the drainage of urine. As a rule, most adults filter approximately 180 liters/day or 125 milliliters (mL)/min. From this filtrate, urine is formed and excreted at rate of 1–2 liters/day, or 40–80 mL/hour. Oliguria is defined as urine output less than 400 mL/day. Normally, the filtrate will have a specific gravity of 1.010 and be protein-free and plasma-like in characteristics. Abnormally, if there are deficiencies in the permeability of the membranes within the filtering system, the filtrate will contain protein, electrolytes, or glucose, which may change the specific gravity and the concentration of the urine.

The process of filtration occurs due to a change in hydrostatic pressure within the glomerulus and the colloid osmotic pressure (oncotic pressure of the plasma proteins in the blood supply).

Typically, the hydrostatic pressure within the glomerulus is higher than the osmotic colloid pressure and the Bowman's capsule pressure, creating a *pressure gradient* favoring filtration. The glomerular filtration rate (GFR) is used clinically to assess the patient's renal function in addition to the blood urea nitrogen (BUN) and creatinine (Cr) levels. The formula for calculation of GFR and creatinine clearance is as follows:

$$\textbf{GFR} = (U_x \times V)/P_x$$

where:

x = substance freely filtered through the glomerulus and not secreted or reabsorbed by the tubules
P = plasma concentration of x
V = urine flow rate in mL/min
U = urine concentration of x

As above, the normal estimated GFR in an adult is 180 liters/day.

Creatinine clearance (mL/min) for adult male [CrCl] $= \dfrac{(140-\text{age}) \times \text{actual weight in kg}}{72 \times \text{serum creatinine (mg/dL)}}$

For women, the estimated **CrCl** above is multiplied by 0.85. Normal **CrCl** is 90–140 mL/min for men and 80–125 mL/min for women.

The significance of both of these figures is in the effectiveness of the renal system with regard to filtration, reabsorption, secretion, and excretion. Initially, blood enters the glomerulus at a pressure of approximately 50 mm Hg. The tissue pressure or pressure within the capillary bed is lower at –10 mm Hg, while the plasma oncotic pressure is also lower at –25 mm Hg.

The glomerular capillary membrane filters several hundred times as much water and solutes than a normal body capillary membrane and is still able to prevent larger molecules such as proteins from filtration. This property is based on the permeability and thickness of the

FIGURE 11.5 *Principles of Filtration*

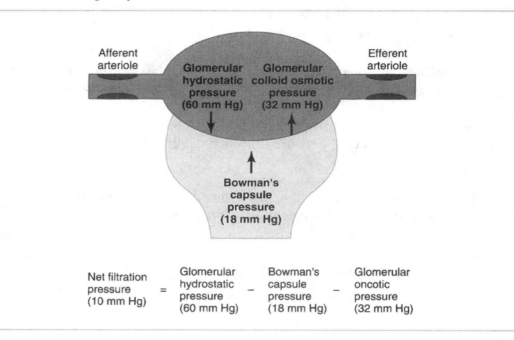

basement membrane. The basement membrane of the glomerulus also is *negatively charged*, which prevents large negatively charged molecules from being filtered. Without this barrier, some proteins such as albumin would be able to pass through the membrane.

The resultant filtrate is stored in the Bowman's capsule temporarily until the process of reabsorption takes place by the tubular system within the nephrons of the kidneys. This process takes the 180 liters of filtrate and reabsorbs the necessary solutes and water back into the blood supply by the peritubular capillaries. The reabsorption takes place through both *passive* and *active* transport of water and solutes. (See figure 11.5.)

Passive/Active Transport, Diffusion, and Osmosis

Passive transport occurs through the pressure gradient created by the hydrostatic pressure and changes in solute concentrations. Passive transport, as the name implies, does not require active energy to support. The two primary processes that occur in passive transport are diffusion and osmosis. **Diffusion** is defined as the spontaneous movement of molecules across a *semipermeable membrane* from higher concentrations of the compound to lower concentrations of the compound. Reabsorption of water from the filtrate produces a higher concentration on the tubular side, resulting in a movement of molecules. One example of this is as water is reabsorbed by the tubules, the concentration within the tubules increases. As a result, molecules such as urea will move from the tubules to the plasma to balance the concentrations.

FIGURE 11.6 *Fundamentals of Pressure Variation*

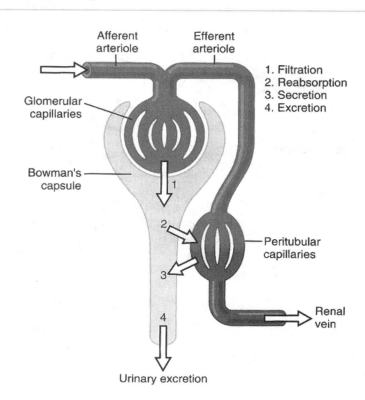

Afferent arteriole

Efferent arteriole

Glomerular capillaries

Bowman's capsule

1. Filtration
2. Reabsorption
3. Secretion
4. Excretion

Peritubular capillaries

Renal vein

Urinary excretion

Osmosis, the other form of *passive transport*, involves the movement of water from an area of lower solute concentration to higher solute concentration. Alternatively, it can be described as the diffusion of water. The most common solute that changes the balance of concentration is sodium. If the concentration of sodium within the tubular system is higher, then water will move from the capillary bed to the tubules to balance the concentrations.

Active transport, as its name implies, requires energy to help move substances such as glucose, amino acids, calcium, phosphate, potassium, and sodium across the semi-permeable tubular membrane. Adenosine triphosphate (ATP) is the source of energy for this process. The reabsorption is achieved by the use of transport molecules in the tubular membrane of the nephron that are designed to move these molecules from the tubules to the capillaries and, finally, back to the venous circulation. Specific thresholds for these carriers can prevent the molecules from being reabsorbed and subsequently excreted in the urine or causing a change in metabolic state (e.g., bicarbonate causing a metabolic acidosis or glucose causing a glycosuria). Because a high degree of energy is required in this transport, the process is very susceptible to hypovolemia and low perfusion states.

FIGURE 11.7 *Passive/Active Transport, Diffusion, and Osmosis*

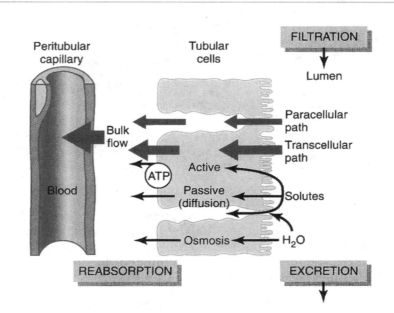

Secretion and Excretion

Another function of the kidneys is the **secretion** of substances from the peritubular capillaries to the tubules. This is referred to as *counter transport* and involves the exchange of substances across the membranes either through passive or active transport. Typically, this exchange is regulated by the needs of the body such as hyper- or hypokalemia states. Drugs may also be secreted in this fashion.

Excretion refers to the elimination of wastes within the renal system. The kidneys selectively filtrate from the circulation system substances such as urea and creatinine, which are by-products of protein metabolism. Other substances that are excreted from the body via the renal system include drug metabolism by-products, bilirubin, and metabolic acids. These substances may significantly change the characteristics of the urine, such as color or pH. Two lab values that consistently are used to measure the performance of the renal system (filtration/reabsorption/secretion) are blood urea nitrogen (BUN) and creatinine (Cr). An increase in these values can be indicative of conditions such as a catabolic state or renal failure.

In summary, the components of the nephrons and their functions are as follows:

- **Proximal tubules:** Reabsorption of sodium, chloride, bicarbonate, glucose, hydrogen, phosphates, and calcium

- **Loop of Henle:** Concentration and dilution of urine

- **Distal convoluted tubule:** Water reabsorption directly via ADH (vasopressin) control and indirectly via aldosterone (which causes reabsoprtion of sodium in the collecting duct)

Hormonal Regulation of Blood Pressure

When the patient's arterial blood pressure falls, the kidneys attempt to maintain circulating blood volume through the regulation of fluid balance and retention of water and alteration in the peripheral vascular resistance. This is done by the initiation of the rennin-angiotensin-aldosterone cascade.

Within the **juxtaglomerular apparatus**, where the distal tubule contacts the afferent arteriole, there are specialized cells called the **macula densa**. These cells sense changes in blood flow and send messages to the arterioles to control the blood flow through constriction or dilation. Without this regulation, blood flow to the kidneys will be reduced in a low-volume state. Additionally, a mean arterial pressure (MAP) less than 60 mm Hg for greater than

FIGURE 11.8 *Hormonal Regulation of Blood Pressure*

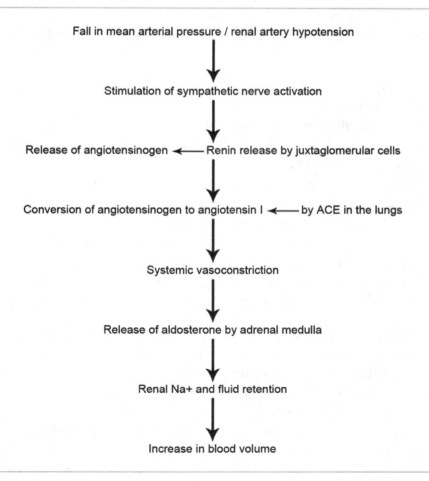

Fall in mean arterial pressure / renal artery hypotension

↓

Stimulation of sympathetic nerve activation

↓

Release of angiotensinogen ←— Renin release by juxtaglomerular cells

↓

Conversion of angiotensinogen to angiotensin I ←— by ACE in the lungs

↓

Systemic vasoconstriction

↓

Release of aldosterone by adrenal medulla

↓

Renal Na+ and fluid retention

↓

Increase in blood volume

40 minutes can cause renal ischemia, which, in turn, can lead to acute tubular necrosis (ATN) or acute renal insufficiency. It is critically important to preserve renal blood flow and oxygenation to prevent nephron damage in the kidney. Therefore, if the patient's own protective mechanisms are unable to respond to these insults, the critical care RN must intervene in a timely manner to protect renal function.

Electrolyte Regulation

The kidneys regulate electrolytes within the body through the filtration, reabsorption, and secretion process. Some of the electrolytes considered essential to the physiology of the body include potassium, sodium, calcium, magnesium, phosphorus, and bicarbonate. The redistribution of these electrolytes is crucial to organ function.

As with most electrolytes, the serum potassium value is actually only a small portion of the body's stores since most potassium in the body is located intracellularly. The normal serum level of potassium is 3.5 to 5.0 mg/dL, depending on the laboratory standards of the testing lab. Despite the fact that the potassium remains primarily intracellular, changes in the extracellular serum levels can accurately predict changes that are occurring intracellularly. Additionally, since both potassium and sodium are cations, a constant competition takes place both intracellularly and extracellularly to remain in balance to protect electrical neutrality at the cell membrane.

Potassium levels are maintained through both diffusion and active transport across the cell membrane. Many factors can influence the distribution of potassium. These may include insulin storage and use, aldosterone secretion, catecholamine secretion, acid-base abnormalities, cell destruction, strenuous exercise, and fluid osmolarity. Of potassium that moves out of the cell through diffusion, 65 percent is reabsorbed under normal conditions via active transport at the level of proximal tubule and another 25 to 30 percent at the loop of Henle. The day-to-day excretion of potassium occurs in the late distal and cortical collecting tubules, based on the body's needs for metabolism. The gastrointestinal tract does excrete a small amount of potassium in fecal material; however, the primary controller of potassium levels within the body is the kidney. Some of the functions of potassium are enzyme activity associated with protein and carbohydrate metabolism for energy production, aiding nerve impulse conduction and muscle contraction, and maintenance of intracellular osmolality.

The most abundant electrolyte within the body is sodium. It is primarily extracellular, in contrast to potassium—which is mostly intracellular. Sodium controls most of the regulation of body water that is retained or excreted by the kidneys. The other primary function of sodium is the transmission of nerve impulses via the active transport mechanism called the "sodium/potassium pump," which occurs at the cellular level. Another secondary function of sodium is the regulation of acid-base balance in the body as it combines with chloride or bicarbonate. The normal value of serum sodium is 135 to 145 mEq/L. Sodium, similar to potassium, is primarily reabsorbed by the proximal tubules and the loop of Henle. The renin-angiotensin-aldosterone system discussed earlier in the chapter explains the process of water retention and the role three organs—the kidneys (renin secretion), adrenal glands (aldosterone secretion), and the posterior pituitary gland (ADH secretion)—play to manage the fluid level in the body. Thirst also plays a role in maintaining a normal hydration state in the body. The thirst center is located in the anterior hypothalamus, and when an individual becomes dehydrated, the neuronal cells cause the sensation of thirst.

Overall, **calcium** is the electrolyte that is most plentiful in the body, with approximately 99 percent stored in the bones. However, calcium is very important to several other functions in the body. These include maintaining the internal integrity of the cell, influencing myocardial contractility, cardiac action potential, neuromuscular activity, cell permeability, coagulation of blood, and strength of bones and teeth. The remaining 1 percent of calcium that serves to carry on these additional functions is located in the extracellular fluid. Mobilization of calcium normally stored in the bone, during extracellular depletion states, requires parathyroid hormone (PTH) to stimulate tubular reabsorption. Secondarily, PTH stimulates phosphate excretion, which serves as an exchange for calcium. Calcium in the intravascular space is either protein bound or circulating in an ionized state. Calcium is measured in both as ionized calcium and total calcium, and the data can be deceptive when the patient has elevated or decreased albumin levels. Ionized calcium may be bound to the albumin and give a false lower serum ionized calcium blood level. When albumin falls, the ionized calcium is freed and creates a rise in the serum ionized calcium level. When this occurs, calcitonin, secreted by the thyroid, will attempt to return the ionized calcium back to the bone, yet another inaccurate reflection of the true availability of ionized calcium. The normal serum calcium level is 8.5 to 10.5 mg/dL. A change of 1 g/dL of serum albumin will result in a serum calcium change of 0.8 mg/dL, which is why all calcium measurements should be done in conjunction with serum albumin. Calcium uptake is dependent upon several factors, including levels of phosphorus, magnesium, and vitamin D, as well as PTH and calcitonin.

Similar to calcium and magnesium, **phosphorus** is primarily stored in the bone and with very little circulating serum levels. The normal phosphorus level is 2.5 to 4.5 mg/dL. Approximately 75 percent of the body's total phosphorus is stored in the bone. The remaining amount is located intracellularly. Intake of phosphorus-rich foods such as milk, poultry, fish, and red meat can significantly impact the phosphorus level in the serum. This is due to the fact that the primary absorption of phosphorus occurs in the gastrointestinal tract but its excretion takes place in the kidney in the distal convoluted tubules. Phosphorus functions to form ATP, which is the functional component in the production of energy for the cell. Active transport cannot occur without ATP. Additional functions of phosphorus include stabilization of the cell membrane, acid-base balance, oxygen delivery at the level of tissues, and bone strength. Within the renal filtrate, phosphorus combines with other ions, sodium and hydrogen, to produce sodium diphosphate ($NaHPO_4$), then later disassociates into the individual components for reabsorption. There is a significant converse relationship between phosphorus and calcium. When one electrolyte is elevated, the other is depleted and vice versa. This complex process involves several other functions, including PTH secretion, vitamin D use, and reabsorption and secretion in the renal tubules. This is also an important concept for discussion of conditions of the renal system and their symptomotology.

Magnesium is another electrolyte that is regulated by the kidney but is primarily stored in the bone and absorbed in the gastrointestinal tract. Approximately 60 percent of the magnesium in the body is stored in the bone, and only 1 percent is in the extracellular fluid, while the balance is in the intracellular fluid. Normal magnesium levels are 1.2 to 2.1 mEq/L. There is a competitive absorption in the gastrointestinal tract for both magnesium and calcium with a preference for whichever electrolyte is in the higher concentration there. Magnesium is critical for the functioning of the intracellular carriers that transport both sodium and potassium across the cell membrane and, therefore, help to balance stores. The effect of a depleted magnesium level is a release of potassium to the extracellular fluid, in turn causing the kidneys to excrete potassium to prevent hypokalemia. The other functions of magnesium include enhancing coronary blood flow in acute myocardial infarction patients, improving ventricular function while decreasing mortality rates, transmission of CNS (central nervous system) messages, maintaining neuromuscular activity, and in the metabolism of proteins and nucleic acids.

Chloride is one of the few electrolytes that is found most commonly in combination with another cation such as sodium or potassium. If the chloride levels are below or above normal levels of 97 to 110 mEq/L, most likely this is due to an imbalance of the other cation or in acid-base balance. Because of chloride's relationship with sodium, this electrolyte plays an important role in balance of serum osmolality and water as well. The competitive nature of chloride and bicarbonate for the sodium cation can also impact acid-base balance through excretion during acidosis and reabsorption during alkalosis. Most of us get our intake of chloride through intake of everyday table salt. Finally, chloride combines with hydrogen produced in the stomach and gastric secretions to form hydrochloric acid. Other functions of the chloride anion involve oxygenation of red blood cells by the release of hydrogen and bicarbonate from carbonic acid within the red blood cells. Hydrogen binds with the hemoglobin molecule, while bicarbonate leaves the intracellular space in exchange with chloride. This movement allows carbon dioxide in the form of bicarbonate to move to the lungs for excretion.

The final solute for consideration in this section is **bicarbonate**. Bicarbonate is an anion, a negatively charged ion, as it is held in the extracellular fluid. The function of bicarbonate is primarily that of acid-base balance, although it is not the sole controller. The normal serum level of bicarbonate is 24 to 28 mEq/L. The two components that assist in the control of acid-base balance are bicarbonate and carbonic acid, which should exist in a ratio of 1 mEq/L of carbonic acid to 20 mEq/L of bicarbonate. Thus, the normal levels of carbonic acid are 1.2 to 2.4 mEq/L. Balance between these two substances is regulated by the kidney through reabsorption and excretion, based on the concentration of hydrogen ions.

The regulation of the electrolytes discussed in this section is a critical function of the kidneys. Many functions within the body, such as respiration, acid-base balance, cardiac activity, etc., are dependent upon levels of these electrolytes in both the intracellular and extracellular spaces. The other physiological functions of the kidneys will be discussed in the following sections.

Excretion of Waste Products

The major waste products excreted by the kidneys are in the form of **BUN, uric acid**, and **creatinine** (Cr). This is done through *selective filtration* of the products from the blood as it circulates through the renal vasculature. These products are primarily by-products of protein metabolism. Other substances such as bilirubin, drug by-products, ammonium chloride, and over 200 additional metabolic waste products are eliminated from the body by the kidneys.

Urea and Creatinine

Physicians typically use these two lab measurements to do a preliminary assessment of renal function. Creatinine and BUN are by-products of protein metabolism and are reabsorbed and excreted within the nephron. **BUN** is a by-product of the breakdown of ammonia within the liver. The serum BUN level can be affected by other factors such as GFR, inadequate metabolism of protein such as in catabolic states, medications, and diet intake of protein. If the kidney is unable to filter adequately, BUN levels will become elevated, which may be an indication of acute tubular necrosis (ATN) or renal insufficiency. It is generally not used as a diagnostic tool in isolation but rather in conjunction with the Cr level, the patient's overall clinical presentation, and other related values such as urine output and other electrolyte levels. An elevation in the BUN that does not have a similar rise in the creatinine is often indicative of other conditions such as dehydration, low renal perfusion state, or increased breakdown of protein as in a catabolic state. The normal BUN ranges from 9 to 20 mg/dL. In general, the BUN-to-creatinine ratio is less than 20:1. A ratio that is 20:1 or greater is indicative of a prenal acute renal insufficiency, such as dehydration or fluid loss state.

Creatinine is a by-product of muscle metabolism. Serum creatinine can be a strong indicator of renal function. Normally, creatinine is *completely filtered* by the kidneys, so an elevation in the blood can be directly related to kidney impairment. It is also directly related to GFR. Normal creatinine is 0.7 to 1.5 mg/dL.

Acid-Base Balance

A combination of regulation of hydrogen ions and maintenance of fluid balance in the body within the renal system assists in maintaining a state of homeostasis in acid-base balance. Other organs, including the lungs, participate in this regulation of acid-base balance, and there are other buffers such as in the blood. The lungs can respond to acid-base changes in a much more rapid fashion than the kidneys. Thus, the lungs are able to respond to critical or emergent situations, while the kidneys function to maintain the balance on a more day-to-day basis.

The kidneys regulate acid-base balance through the *reabsorption of bicarbonate and secretion of hydrogen.* The reabsorption of bicarbonate takes place primarily in the proximal tubule but also occurs in the distal tubules. Secretion of hydrogen occurs passively in the proximal tubule and actively in the distal tubule. Both occur with the exchange of sodium ions. Bicarbonate is synthesized in the distal tubule by excreting hydrogen in the urine at the same time that the sodium and bicarbonate are delivered to the extracellular fluid. As above, this occurs through ionization of carbonic acid. Buffering also takes place with the combination of ammonia (NH_3^+) and phosphate (HPO_4^{-2}) before excretion without lowering the pH, and the molecules are transported to the tubular filtrate and excreted in the urine.

In an acidotic state, the kidney will increase hydrogen ion secretion in the distal tubule, while all bicarbonate is reabsorbed by the proximal tubule. In akalemia, the opposite occurs with decreasing hydrogen ion secretion while bicarbonate is excreted, causing the urine to become more alkaline.

Fluid and Water Regulation

One of the most important physiological functions of the kidneys is the regulation of fluid and water to help maintain homeostasis in the body. Without this regulatory effect, there could potentially be two diverse fluid states: fluid overload or severe dehydration.

To begin the discussion of this regulatory effect, the concept of *fluid compartmentalization* must be explained. Within the body are two distinct compartments: the intracellular and the extracellular. Between these two compartments are membranes that serve to separate the two spaces and filter both fluids and solutes. These membranes are semipermeable. The semipermeable membrane has openings that allow molecules of specific sizes or weights to pass through and prevents movement of other molecules. The specificity of the membrane permeability is based on its location in the body. Within the extracellular space there are also two subcompartments: the *intravascular* and the *interstitial* compartments. About 40 percent of the patient's body weight is in the intercellular space. Five percent is in the intravascular space and the rest (15 percent) is in the extracellular spaces of the tissues (remember that 60 percent of the body weight is composed of water).

The composition of the fluids within these compartments varies slightly. Movement of the molecules must occur simultaneously with the fluids within the spaces. The *intercellular space* is primarily electrolytes such as sodium, potassium, magnesium, etc.; water; and proteinate. The *extracellular space* includes organic acids, phosphates, and similar substances. The substances disassociate into ions that are either positively or negatively charged when dissolved in water. Movement of electrolytes within the nephron has been discussed earlier in the chapter. One factor that impacts fluid movement is the dissolution of these electrolytes in water and the creation of ions that are either negatively or positively charged. The electrical charges influence the movement through the semipermeable membranes and the maintenance of homeostasis.

In discussing fluid movement between these spaces, it is also important to understand the concepts of isotonic, hypertonic, and hypotonic. These terms describe the differences between concentrations of solutions on two sides of a membrane. The term *isotonic* refers to a state when the concentrations on both sides of the membrane are the same. *Hypertonic* refers to when the solution outside the cell has a higher concentration of solutes than the solution inside the cell. Finally, *hypotonic* refers to when the concentration of the solution outside the cell has a lower concentration of solutes than the solution inside the cell. The key to understanding these terms is that, in medicine, they refer to the solute concentration of the solution outside the cell; hence, when you have a hypertonic state, the solution *outside* the cell is more concentrated. These concepts are important in helping understand the movement of water between compartments. The measurement of this concentration or the number of particles in a solution is called osmolality.

In an isotonic solution, water will remain constant on both sides of the membranes because the concentrations of solutes on both sides of the membrane are equal and there is no osmotic gradient. Infusing hypertonic solutions, such as 3 percent saline, into the body will result in a fluid shift from inside the cells and into the extracellular space, causing a withering of the cell itself. Infusions of this nature may be of some value if the goal is getting fluid to move from the cells and into the intravascular space and bolstering blood pressure due to

FIGURE 11.9 *Secretion of ADH*

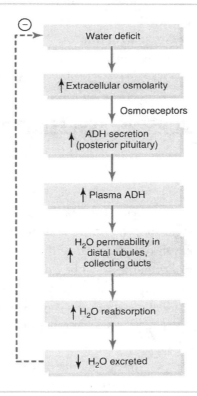

elevation of blood volume. Using hypotonic solutions would have the reverse effect, causing fluid to shift from the extracellular compartment to the intracellular compartment.

Using the above concepts and the fact that hydrostatic pressures force blood through the vasculature of the renal system, one can hypothesize a solute gradient is used in the process of secretion, filtration, and reabsorption in the nephron. Water movement is typically a function of the concentration of plasma proteins in the intravascular space and the solute content of both the extracellular and intracellular fluids. A decrease in plasma protein will cause the fluid to move into the interstitial space, causing interstitial edema. In reverse, an increase in the plasma proteins would cause the movement of fluid from the interstitial space into the intravascular space. In hypotensive states, the body may try to preserve volume by pulling fluid from the cells into the intravascular space, though at a risk of depleting the cells of fluids that are needed for normal function.

Antidiuretic Hormone (ADH)

ADH, also known as vasopressin, is a hormone secreted by the anterior pituitary gland in response to the need to regulate the extracellular fluid balance. The secretion of ADH by the pituitary gland results in the stimulation of water reabsorption by the distal tubules and collecting ducts. The effect of this is an increase in the volume of extracellular fluid and excretion of hypertonic (concentrated) urine. There are stimulants for the release of ADH, one of which is physical or emotional stress. Intracellular dehydration will also stimulate the sensation of thirst, which in turn encourages the individual to drink fluids to return the body to the appropriate water balance. If the body is unable to compensate for the loss in this manner, ADH release will be stimulated by an increase in serum osmolality. As above, this causes the kidneys, specifically the distal tubules, to reabsorb water. When the serum osmolality is corrected, ADH secretion will be inhibited. ADH secretion is also inhibited during water intoxification.

KEY COMPONENTS OF NURSING ASSESSMENT RELATED TO THE RENAL SYSTEM

Patient History

A complete history and physical are essential for patients with renal dysfunction. Detailed information should be obtained regarding chief complaint and the history of the present illness. This should include onset and length of symptoms and any factors that influence the symptoms. The clinical manifestations of the illness will be due to the pathophysiology of the renal dysfunction. Some of the signs and symptoms include decreased urinary output, edema, flank pain, nausea, vomiting, bitter or metallic taste in the mouth, dry itchy skin, bruising, fatigue, decreased level of consciousness, shortness of breath, and weight gain. Medication history, both prescribed and over-the-counter, including herbal and dietary supplements, is important and must include recent antibiotic therapy, contrast media that may have been administered during diagnostic procedures, or nonsteroidal anti-inflammatory drugs. All of these medications have the potential to cause renal dysfunction. Any recent injuries or strenuous exercise should also be investigated, as these have the potential to cause rhabdomolysis. Rhabdomolysis can be the result of muscle damage and the release of myoglobin into the bloodstream, which can block structures of the kidneys. The patient should be questioned regarding any recent weight gain, which may indicate water overload and potential renal dysfunction. Excessive nausea and vomiting or loss of appetite caused by changes in taste may indicate uremia. A family history is also helpful to ascertain if there are similar symptoms in relatives that may help to identify the condition. The history should be taken simultaneously while completing the physical exam in critically ill patients. Illnesses that may be of significance in the family history are hypertension, diabetes, renal diseases such as polycystic kidneys, heart failure, or headaches.

The Physical Examination

An *initial set of vital signs* should be completed, including admission weight. These should be compared to the patient's normal values. *Orthostatic blood pressures* will assist in identification of dehydration and should be done if the patient can tolerate the position changes.

The initial assessment should begin with checking the airway, breathing, and circulation. Once the patient is determined to be stable and not to require any immediate intervention, further assessment should be obtained. The nurse should observe for *signs of volume depletion or overload,* which might include poor skin turgor, swollen extremities, distended neck veins (done initially while the patient is flat, then at a 45- to 90-degree angle), peripheral vein distention, and dry oral cavity. Measurements in the degree of edema need to be consistent, with 1+ indicating minimal pitting and 4+ indicating severe pitting edema. Edema should be noted to be peripheral or extended to larger areas such as the sacrum in a reclining patient.

Heart and lung sounds should be auscultated. Any cardiac murmur or arterial bruit auscultated (carotid, aortic, or renal artery) may be indicative of fluid overload or stenosis. The most common extra heart sound heard in a patient with fluid overload is the third heart sound or S3. Also auscultation for a pericardial friction rub should be done. Uremia may cause pericarditis. Any extra lung sounds such as rales are probably indicative of fluid overload. The patient should be observed for *dyspnea or tachypnea.*

The physician may add to the physical assessment with the palpation of kidneys where masses or unusual shaping of the kidney would be noted. Percussion is used to detect pain or air, fluid, or solid accumulation, particularly in the retroperitoneal area, which could be indicative of infection or traumatic injury.

Other *hemodynamic monitoring* devices may be used to gather additional information. This may include an arterial line or pulmonary artery or SVO_2 catheter. If possible, a central line should be inserted to provide information about the patient's fluid status with the measurement of a central venous pressure (CVP). The CVP is indicative of the right atrial filling pressure and is a measurement of preload of the right ventricle. In the majority of cases, the mean arterial pressure and central venous pressure are sufficient to provide adequate information in patients with real or potential renal disorders. The pulmonary artery catheter is used if the patient has comorbidities such as cardiovascular disorders, while the SVO_2 is helpful in patients with possible sepsis. Patients in the critical care unit should always have careful intake and output monitored.

Diagnostic Testing

The two most familiar diagnostic tests done in patients with renal dysfunction are **BUN and creatinine levels**. These two serum tests when used in conjunction will give the practitioner excellent information about renal function. However, these tests are not used in isolation, and other serum testing should include the standard chemistry panel with the **major electrolytes, osmolality, albumin, hemoglobin**, and **hematocrit**. The calculation of the **anion gap**, which looks at the difference between measurable cations (sodium and potassium) and anions (chloride and bicarbonate), will provide information regarding acid-base balance, especially since renal failure can manifest as a metabolic acidosis. A normal anion gap is 10 to 15 mEq/L. An elevated anion gap indicates the presence of increased metabolic acidosis.

Additional testing should include a **standard urinalysis** and, if indicated, a urine culture. A random urine specimen can also be collected for a **urine osmolality**, sodium, potassium, urea, and Cr. The urinalysis will perform a screening for the presence of blood, glucose, and protein. An abnormal urinalysis for any of these components should be followed up with a repeat urinalysis and further testing as indicated. This will provide information regarding the ability of the kidneys to reabsorb solutes or if tubular damage is resulting in hematuria.

In addition to serum testing, radiological testing should be completed to ascertain if there is mechanical, vascular, or traumatic injury to the renal system. Imaging tests that may be ordered by the physician include a flat film of the kidneys, ureters, and bladder (KUB); intravenous pyleogram; renal angiography; abdominal computerized tomography; and renal ultrasound. Advanced testing, such as magnetic resonance imaging or guided renal biopsy, may be indicated for complex disease states.

CONDITIONS/DISORDERS OF THE RENAL SYSTEM

Acute Kidney Injury (AKI)

Rather recently, the term *acute renal failure* has been replaced with the term *acute kidney injury* (AKI). AKI is a clinical condition that occurs in a rapid fashion and is commonly diagnosed by a decrease in glomerular filtration rate, an increase in BUN and Cr, and subsequent retention of metabolic waste products. Oliguria (less than 400 mL of urine output in a 24-hour period) is a clinical symptom that assists in the diagnosis. The mortality associated with AKI is significant, despite technological advances in critical care, particularly if not recognized early or if the patient is unresponsive to traditional treatment. The mortality rate can be as high at 85 percent. Even to the nephrologists, the pathophysiology of AKI is variable and not well understood. Dialysis remains the treatment of choice in AKI, provided that the patient meets criteria for dialysis.

Acute kidney injury can be classified into three major categories based on the clinical events that cause the condition: prerenal, intrarenal, and postrenal. However, in many cases, there may be multifactorial causes of acute renal failure. Examples of these may be septic patients who also have a comorbidity of heart failure, patients who receive contrast media who are also on anti-inflammatory medications, and diabetic patients who suffer from obstructive renal calculi.

Prerenal conditions are those that cause reduced blood flow to the kidneys. The result of these conditions is *renal hypoperfusion and a decrease in the glomerular filtration rate.* A cascade of events occurs in prerenal conditions. This begins with vasoconstriction of the vasculature which supplies the critical filtering components (tubules) of the kidneys, followed by a reduced filtration of the blood and reduced urine excretion. If treatment is initiated to counteract the hypoperfusion, such as vasopressors, increased fluid volume, or removal of nephrotoxins through dialysis, there is a strong likelihood that the condition can be reversed. Prerenal azotemia may affect as many as 70 percent of all critically ill patients. In the septic patient, the cause of the hypoperfusion is due to the systemic inflammatory response. Examples of other causes of prerenal acute renal failure include hemorrhage, excessive diarrhea or vomiting, myocardial infarction, thrombosis of the renal artery, and anaphylactic shock. In prerenal failure (azotemia), the BUN and creatinine ratio is greater than 20:1. (This number can be obtained by dividing the BUN by the creatinine.)

Intrarenal conditions may be also described as intrinsic, primary, or parenchymal. Intrarenal damage is that which occurs in the nephron of the kidney either at the site of the glomeruli or in the tubules. Another name for this condition is acute tubular necrosis (ATN). This condition will be discussed at length in the following section. Approximately 25 percent of renal failure is due to an intrarenal cause. The mortality/morbidity of ATN is such that 50 percent of patients die as a result of the condition, 25 percent require long-term chronic dialysis due to a lack of kidney regeneration, and 25 percent recover with no long-term effects. Some potential causes of intrarenal acute renal failure are malignant hypertension, acute glomerular nephritis, nephrotoxicity from heavy metals, and acute pyelonephritis. In intrarenal failure, the BUN and creatinine ratio is less than 20:1.

Finally, **postrenal** conditions are those that are due to obstruction in the urine flow in the key components beyond the kidney, such as in the ureters or bladder. An example of this may be a renal calculi or tumor. A very small portion of patients actually show evidence of this type of renal failure. The treatment for this condition is to relieve the obstruction as quickly as possible.

In the critical care unit, it is important to manage the patient to reduce the likelihood of renal failure. It is the only truly effective remedy for AKI. In order to achieve this, the patient must be constantly assessed for the risk of AKI. Care should be taken to avoid the use of nephrotoxic medications, particularly in the elderly population. Antibiotics should be evaluated for the risk/benefit to the patient, recognizing that aminoglycocides, as well as other antibiotics, pose a considerable risk for renal failure. Caution should be taken when using contrast mediums, including evaluation of the creatinine clearance and pre-treatment with infusion of bicarbonate solutions to prevent kidney damage. Prevention of hypovolemia or vasoconstriction of critical renal vasculature should be undertaken early in the course of the symptoms.

Medical management of the patient in acute renal failure should focus on the following parameters: *fluid balance, electrolyte regulation, treatment of the causative factor, and promoting regeneration of functional kidney structures.* Secondarily, treatment of other symptoms such as decreased neurological function, skin conditions, and gastrointestinal disorders should also be considered important to the patient's recovery and should not be overlooked.

Fluid balance can be treated with a variety of interventions based on etiology of the AKI. Administration of fluids intravenously at a rate that will replace lost volume, as well as to maintain the perfusion to critical organs, is necessary. In septic conditions, this may require large, rapid infusions of crystalloid solutions. Individual requirements may vary based on fever, blood loss, and other factors affecting perfusion. Colloids may be needed to expand intravascular volume in conditions where the mean arterial pressure, cardiac index, and/or pulmonary artery wedge pressure are low. These infusions may also be required to assist in the shift of fluid from the extracellular space to the intravascular space. Constant evaluation of hemodynamic parameters and serum electrolyte levels is necessary to judge the adequacy of the infusions. In cases where fluid administration does not significantly increase perfusion, vasopressor therapy may be required to elevate mean arterial pressure. Occasionally, combination therapy of dopamine and furosemide therapy may reverse the oliguria.

In conditions where the patient is experiencing circulatory overload or interstitial edema, fluid restriction may be required. Monitoring of daily weights and accurate intake and output will provide information in regard to the fluid status. In addition to fluid restriction, patients with intrarenal acute renal failure may require diuretic therapy (recognizing that in some cases diuretic therapy will worsen the AKI) and in advanced stages hemodialysis to acutely remove fluid, especially if there is cardiac or pulmonary compromise.

Management of electrolyte balance is also critical in the prevention of other complications that may occur as a result of AKI. **Hyperkalemia** occurs as a result of the inability of the kidney to excrete potassium. Clinical manifestations of hyperkalemia include ECG changes such as peaked T waves, lengthening of the QRS interval, and subsequently ventricular tachycardia. Levels may rise quickly to measurements of 6.0 mEq/L or higher. All potassium supplements are held, and if the patient is continuing to produce urine, diuretics may be ordered. If hyperkalemia requires immediate treatment, administer 100 mL of 50 percent glucose (D50) and 20 units of IV insulin with 1 ampule of calcium gluconate (for cardioprotection). The insulin forces the potassium out of the intravascular space and back into the intracellular space. Additionally, infusion of sodium bicarbonate (40–160 mEq) will promote excretion of potassium in the urine. Finally, oral, rectal enema, or nasogastric tube administration of sodium polystyrene sulfonate (Kayexalate) will have an effect of binding with potassium in the bowel, which would then be excreted in the stool; this is often administered in 15 or 30 doses.

Sodium imbalances may be categorized as hyponatremia or hypernatremia. Hypernatremia is essentially always the result of a free water deficit and requires adjustment in the amount of free water being administered to the patient. In contrast, hyponatremia is more complex. A full discussion of hyponatremia is beyond the scope of this review, but the critical care RN should understand that hyponatremia may be categorized as hypovolemic, euvolemic, or hypervolemic. Each of these categories has a different clinical treatment. Hypovolemic hyponatremia is treated with intravenous fluid administration. Euvolemic hyponatremia is treated with fluid restriction, where hypervolemic hyponatremia is treated with diuretic therapy. Hypertonic saline (3 percent NS) is generally reserved for symptomatic patients with hyponatremia, but its use is decided by the treating physician.

Hypocalcemia and **hyperphosphatemia** occur in acute renal failure. Calcium and phosphorus have a converse relationship. Depletion of one causes elevation of the other in the serum, as reabsorption of calcium promotes excretion of phosphorus. The clinical manifestations of this condition are nervous system excitement and irritability and tetany. The treatment for hyperphosphatemia is a polymeric phosphate binder like sevelamer (RenaGel or Renvela). It binds phosphate in the GI tract, preventing its absorption. Calcium supplements such as Tums or calcitriol can also be administered.

Diet restrictions may also be initiated with regard to protein, potassium, sodium, and phosphorus. Patients need to be encouraged to take energy-rich foods such as carbohydrates to promote necessary healing. Patients who are significantly malnourished may require total parenteral nutrition.

Chronic Renal Insufficiency (CRI)

Similar to acute renal failure, chronic renal failure is now referred to clinically as **chronic renal insufficiency (CRI)**. Patients may be admitted to the critical care unit with a history of CRI. This condition is the result of the progressive and primarily irreversible death of functional nephrons in the kidney. As mentioned earlier, the kidney may function normally despite damage or the loss of thousands of nephrons. One kidney may have up to 1 million nephrons. When there is approximately 90 percent loss of functional nephrons, the patient will have evidence of CRI, which leads to end stage renal disease (ESRD). Currently, the treatment for CRI is dialysis. This can be in the form of either peritoneal dialysis or hemodialysis. Many years ago, glomerularnephritis was the most common etiology behind CRI; however, diabetes and hypertension have become the leading causes of CRI. Other causes of chronic renal insufficiency are renal vascular disorders, pyelonephritis, nephrotoxins, and congenital disorders.

Typically, the occurrence of chronic renal failure begins with an insult to the functional units of the kidneys, causing destruction of a significant number of nephrons. As a response, the remaining functional nephrons become hypertrophic, and vasodilation occurs. Subsequently, the glomerular pressure and filtration increases. This is a temporary situation, as, over time, further injury to the surviving nephrons occurs. The exact cause of the additional injury is hypothesized to be the constant stress of vasodilation and increased arterial blood pressure causing stenosis of the functional nephrons.

There are four stages of this progressive nephron loss: diminished renal reserve, renal insufficiency, end stage renal disease, and uremic syndrome. In the first stage, the function of the kidneys is mildly reduced, and the patient does not demonstrate significant symptoms of kidney failure. As the nephron loss increases, the patient develops renal insufficiency where there is evidence of impairment of the renal function, and azotemia develops. The kidneys are unable to concentrate urine efficiently. At 90 percent nephron loss, the patient has end stage renal disease and must undergo dialysis to filter water and solutes adequately. Transplantation is considered if the patient is an appropriate candidate. The final stage is called uremic syndrome. The failure of the kidneys to function adequately causes a build-up of waste products and uremic waste.

Typically, the result of chronic renal failure is the inability of the kidney to adequately filter electrolytes and water, which causes a buildup in waste solutes and water retention. Over time without treatment, the patient could show evidence of serious pulmonary consequences of increased fluid retention, such as pulmonary edema. Sodium and water is excreted in larger quantities into the intravascular space by the kidneys, causing water retention. The renin-angiotension secretion that is stimulated in response to the fluid overload causes hypertension. The BUN and Cr also rise dramatically, as these products are not reabsorbed adequately by the viable nephrons. The effects are a vicious circle and continually worsen, causing a pattern of unrelenting symptoms.

Another condition that is commonly seen in patients with CRI is anemia. The cause of anemia of this type is that the damaged kidney fails to secrete erythropoietin, which normally stimulates the bone marrow to produce red blood cells. The shortened RBC lifespan also contributes to the anemia. This is treated with the exogenous administration of erythropoietin.

Chronic renal failure can also lead to a condition where the bones are demineralized from the rise in phosphates in the serum caused by the decreased GFR. Phosphates bind with calcium; thus, ionized calcium in the serum is decreased, and the secretion of parathyroid hormone occurs. Subsequently, calcium is released from the bones. Similarly, chronic renal failure also causes a condition called osteomalacia, where the bones are literally partially absorbed and become weakened from the lack of calcium. The kidneys assist in the conversion of vitamin D along with the liver. An inability to produce active vitamin D prevents the reabsorption of calcium in the intestines and availability of calcium to the bone.

Acute Tubular Necrosis (ATN)

Acute tubular necrosis (ATN) is an acute renal disorder classified as *intrarenal* and is the most common form of this type. With as high as 75 percent of all cases being of this type, the majority of hospital-acquired renal failure is ATN. Damage occurs to the renal tubular epithelium as a result of nephrotoxins or ischemic injury. If left untreated or if it is severe, the damage may spread to the basement membrane. As described above in acute renal failure, the kidneys are unable adequately to concentrate urine, maintain acid-base balance, or regulate wastes.

There are many potential causes of ATN. The two types of ATN are described as **ischemic and toxic**. In situations where there is serious hypoperfusion to the kidneys, damage to the tubular cells membranes occurs. Subsequently protein casts form, and these as well as cellular debris obstruct the tubules. The *ischemia* and the obstructions further reduce flow to the kidneys, and the ability of the afferent and efferent arterioles to autoregulate is seriously limited. Examples of ischemic ATN are hemorrhage, burns, sepsis, myocardial ischemia, pulmonary emboli, and obstetrical complications such as placenta previa or abruptio. The other type of ATN is *nephrotoxic*. There are drugs, bacterial endotoxins, and chemical agents that can cause damage to the renal tubular cells. In this type of ATN, the basement membrane is not typically damaged and therefore can be reversed more frequently. Toxic agents that can cause this type of ATN are rhabdomyolysis, gram negative sepsis, aminoglycosides, contrast media, and street drugs.

ATN is classified into *four phases* based on the clinical course of the condition. Initially, the **onset phase** is difficult to detect as it occurs prior to cell injury. GFR is reduced due to hypoperfusion and decreased glomerular ultrafiltration pressure. This phase can last from a few hours to several days. If treatment is initiated during this phase, most likely there will be no permanent injury. The **second phase** is the oliguric/anuric phase. Oliguria most commonly occurs in ischemic ATN, whereas nonoliguric ATN occurs in toxic exposure. This phase can last 5 to 8 days in the patient with anuria and 10 to 16 days in the oliguric patient. Mortality can be as high as 66 percent with oliguric ATN. The **third phase** is the diuretic phase where the patient has polyuria with urine outputs of up to 4 L/day. In this stage, tubular function returns slowly, and reabsorption by the kidney may not increase as quickly as the GFR. Fluid volume must be monitored closely to prevent hypovolemia. The **final stage** of ATN is the recovery phase. During this stage, tubular function slowly returns to a normalized state. The period of recovery may be up to two years. In approximately 5 percent of cases of ATN, the patient may continue to require long-term hemodialysis, while 33 percent of patients will be left with renal insufficiency.

Critical Electrolyte Imbalances

Hyperkalemia

Elevated potassium levels above 5.5 mEq/L are one of the most significant electrolyte imbalances due to the effects on the myocardium. Acute and chronic renal failure are the primary causes of hyperkalemia due to the nephron's inability to excrete the potassium ion. Decreased renal perfusion can also reduce the excretion of potassium due to the limited availability of sodium for exchange. Other causes of hyperkalemia include acute cellular destruction and potassium release due to burns, trauma, acidosis, rhabdomyolysis, etc.; adrenal cortical insufficiency; and excessive intake or infusion of potassium chloride.

It is imperative that the critical care nurse monitor the potential cardiac effects of hyperkalemia, including continuous cardiac monitoring of QRS width, ST segment changes, and PR intervals. Asystole may be the result of a significantly elevated potassium level, and resuscitating a patient with this condition is extremely difficult. Obtaining the patient's medical history relating to electrolyte imbalance, including medical conditions and medication history, is necessary to ascertain the potential cause of the hyperkalemia. Early ECG changes seen in hyperkalemia are peaked T waves, first-degree heart blocks, and widened QRS.

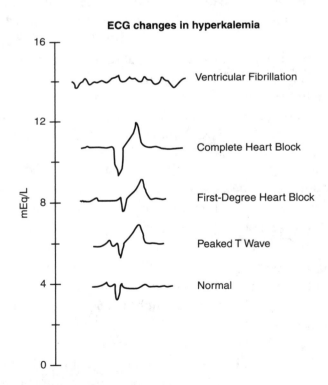

ECG changes in hyperkalemia

Treatment of this condition is the administration of IV glucose (one ampule of D50), insulin, and bicarbonate to force the movement of potassium back into the intracellular space for excretion by the kidneys. Kayexalate and sorbitol administration by oral or rectal routes should be done to remove the potassium more permanently via binding from the gastrointestinal tract. Administration of IV calcium chloride or gluconate to improve cardiac contractility is also indicated unless contraindicated, such as in patients who take digoxin.

Hypokalemia

One of the most common causes of hypokalemia is the continued symptom of prolonged vomiting and/or diarrhea where the intake of potassium is considerably lower than the output. Other conditions that may cause hypokalemia include diuretic therapy without adequate potassium replacement, renal tubular acidosis, liver disease, and alkalosis.

Clinical manifestations of hypokalemia include weakness, muscular tenderness, respiratory changes, and ECG changes. With potassium levels below 3.5 mEq/L, the patient may experience depressed ST segments, flattened T waves, presence of a "U" wave, and ventricular dysrhythmias such as PVCs, PACs, PAT, and AV blocks.

The treatment for hypokalemia is the administration of either IV or oral potassium supplements. For intravenous potassium in severe cases of hypokalemia, it is recommended that the patient have central venous access and administration be done over several hours. During this time, it is important for the critical care nurse to monitor to ensure that the patient does not develop hyperkalemia due to overcorrection.

Hypernatremia

Patients who show evidence of water retention and increased extracellular fluid volume will develop hypernatremia due to the inability to excrete sodium. In patients with normal renal function, this condition is most likely due to a lack of ADH secretion or neurohypophyseal insufficiency, such as in diabetes insipidus. For patients who do not have normal renal function, the cause is typically the inability of the renal tubules to respond to ADH secretion. The patient with hypernatremia will present with excessive weight gain, potential shortness of breath due to fluid overload, lethargy, muscle weakness, decreased urine output, and thirst.

METHODS OF DIALYSIS

There are three methods of dialysis, two of which have been used for many years and one that has been recently developed.

Hemodialysis

Hemodialysis requires vascular access, which can either be done as an acute intervention or through long-term chronic intervention. In the critical care unit, most often the vascular access is inserted on an emergent basis by a physician who is trained in inserting central lines. Common sites for these line insertions are the internal jugular, subclavian, or femoral veins. The catheter used is a dual lumen catheter with a venous port (blue) for pulling blood flow and an arterial port (red) for returning the filtered blood.

FIGURE 11.10 *Principles of Dialysis*

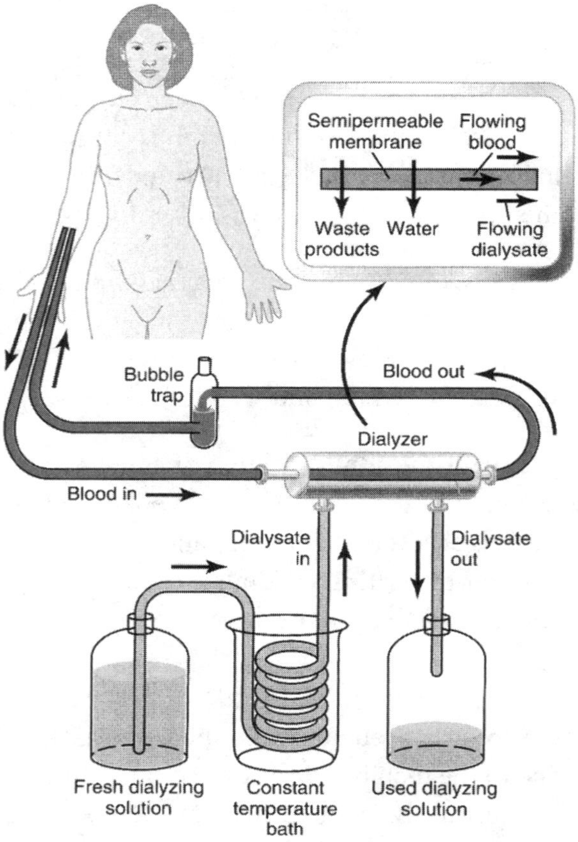

More chronic or long-term access can be obtained through a variety of *fistulas* or *grafts*. With these devices, both the venous and arterial vasculature is accessed on a more permanent basis. The types are arteriovenous fistula, arteriovenous grafts, and arteriovenous shunts. An arteriovenous fistula grafts an artery with a vein, such as the radial artery with the cephalic vein, by creating an opening in both and anastomosing the two together. In an arteriovenous graft, a tube is surgically implanted in the limb and tunneled in both the artery and the vein. Finally, the arteriovenous shunt requires a cutdown to be performed on both the artery and the vein, and a device is inserted in each and run through the skin externally between the two. Blood flows through the device via a T-connector where the dialysis connection occurs. This last device is not currently an access of choice due to frequency of complications such as thrombosis, infection, and skin erosion.

The treatment of hemodialysis works very similarly to the normal functional kidney. It takes the patient's blood and filters water, electrolytes, and toxins using the principles of osmosis, diffusion, and convection/ultrafiltration. A hollow fiber tube with seimpermeable membranes, called an extracorporeal dialyzer, is used to separate these components from the blood.

A solution known as dialysate bathes the membranes and performs exchange of the blood and the bath through osmosis and diffusion to pull fluid, electrolytes, and toxins from the blood. Because the blood circulation does not have enough pressure to move the blood through the filtration device, a pump is used to provide a consistent flow of blood to the dialyzer.

Typically, this treatment takes three to four hours and in acute renal failure is performed daily, often at the bedside of the critical care patient. The dialysis patient must receive regional heparinization to prevent clotting of blood before it enters the dialyzer and while it is outside the body. The patient must be closely monitored for hemodynamic stability during the treatment. Inadvertent disconnect during the treatment can cause severe blood loss, so the patient must be maintained on a 1:1 observation by the dialysis nurse.

Peritoneal Dialysis

Peritoneal dialysis is done through an abdominal catheter that is placed surgically through the abdominal wall into the peritoneal space. The catheter has multiple holes at the end, which allow rapid infusion of dialysate into the abdominal wall. The peritoneal membrane, which covers the abdominal organs and overlies the capillary beds supporting the organs, serves as the filtering device. Under aseptic conditions, dialysate solution is infused into the abdominal cavity and left to dwell for a specific period of time. During this time, electrolytes and water are exchanged through the peritoneal membrane and filtered. After the dwelling time, the solution is drained from the abdomen. Recent abdominal surgery or past surgical interventions with history of adhesions or scarring are contraindications for peritoneal dialysis. Peritoneal dialysis is used for chronic renal failure and can be done in the patient's home after proper training. It can also be used for patients who are unable to tolerate hemodialysis due to hemodynamic instability.

Continuous Renal Replacement Therapy (CRRT)

Continuous renal replacement therapy (CRRT) is a new trend in acute care dialysis and requires specialized training, but it can be done by the critical care nurse. CRRT mimics the functioning of the nephron in regulation of water, electrolytes, and other solutes. The process is, as the name implies, a continuous treatment that occurs over the 24-hour period at a rate that is slower than that of the hemodialysis machine. Following are the five types of CRRT:

SCUF	Slow continuous ultrafiltration
CAVH	Continuous arteriovenous hemofiltration
CAVHD	Continuous arteriovenous hemodialysis
CVVH	Continuous venovenous hemofiltration
CVVHD	Continuous venovenous hemodialysis

The indications for using this type of system versus the conventional hemodialysis are multi-fold and include the following: 1) involves a slower process, which the patient who is hemodynamically unstable can tolerate more easily than hemodialysis, 2) does not require the renal nurse to manage the system, and 3) cytokines can be removed more readily with high-permeability membranes. All of these therapies use a specialized hemofilter.

SCUF is used for the removal of large amounts of fluid to achieve fluid balance. No dialysate or replacement fluids are used with this therapy if electrolytes or solutes are filtered. Patients who have been unresponsive to diuretic therapy may benefit from fluid removal using this treatment, particularly if there is pulmonary compromise due to the fluid overload.

CAVH uses an arterial access and an ultrafiltration pump to create a pressure so that convection and ultrafiltration can be used to remove water and waste products. Physiological replacement fluids are used to replace the majority of ultrafiltrate extracted during this therapy, since the focus on this therapy is removal of solutes. This is usually done prefilter or postdilution. The rate of exchange in either SCUF or CAVH is dependent on the membrane area, fiber diameter area, hematocrit, serum osmolality, pressure gradient, and blood flow.

Similarly, CAVHD requires an arterial access and adequate arterial hydrostatic pressure to move the blood through the filtering device. It is different than CAVH, as dialysate solution is infused via a volumetric pump into the dialysis filter countercurrent to the blood flow to remove solutes and fluid. Blood is returned to the patient through a venous catheter after it flows through the hemofilter. The use of replacement fluid is optional, as the purpose is primarily to remove waste or solutes.

In both CVVH and CVVHD, as the name implies, there does not need to be an arterial access. However, a roller pump is needed, as the venous circulation does not create the force necessary to create the flow through the system. In CVVHD, dialysate solution is infused countercurrent into the hemofilter to increase filtration of both fluids and solutes. In CVVH, the dialysate is infused into the blood. Prefilter replacement fluid may also be infused in either treatment.

SPECIAL CONSIDERATIONS FOR THE CRITICALLY ILL PATIENT WITH RENAL SYSTEM DISORDERS

The critical care nurse is responsible for the ongoing monitoring of and intervention with all patients under her care. The patient with renal disorders poses some additional challenges with regard to fluid balance and electrolyte disturbances due to inefficient functioning of the filtering system of the kidneys. Nursing diagnoses that would apply to these conditions include fluid volume excess related to renal dysfunction, fluid volume deficit related to absolute loss, anxiety related to the fear of long-term dialysis therapy and lifestyle changes, knowledge deficit due to new diagnoses, and potential for infection related to venous or arterial access devices.

FIGURE 11.11 *Putting It All Together: Hemodynamics and Fluid Balance*

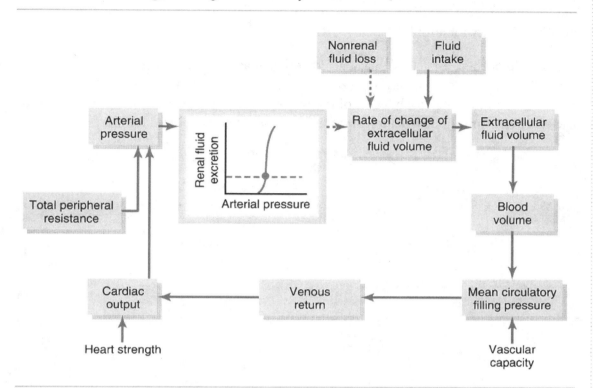

During the initial admission history and physical assessment of the critically ill patient with a real or potential renal disorder, it is imperative to get a clear understanding of the signs and symptoms that precipitated the condition. This includes history of cardiovascular diseases such as hypertension, congestive heart failure, or artherosclerosis. Diabetics are more prone to renal disorders due to vascular alterations as well. Changes in urine output, such as reduced or excess urine, appearance of urine, or patterns of urination, should be noted.

Pharmacological management of renal patients includes the following classes of drugs: diuretics, methylxanthines, antiinfectives, cardiovascular drugs, anticonvulsants, electrolytes, and analgesics. Diuretics are commonly administered to address fluid excess in attempt to reduce the likelihood of dialysis treatments, balance outputs, and to assist the kidney in excretion of filtrate. Conditions such as hyperphosphetemia may require phosphate-binding drugs such as Renagel, while an erythrocyte-stimulating drug such as Epogen may help the bone marrow increase production of red blood cells. Antiinfectives will be ordered to prevent or treat line, urine, or lung infections. Cardiac drug classifications also include beta-blockers, ACE inhibitors/ARB, calcium channel blockers, and antidysrhythmics. These medications may be required to treat the cardiac symptoms that may arise from electrolyte disturbances or uremic conditions. Intravenous or oral electrolytes will be used to supplement hypo-states. Patients in renal failure may need to have medication dosages altered based on metabolism and site of absorption and excretion in the kidneys, particularly for antibiotics.

Another important aspect of pharmacological management is related to the patient on hemodialysis. Many drugs are dialyzed during treatments and therefore should not be administered until after completion of the treatment. Patients who are on hemodialysis or CRRT will require anticoagulation and therefore should be monitored for bleeding.

Review Questions

1. What electrolyte abnormality produces a U wave, ST depression, and T wave changes on the ECG?

   A. hyperkalemia

   B. hypocalcemia

   C. hyperphosphatemia

   D. hypokalemia

2. End stage renal disease (ESRD) is characterized by

   A. nephron loss of approximately 90 percent.

   B. serum creatinine > 3.0.

   C. BU > 100.

   D. inability to concentrate urine.

3. A patient in the ICU presents with the diagnosis of acute renal failure. During your shift, you note the ECG to have tall peaked T waves that progress to a widening QRS. What electrolyte imbalance produces these findings?

   A. hypokalemia

   B. hyperphosphatemia

   C. hyperkalemia

   D. hyperchloremia

4. You are caring for a patient in the ICU who has a urinary catheter in place. You note that there has been no drainage out of the catheter in the last two hours. What is your **first** action?

   A. Check for patency.

   B. Call the physician for further orders.

   C. Remove the catheter.

   D. Give the patient an IV fluid bolus.

5. Anemia caused by chronic renal failure is associated with

   A. acute blood loss.

   B. decreased erythropoietin production by the kidneys.

   C. malnutrition.

   D. hemolysis.

6. You are caring for a patient with chronic renal insufficiency. The morning labs show a sodium level of 119 mEq/dL. What neurologic signs or symptoms may occur?

   A. seizures

   B. weakness

   C. nystagmus

   D. torticollis

7. The normal anion gap is

   A. less than 1 mEq/L.

   B. 5 to 10 mEq/L.

   C. 10 to 15 mEq/L.

   D. greater than 20 mEq/L.

8. You are caring for a patient who has been hypotensive with a MAP < 60 mm Hg for three hours. This patient is at risk for developing what type of renal failure?

   A. prerenal failure

   B. intrarenal failure

   C. postrenal failure

   D. chronic renal failure

9. Which of these clients would the nurse monitor for potential prerenal failure?

    A. a client with diabetes with hemoglobin A1C of 5.0 percent

    B. a client with dementia with albumin of 5.5 g/dL (55 g/dL)

    C. a client with heart failure with a BNP of 704 pg/mL

    D. a client with stroke with a BUN of 20 mg/dL (7.1 mmol/L)

10. What is the most sensitive indicator that a patient is retaining fluid in the ICU?

    A. intake and output

    B. daily weight

    C. patient assessment

    D. urine electrolytes

REVIEW ANSWERS AND EXPLANATIONS ON FOLLOWING PAGE ▶ ▶ ▶

Review Answers and Explanations

1. D

Patients with low potassium levels can present with acute ECG changes including a U wave, T wave changes, and ST depression. These changes are due to delayed ventricular repolarization.

2. A

Patients are classified as ESRD when they have 10 percent or less of the normal renal function. When a patient's kidney function is 10 percent or less, the patient will require dialysis or kidney transplant.

3. C

Typically patients with a potassium level around 6 mEq/L will start to display ECG changes, including tall peaked T waves. These changes will progress as the potassium rises to a prolonged PR interval, absent P waves, and a widening of the QRS complex.

4. A

A full assessment must be completed on patients who have an acute onset of no urine output. This assessment should include checking patency of the urinary catheter prior to any other interventions.

5. B

Patients with chronic renal failure have a decreased production of red blood cells. This decreased production is due to the inability of the kidneys to secrete the hormone erythropoietin.

6. A

Hyponatremia causes an extracellular hypo-osmolarity that causes free water to shift from the vascular space to the intracellular space. Cellular edema is well tolerated in most tissues except for the brain, due to cerebral edema and the rigid confines of the skull. This cerebral edema causes neurological findings such as seizure activity.

7. C

The anion gap is the difference between routinely measured anions and cations in the serum. The normal value is between 10 and 15 mEq/L.

8. A

Hypotension causes decreased renal blood flow, resulting in ischemia and cell death. This ischemic event will cause a cascade of events, including free radical production, cytokine release, endothelial activation, leukocyte adhesion, activation of the coagulation pathway, and apoptosis and these cause further damage to the organ. The damage would manifest as prerenal failure.

9. C

Prerenal causes include heart failure due to low renal perfusion. An elevated BNP (normal less than 100 pg/mL) indicates CHF. (A) Hemoglobin A1C of 5.0 percent is within normal range; it is not a risk for renal failure. (B) Albumin of 5.5 g/dL (55 g/dL) is within normal range. (D) BUN of 20 mg/dL (7.1 mmol/L) is within normal range.

10. B

Daily weights should be used in the ICU setting to trend fluid status. Weight is one of the most sensitive indicators of fluid retention.

Multiorgan System 12

The multiorgan portion of the CCRN exam makes up 14 percent of the total number of questions.

This chapter covers a wide variety of conditions that affect multiple organ systems. These conditions make patients very complex to care for, increase their length of stay in an Intensive Care Unit, increase the morbidity and mortality rates, and increase the cost of providing care. Topics covered include *traumatic injury, distributive shock, systemic inflammatory response syndrome (SIRS), multiorgan dysfunction syndrome, toxic exposure, toxic ingestions and inhalations,* and *asphyxia.* Clinical manifestations and collaborative care will be discussed for each topic. The purpose of this chapter is to provide specific information necessary for the critical care RN to provide care for this vast group of conditions.

MULTISYSTEM TRAUMA: ADULT

Mechanism of Injury

The four most common mechanisms of injury are blunt trauma, penetrating trauma, burns, and toxic exposure.

- **Blunt**—The *transmission of energy causes the injury.* This is the most common type of injury. Falls, crush injuries, motor vehicle crash, assault, motorcycle crash, bicycle crash, and sports injuries are examples. The forces involved are acceleration, deceleration, shearing, and crushing. Blunt trauma may also cause asphyxia.

- **Penetrating**—An *object causes the injury as it passes through body tissues.* Gunshot wounds, shotgun wounds, stab wounds, and impalements are examples. The forces involved are velocity and mass.

- **Burns**—*Chemical, electrical, or thermal energy causes tissue injury.* Other less common mechanisms of injury include bites, stings, inhaled and ingested poisons, and toxic exposure.

- **Toxic exposure**—*Inhaled or injected toxins cause injury.* These include poisons, bites, stings, and contact with irritating substances affecting skin and/or mucous membranes.

Clinical Manifestation

Clinical manifestation is specific to the mechanism of injury and is different in every patient. Examples of factors that affect clinical manifestation include age, gender, preexisting illnesses, time between injury and treatment, and substance abuse.

Resuscitation and Collaborative Care

Injured patients need an organized and rapid approach to assessing their injuries, regardless of the mechanism of injury. The American College of Surgeons Committee on Trauma recommends performing a primary and secondary survey on all injured patients to identify and treat all life-threatening and non-life-threatening injuries. The primary survey includes ABCDE. During this assessment, all *life-threatening injuries* are identified and treated. The survey does not proceed until an identified issue is addressed (e.g., patient not breathing—intubation and ventilation).

A = Airway:	Does the patient have a patent airway? Is subcutaneous emphysema present?
B = Breathing:	Is the patient able to breathe effectively? What color are the mucous membranes? Is there thoracic penetration or flail chest?
C = Circulation:	What is the patient's volume status? Are there obvious long bone or pelvic fractures? Stop obvious bleeding. Check peripheral pulses and capillary refill. Draw labs, including ABGs and type and cross.
D = Disability:	Check level of consciousness, pupils, motor and verbal response. Assess for spinal cord injury.
E = Exposure:	All clothing and jewelry must be removed. Assess skin temperature; cover patient after primary survey is complete to prevent hypothermia.

Once the primary survey is complete (i.e., all life-threatening injuries have been identified and treated), the secondary survey begins. This may be delayed by a trip to the operating room, angiography suite, or interventional radiology. The secondary survey is a systematic head-to-toe assessment to identify all injuries the patient has sustained. During the secondary survey, a patient history, injury history, and further diagnostic studies are obtained. Information may be obtained from the patient, prehospital providers, and/or friends and family when available. During this time, a definitive plan for care of the patient is formulated.

Fluid Resuscitation

Most injured patients need some degree of fluid resuscitation. The goal of fluid resuscitation is to restore adequate circulating fluid volume and oxygen delivery to the tissues. Remember that vital signs are just one piece of the puzzle. In the setting of an injured patient, urine output, capillary refill, and level of consciousness are often more sensitive indicators of the adequacy of resuscitation. Crystalloids and blood products are the resuscitation fluids of choice for injured patients. Colloids such as dextran and hetastarch do not have hemoglobin-carrying capacity, and research has not shown that colloids are more effective than crystalloids in resuscitating injured patients. Potential adverse effects of the above mentioned colloids include large fluid shifts, anaphylaxis, and coagulopathy.

Crystalloids

Crystalloid solutions are clear fluids made up of water, glucose, and electrolytes (e.g., normal saline, lactated Ringer's, etc.). The formula to determine the volume of crystalloid to be administered initially is three milliliters of crystalloid for each milliliter of blood lost (3 mL crystalloid: 1 mL blood loss). In the setting of resuscitation, crystalloids are categorized as shown in table 12.2.

Blood and Blood Products

Transfusion of blood and blood products during resuscitation is limited to hemodynamically unstable patients who have lost blood and need volume expansion and oxygen-carrying capability. In an emergency situation, when there is no time to obtain a type and cross match for blood products, type-specific or O-negative blood may be administered. Replacement of coagulation factors, such as platelets, fresh frozen plasma (FFP), or cryoprecipitate, should occur only in the presence of active bleeding or if interventional procedures are to be undertaken emergently. Autotransfusion is sometimes used in patients with chest injuries. It is not useful in patients with abdominal injuries due to potential contamination of blood from spilled gastric contents.

TABLE 12.1 *Parameters That Reflect Adequacy of Resuscitation*

Parameter	Normal	What it indicates
Lactate	0.3 to 2.2 mmol/L	A rising lactate indicates inadequate tissue perfusion and oxygenation.
Base Deficit	−2 to +3 mEq/L	An increasing base deficit (> −2) indicates decreased perfusion and oxygenation.
Urine Output	30 mL/hr in an adult	Less than 30 mL/hr indicates inadequate circulating volume or kidney perfusion.
Capillary Refill	< 2 seconds	Prolonged capillary refill indicates decreased perfusion to the extremities.

TABLE 12.2 *Addressing Tonicity for Resuscitation*

	Solutions	Contents	Uses	Effect	Miscellaneous
HYPOTONIC	D5W (5% dextrose in water)	Dextrose and free water, no electrolytes	Not used to resuscitate injured patients who are volume depleted.	Cause leakage of fluid into interstitial and intracellular spaces.	Monitor patient for fluid overload, total body edema, and hyperglycemia.
ISOTONIC	NS (0.9% normal saline)	Sodium and chloride	Used for volume replacement in hypovolemic patients, used with blood transfusions, and used to replete low serum sodium.	No significant fluid shifts across cellular membranes or vessels.	Monitor patient's serum sodium during infusion to prevent hypernatremia. Monitor patient for fluid overload.
	LR (lactated Ringer's)	Sodium, chloride, potassium, calcium, and lactate, similar to concentration in human plasma	Used to resuscitate volume-depleted trauma and burn patients. Can also be used to replete volume lost from vomiting, dehydration, or diarrhea.	No significant fluid shifts across cellular membranes or vessels.	Lacks the magnesium and phosphate in human plasma.
HYPERTONIC	3% normal saline	Saline	Used cautiously in patients due to sodium load. Useful to treat cerebral edema.	Draws fluid from cells and interstitial spaces into vessels.	Monitor, serum sodium, monitor for fluid overload. Generally requires central venous access.
	D5 ½ NS (5% dextrose and 0.45% normal saline)	Dextrose, sodium, and chloride	Commonly used as a maintenance fluid, not a resuscitation fluid.	No significant effect on intravascular volume, increases total body edema.	Monitor patient for hyperglycemia and total body edema.
	D5 NS (5% dextrose and 0.9% normal saline)	Dextrose, sodium, and chloride	Commonly used as a maintenance fluid, not a resuscitation fluid.	No significant effect on intravascular volume, increases total body edema.	Monitor patient for hyperglycemia and total body edema.

- Platelets: Generally given if platelet count falls below 50,000 and there is evidence of bleeding.

- Fresh frozen plasma: Administered if PT/INR or PTT is higher than 1.5 times control.

- Cryoprecipitate: Given for fibrinogen levels < 0.8 g/L.

Additional aspects of collaborative care for injured patients involve continued monitoring and treatment of deficits in oxygenation, ventilation, circulation, perfusion, mobility, skin integrity, nutrition, and pain. It is also essential to maintain patient safety at all times, assess and treat the patient and family's psychosocial status, and initiate discharge planning and teaching when it is appropriate.

Sequelae of Multisystem Trauma

The following is a list of potential complications of multisystem trauma and their causes. The nurse plays an integral part in the prevention of and early recognition of the signs and symptoms of these potentially fatal conditions.

Pressure Ulcers

Inadequate tissue perfusion, direct trauma to tissue, and edema resulting from prolonged bed rest

Atelectasis/Pneumonia

Chest trauma, pain, head injury, inhalation injury, aspiration, prolonged immobility or bed rest, intubation, multiple transfusions, massive fluid resuscitation

Deep Vein Thrombosis (DVT)

Endothelial injury (traumatic or iatrogenic), venous stasis (due to hypovolemia, immobility, etc.), prolonged immobilization

Pulmonary Embolism/Fat Embolism

Fractures, particularly long bone fractures such as to the femur; head and/or spinal cord injury; hypotension; hypovolemia; shock; prolonged immobilization; and any risk factor for DVT

Hypovolemic Shock

Massive blood loss or continued bleeding, significant dehydration due to cutaneous loss in severe large surface area burns or large open wounds

Infection/Sepsis

"Dirty wounds," open wounds, indwelling lines and catheters, depressed immune system, advanced age, history of immunosuppression or diabetes, malnutrition, massive blood transfusion

Acute Respiratory Distress Syndrome (ARDS)

Head injuries, multiple major fractures, pulmonary contusion, massive transfusion, immunosuppression, ongoing shock, aspiration

Acute Kidney Injury (AKI, previously referred to as Acute Renal Failure)

Long periods of hypoperfusion or hypovolemia, renal trauma, vasopressors, antibiotics, contrast medium, rhabdomyolysis, transfusion reactions, preexisting renal disease, obstruction of the renal tubular system (e.g., nephrolithiasis), patients with history of severe diabetes and/or severe hypertension

Disseminated Intravascular Coagulation (DIC)

Shock, massive transfusion or mismatched blood, sepsis, near drowning, hypothermia, venomous bites, crush injuries

Systemic Inflammatory Response Syndrome (SIRS)

Widespread inflammation including organs and systems not involved in the initial injury, increased temperature, increased WBC, increased metabolic rate

Multiple Organ Dysfunction Syndrome

Hemorrhage, massive blood transfusion, shock, sepsis, prolonged tissue hypoxia, toxic exposure

DISTRIBUTIVE SHOCK

The definition of distributive shock is decreased tissue perfusion resulting from decreased vascular tone and a pooling of unoxygenated blood in the tissues. Distributive shock may occur as a result of several etiologies that lead to systemic vasodilation: anaphylactic, neurogenic, and septic.

Anaphylactic Shock

Antigens are protein-based molecules that are introduced into the body via injection, ingestion, the skin, and/or breathing. When these antigens are taken in, there is a chance that they will cause a severe hypersensitive immunological reaction and a life-threatening event. The initial contact of antigens with the body is called a *primary immune response*. Subsequent exposure causes a *secondary immune response* and potentially, anaphylaxis. *Antibodies* in the blood are formed and trigger a cascade of chemical events and reactions with the mast cells and basophils. These chemical reactions cause vasodilation, increased capillary permeability, bronchospasms, excessive mucous secretion, inflammatory response, and constriction of smooth muscle. Subsequently, circulating volume is decreased, and oxygenation is not adequate. With the decrease in circulating volume, venous return and stroke volume are also decreased. The ultimate result is decreased tissue perfusion and impaired cellular metabolism.

It is critical that an immediate response is directed toward removal of the antigen; protection of the airway and circulation; administration of medications such as *epinephrine, diphenhydramine, corticosteroids,* and *bronchodilators*; and fluid replacement to prevent further deterioration in the patient's condition and potential death.

Neurogenic Shock

Neurogenic shock is the result of impairment to the SNS and, similar to the other shock states, results in decreased tissue perfusion. It is the least common form of distributive shock. Etiologies of neurogenic shock are trauma, anesthesia, and spinal shock.

The clinical symptoms that the patient manifests as a result of neurogenic shock include alterations in level of consciousness, bradycardia, lack of sweating, apnea, paralysis, hypotension, and decreased urine output. Hemodynamically, the patient evidences decreased CVP, systemic vascular resistance (SVR), CO, CI, and oxygen saturation. The loss of sympathetic tone results in arterial and venous vasodilation and impaired thermoregulation. The cascade continues with decreased venous return, stroke volume, and cardiac output.

Treatment of neurogenic shock is careful fluid resuscitation, and vasopressors may be needed to support blood pressure. Hypothermia is treated with warming measures such as warming blankets and should be done slowly so as to prevent rapid changes in the patient's core temperature. Aggressive pulmonary management is required, particularly in the patient who has evidence of paralysis. Treatment of the underlying condition is also needed and may require stabilization of traumatic injuries and immobilization of spinal injuries.

Sepsis and Septic Shock

Septic shock is one type of distributive shock that involves all organ systems. Critically ill patients are at increased risk for developing sepsis and septic shock. Technology has enabled us to prolong the life of patients who previously would have died from their initial insult. Blood, urine, and or sputum cultures will be positive for bacterial growth. The most commonly implicated organisms are either gram negative bacilli, such as *E. coli*, or gram-positive cocci, like methicillin-resistant *Staphylococcus aureus* (MRSA). The list of potential infectious agents is significantly broadened in immunocompromised and transplant patients. The emergence of antibiotic-resistant bacteria has also contributed to the rising rates of sepsis and septic shock. Septic shock due to viral pathogens is uncommon in adults. Many cases of septic shock are from hospital-acquired or nosocomial infections. These pathogens commonly enter the body through the pulmonary, urinary, or gastrointestinal tract. Line sepsis involves infection of an indwelling IV catheter. Generally, if "line sepsis" is being considered, the medical team will provide antibacterial coverage for gram positive organisms with vancomycin until speciation and antibiotic sensitivities are known from the cultures sent. Central venous lines and pulmonary artery catheters necessary for care of critically ill patients are commonly implicated. To decrease a patient's risk of developing line sepsis, it is imperative to use sterile techniques during insertion of all indwelling lines. Also, meticulous nursing care after line insertion helps prevent infection. The use of antibiotic-coated and impregnated catheters has been found to have little effect on reducing the rate of line sepsis. As soon as line sepsis is suspected, the line must be removed.

Clinical Manifestations

There is a continuum of infection that involves sepsis, severe sepsis, and septic shock. The clinical manifestations of the "sepsis continuum" are listed below.

TABLE 12.3 *Sepsis Definitions*

Systemic Inflam-matory Response Syndrome (SIRS) ($\geq$2 criteria)	+	Infection T >38 °C (100.4 °F) or <36 °C (96.8 °F) HR >90 RR >20 or pCO_2 <32 mm Hg WBC >12K, or <4K, or >10% Bands		=	Sepsis
Sepsis	+	One or More Organ Dysfunction*		=	Severe Sepsis
		*Elevated lactate ($\geq$4) ALI/ARDS (P/F ratio <300 Thrombocytopenia (PLR <1,000)	Oliguria (<0.5 cc/kg/hr despite adequate fluid) ARF (Cr. Increase > 0.5) Bilirubinemia (<4) Coagulopathy (INR >1.5)		
Sepsis	+	Hypotension (shock)* (despite IVF of 30 ml/kg) or requiring pressors		=	Septic Shock
		*SBP $\leq$90 mm Hg OR MAP <65 mm Hg OR SBP decrease $\geq$40 mm Hg from baseline			

Collaborative Care

The priorities of care for the patient with sepsis and septic shock are *identification and treatment of the infecting pathogen*. Treatment goals are directed toward maintaining oxygenation, ventilation, circulation, perfusion, skin integrity, nutrition, and pain control. It is also important to ensure patient safety, prevent hazards of immobility, and address any psychosocial issues the patient and family might have. Clinically, the patient may be intubated and mechanically ventilated, may have a central venous catheter to monitor fluid/volume status and cardiac output, and potentially need vasoactive and/or inotropic support. Broad spectrum antibiotic coverage may be initiated prior to obtaining culture results, then streamlined when the pathogens are positively identified. Based on the 2012 Surviving Sepsis Campaign (SSC), the following actions must be completed within 3 hours of recognition that the patient is septic:

- Measure lactate level (send specimen in ice)

- IV antibiotic within the first hour of recognition of septic shock (1B) and severe sepsis without septic shock

- Administer 30 mL/kg of crystalloid (NS, LR) for hypotension or lactate ≥4mmol/L

- Maintain a MAP >65 mm/Hg

Use norepinephrine as the first choice vasopressor. Use epinephrine (added to and potentially substituted for norepinephrine) when an additional agent is needed to maintain blood pressure. Vasopressin 0.03 units/min can be added to norepinephrine to raise MAP to target, or norepinephrine can be decreased.

The SSC bundle recommends that the following be completed within 6 hours from the time sepsis is diagnosed or suspected:

- Apply vasopressors to maintain a mean arterial pressure (MAP) ≥65 mm Hg

- In the event of persistent arterial hypotension despite volume resuscitation (septic shock) or initial lactate ≥4 mmol/L (36 mg/dL):

  – Measure central venous pressure (CVP)(Normal: 2–6 mm Hg)

  – Measure central venous oxygen saturation ($ScvO_2$)(Normal: > 75 percent)

- Remeasure lactate if initial lactate was elevated. Targets for quantitative resuscitation included in the guidelines are CVP of ≥8 mm Hg, $ScvO_2$ of ≥70 percent, and normalization of lactate (grade 2C).

Systemic Inflammatory Response Syndrome (SIRS)

A syndrome characterized by a widespread inflammatory response to an insult.

Clinical Manifestation

Two or more of the following are present: T > 38 °C or < 36 °C, HR > 90 beats per minute, RR greater than 20 per minute, WBC > 12,000 cells/mm^3, less than 4,000 cells/mm^3 or > 10% bands on differential. There is often no infectious pathogen identified. When SIRS is caused by documented infection, it is called sepsis.

Collaborative Care

Treatment goals are similar to those of septic shock and center around restoring adequate oxygenation and tissue perfusion. Because no infectious source is usually identified, administration of antibiotics has no effect on SIRS, although some clinicians may consider starting empiric antibiotics if the suspicion of infection is high.

Multiple Organ Dysfunction Syndrome (MODS)

At the end of the shock continuum, organs begin to fail due to continued lack of adequate oxygenation and perfusion. MODS is defined as progressive physiologic failure of two or more separate organ systems in an acutely ill patient such that homeostasis cannot be maintained without intervention. MODS is the major cause of death in patients cared for in critical care units.

- The failure of one organ causes the failure of subsequent organs. The lungs often fail first and are followed by the liver, GI tract, kidneys, hematologic system, and finally the heart. Early identification and meticulous monitoring of patients at risk for developing MODS is the best way to decrease morbidity and mortality.

- The treatment of MODS is largely supportive. The mortality rate of MODS approaches 75 percent despite intervention.

TOXIC EXPOSURE

Chemical Exposure: Nerve Agents

Nerve agents are organic chemicals (organophosphates) that disrupt the mechanism by which nerves transfer messages to organs. The disruption is caused by blocking acetylcholinesterase, an enzyme that normally relaxes the activity of acetylcholine, a neurotransmitter. Nerve agents are classified as **G-agents** (sarin, somon, and tabun) or **V-agents** (VX). These agents can be absorbed either through the respiratory tract or through the skin. They are easily vaporized or aerosolized, enabling them to spread over large areas.

Clinical Manifestations

Sarin has no odor; therefore, patients may not initially be aware of exposure. Soman has a fruity or camphor-like odor, and tabun has a very faint fruity odor. These odors are not unusual, so patients exposed to either soman or tabun may not initially be aware of exposure. Signs and symptoms of exposure to **G-agents** develop within seconds to hours of exposure. Patients with *minimal to moderate exposure* present with non-life-threatening symptoms that include runny nose, watery eyes, small pinpoint pupils, eye pain, blurred vision, drooling, excessive sweating, cough, chest tightness, tachypnea, diarrhea, increased urine output, confusion, drowsiness, weakness, headache, nausea, vomiting, abdominal pain, tachycardia or bradycardia, and hypotension or hypertension. With *significant expo-sure,* signs and symptoms are life threatening and include change in level of consciousness ending in unconsciousness and seizure, paralysis, respiratory failure, and death. Patients exposed to **V-agents** display the same signs and symptoms as those exposed to G-agents.

Collaborative Care

Initial care for patients exposed to both G- and V-agents includes *removal of all clothing and thorough decontamination.* Health care professionals involved in decontamination pro-cedures must wear full body protection to avoid exposure to both G- and V-agents. Early administration of *atropine and pralidoxime (Protopam)* within minutes of exposure has been shown to be effective to block acetylcholine receptors, thereby preventing further nervous system effects.

Blood Agents

This is a group of toxins that are carried by the blood and travel throughout the body, ultimately affecting every body system. These agents exert their effect at the cellular level (e.g., cyanide).

Clinical Manifestations

Even minimum exposure to cyanide, either by breathing, absorption via the skin, or inges-tion, causes *immediate signs and symptoms,* including tachypnea, restlessness, dizziness, weakness, headache, nausea, vomiting, and tachycardia. Cyanide smells like bitter almonds, but it is sometimes difficult to detect. After exposure to large amounts of cyanide via any of the above mentioned portals, the patient immediately develops seizures, hypotension, bradycardia, and unresponsiveness. Patients who are exposed to large amounts of cyanide immediately develop acute lung injury, which leads to respiratory failure and death. Patients exposed to small or moderate amounts of cyanide can survive but may have long-term cardiac and brain damage.

Collaborative Treatment

Decontamination is the initial step in treatment of patients exposed to cyanide. Health care workers involved in the decontamination must wear full body protection to avoid exposure to cyanide. All of the patient's clothing must be removed and the body thoroughly cleansed with soap and water. Pharmacologic treatment of cyanide poisoning includes the administration of amyl nitrate, IV sodium nitrate, and sodium thiosulfate. When available, a newer treat-ment of cyanide poisoning involves administration of hydroxocobalamin. This reacts with cyanide in the bloodstream to create cyanocobalamin, which is eliminated by the kidneys.

Vesicant or Blister Agents

Exposure to vesicant or blister agents such as HD (sulfur mustard), HN (nitrogen mustard), L (Lewisite), or CX (phosgene) may not immediately be apparent to the patient, as none of these agents has an identifying odor.

Clinical Manifestations

Patients exposed to mustard gas may not develop signs and symptoms 2 to 24 hours after exposure, depending on the amount of agent the person is exposed to. Initially, the patient's skin becomes red and itchy; then it turns yellow and blisters. Within an hour of exposure, the patient may experience nonspecific symptoms of skin irritation, pain, swelling, and tearing. Severe exposure may produce blindness lasting up to 10 days. Respiratory signs and symptoms mimic those of a cold and include runny nose, sneezing, hoarseness, bloody nose, sinus pain, shortness of breath, and cough. Exposure to phosgene causes immediate cutaneous pain with accompanying blanching surrounded by red rings (within 30 seconds of exposure). Hives appear within 30 minutes, and after 24 hours the blanched areas turn brown, the skin dies, and a scab is formed. Pain and itching continue until the wound is healed. Phosgene in the eyes causes severe eye pain and temporary blindness along with tearing. Respiratory symptoms of phosgene exposure include immediate signs of upper respiratory tract irritation, runny nose, hoarseness, and sinus pain along with shortness of breath, cough, and, with large exposure, pulmonary edema. Data on Lewisite exposure has been obtained largely from animal models.

Collaborative Care

Initial treatment of patients exposed to vesicant or blistering agents involves *decontamination*, including the removal of all clothing. Health care professionals involved in the decontamination effort must wear protective body suits to avoid exposure to the agents. There are *currently no antidotes* for exposure to vesicant or blistering agents, and the care is largely supportive.

Pulmonary or Inhaled Agents

Chemicals that cause rapid and severe irritation to the respiratory tract include ammonia, chlorine, phosgene, ricin, and carbon monoxide.

Clinical Manifestations

The severity of signs and symptoms is directly related to the amount and duration of exposure. Immediate symptoms are manifested in three categories: muscarinic, nicotinic, and central nervous system. **Muscarinic** manifestations include bradycardia, hypotension, rhinorrhea, bronchorrhea, bronchospasm, cough, respiratory distress, increased salivation, nausea, vomiting, diarrhea, abdominal pain, urinary and fecal incontinence, blurred vision, miosis, diaphoresis, and increased lacrimation. **Nicotinic** effects include muscle fascicula-tions, cramping and weakness, diaphragmatic failure, hypertension, tachycardia, mydriasis, and pallor. **Central nervous system** manifestations include altered mental status, anxiety, emotional lability, restlessness, confusion, ataxia, tremors, seizures, and coma. Symptoms of **carbon monoxide poisoning** vary widely depending on the level of exposure and can include headache, dizziness, nausea, flulike symptoms, fatigue, shortness of breath on exertion, impaired judgment, chest pain, confusion, depression, hallucinations, seizures, impaired memory, and cherry red skin. Carboxyhemoglobin level is obtained to measure the severity of exposure and to trend improvement with treatment.

Collaborative Care

Decontamination is the first priority of care in patients exposed to ammonia, chlorine, and phosgene. All clothing must be removed and the body washed thoroughly with soap and water to limit further exposure. There is *no antidote* for ammonia, chlorine, or phosgene exposure; hence treatment is symptomatic. Patients with high levels of exposure to inhaled agents may be intubated, mechanically ventilated, and admitted to an intensive care unit. The patient's condition may warrant use of hemodynamic monitoring and support of circu-lation with the use of vasoactive and/or inotropic agents.

Biologic Exposure

Biologic agents are categorized into two categories, A and B. **Category A** includes anthrax, botulism, plague, smallpox, tularemia, and viral hemorrhagic fevers. These agents are easily spread person to person and have a high mortality rate. **Category B** includes brucellosis and ricin. Category B agents are moderately easy to transmit person to person and cause increased morbidity, but low mortality, after exposure.

Clinical Manifestations

Anthrax is a spore-forming bacteria that is not easily spread from person to person. There are three routes of exposure to anthrax, all with different manifestations. **Cutaneous expo-sure** is the most common (95 percent of all exposures). The spore enters the body via a cut in the skin. Within two days of exposure, a small raised itchy bump resembling an insect bite is noted; this bump evolves into a vesicle, eventually becoming a painless ulcer with a black necrotic center. **Inhalation** of the spore initially presents with signs and symptoms of the common cold, including malaise, sore throat, low-grade fever, and muscle aches. The symptoms quickly progress to acute respiratory failure and shock. **Gastrointestinal expo-sure** is generally due to eating meat contaminated with the anthrax spore. Signs and symp-toms resemble those of acute inflammation of the gastrointestinal tract, including anorexia, nausea, and vomiting, bloody stools, and uncontrolled diarrhea.

Botulism (*Clostridium botulinum*) is not spread from one person to another. Exposure can be either *food-borne* (from eating meat, canned fruit jam, honey) or from a wound infected with the toxin-producing bacteria. Signs and symptoms may not be apparent for up to two weeks after exposure but most commonly appear within 12–36 hours of exposure. The botulism toxin is a *muscle-paralyzing agent.* Symptoms include double or blurred vision, drooping eyelids, slurred speech, dysphagia, dry mouth, and muscle weakness that always involves the shoulders first and progresses downward.

Plague (*Yersinia pestis*) is a bacteria common to rodents and their fleas. Plague can be bubonic, pneumonic, or septicemic. **Bubonic plague**, the most common, is contracted via a flea bite or through a cut in the skin. Exposure is manifested by swollen and very tender lymph nodes accompanied by painful swollen glands, called *buboes,* approximately two to six days after exposure. It is not spread person to person. **Pneumonic plague** is contracted by inhaling aerosolized particles or droplets from very close contact with an infected person or animal. Signs and symptoms include headache, fever, weakness, aggressive pneumonia with shortness of breath, chest pain, and cough with watery and/or bloody sputum. Within two to four days of exposure, respiratory failure and shock develop. **Septicemic plague** is not spread person to person and is commonly a complication of the other two forms of plague but can occur on its own. The signs and symptoms are similar to those of bubonic and pneumonic plague without the development of buboes. Abdominal pain and internal bleeding may occur with septicemic plague.

Smallpox is caused by two viruses, *Variola major/minor,* and has been eradicated in the United States except for laboratory stockpiles. *Variola minor* produces very mild signs and symptoms, is rare, and is much less serious. *Variola major* has four subcategories: *ordinary,* the most frequent type (90 percent of all exposures); *modified,* a mild form in previously vaccinated individuals; and *flat* and *hemorrhagic,* both of which are severe and fatal. Clinical manifestations include fever (greater than or equal to 101 °F), followed by a rash with firm, deep-seated vesicles or pustules that are all at the same stage of development. The incubation period is approximately 1 to 17 days, and it is not contagious during this time. Smallpox is highly contagious once the rash appears. The rash starts as small red spots in the mouth and on the tongue that spread to the face, arms, legs, hands, and feet. Within 24 hours of appearance, the mouth and tongue rash becomes pustules.

Exposure to **tularemia** or rabbit fever is most common from an infected tick bite; the bacteria is found in rodents and rabbits. Tularemia can also be transmitted from touching the dead animal or eating or drinking from infected sources. The bacteria can also be inhaled. Exposure to a small amount of bacteria can cause symptoms in approximately three to five days. Clinical manifestations include chills, enlarged groin or underarm lymph nodes, fever, headache, joint stiffness, muscle pain, red spots on the skin that enlarge over time and progress to an ulcer, shortness of breath, sweating, and weight loss and pneumonia.

Hantavirus is a zoonotic disease that is transmitted from deer rats to humans via excretions when they are aerosolized and inhaled. It is caused by the **Sin Nombre virus** and was first identified in 1993. The challenge with identification of the condition is that it typically develops 1–6 weeks after exposure and the early symptoms are similar to those of the flu, including fever, cough, muscle aches, and fatigue. However, it can quickly progress to severe respiratory symptoms, including pulmonary edema and acute respiratory failure. Patients may require advanced modes of ventilation or more sophisticated treatments, such as extra corporeal membrane oxygenation (ECMO).

Collaborative Treatment

Diagnosis of exposure to **anthrax** is by history. Early treatment (within seven days) of cutaneous exposure with tetracyclines, fluoroquinolones, or penicillins is usually curative. Lack of treatment carries a 20 percent mortality rate. Exposure by inhalation carries a 75 percent mortality rate, even with aggressive treatment with antibiotics, intubation, mechanical ventilation, and circulatory support. Gastrointestinal exposure has up to a 60 percent mortality rate with aggressive treatment, as mentioned above. There is currently a vaccine available for anthrax, but it is only recommended for active duty military personnel, persons working directly with anthrax spores in the laboratory, or persons who work with animals or animal hides that can potentially be infected. Vaccination of the general public is not currently recommended.

Diagnosis of exposure to **botulism** is presumptive and based on the patient's history. Treatment for presumed exposure must be initiated long before the confirmatory laboratory tests are available. These tests include culture of feces, gastric secretion, vomitus, serum, and/or wounds. Treatment includes an antitoxin stored at the Centers for Disease Control and Prevention that reduces the severity of the symptoms if given early in the postexposure period. Persons exposed to the botulism toxin usually survive after weeks to months of supportive treatment, including aggressive intensive care unit treatment with intubation, mechanical ventilation, and circulatory support.

The diagnosis of exposure to **plague** relies on the patient's history. Laboratory tests include bronchial washings and blood and tissue from the patient. *Immediate treatment with antibiotics* for patients with pneumonic plague is essential for survival. Streptomycin, gentamycin, the tetracyclines, or chloramphenicol is recommended for treatment. Intensive care unit treatment with intubation, mechanical ventilation, and circulatory support is essential, as death occurs within four days without appropriate treatment. Plague has not been reported east of the Rocky Mountains in the United States.

Exposure to **smallpox** is fatal if left untreated; those who survive exposure are left with deep scars, possible blindness, and arthritis. Treatment is supportive with intravenous fluid, pain medication, and antipyretics. Antibiotics are given only to treat secondary infections. A vaccine is currently available but is not recommended for the general public.

Collaborative treatment for **tularemia** includes blood and sputum cultures, a thorough history of potential for exposure, and treatment with antibiotics. The tetracyclines and fluoroquinolones are given orally, and streptomycin or gentamycin can be given intramuscularly or intravenously. Inhaled tularemia can evolve into a life-threatening pneumonia if not treated.

Treatment for **hantavirus** should be aggressive and focused on maintaining oxygenation and tissue perfusion, including ventilator support. Infusion of intravenous ribavirin may be indicated, but this often is not effective once the patient has reached the cardiopulmonary phase of the disease. Environmental controls and eradication of the mouse population should be attempted to prevent further spread of the disease.

Nuclear/Radiation Exposure

There are two types of radiation, *ionizing and nonionizing.* Nonionizing does not cause tissue damage and will not be discussed here. Ionizing radiation causes an immediate effect on human tissues. In the event of a radiation or nuclear event, everything, including soil and water, at the site of the blast would be vaporized. The vapors mix with radioactive material, eventually cool, and fall back to earth as dust; this is referred to as the "fallout" and can be carried over a large area. Anything the fallout lands on becomes contaminated with radiation. Injury to humans and animals can be from the blast itself or from exposure to radioactive fallout and its contaminants.

Acute Radiation Syndrome (ARS)

Acute radiation syndrome occurs when the *entire body is exposed to a high dose of radiation* over a short period of time. Persons at the site of nuclear blasts or accidents are most likely to develop ARS. There are four stages of ARS: the prodromal stage, the latent stage, the manifest illness stage, and the recovery/death stage.

Clinical Manifestations

In the **prodromal stage** of ARS, symptoms can appear almost immediately, including nausea, vomiting, and diarrhea, and last minutes to days. In the **latent stage,** the exposed person looks and feels healthy for the next few hours to weeks. After this brief respite from symptoms, the **manifest illness stage** begins and lasts hours to months. Symptoms of this stage include anorexia, fatigue, fever, nausea, vomiting, diarrhea, temporary blindness, and possibly seizures and coma. Skin manifestations range from red, itchy skin to severe burns, depending on the level of exposure. The skin may also take months to heal. The final stage of ARS is the **recovery/death stage**, which may take years to complete.

Collaborative Care

Treatment is based on the severity of exposure and the signs and symptoms the patient exhibits. Survival depends on the severity of exposure and the syndrome with which the patient presents. Survival of patients with **bone marrow syndrome** decreases as the dose of radiation increases; the cause of death in this group is bone marrow destruction and hemorrhage. Patients presenting with **GI syndrome** are not likely to survive. Death is within two weeks of exposure from irreparable changes to and destruction of the GI tract and bone marrow. Patients develop infection, dehydration, and electrolyte imbalance. Patients presenting with **CV/CNS syndrome** usually die within three days of exposure from circulatory collapse, increased intracranial pressure secondary to cerebral edema, vasculitis, and meningitis. Initial care of patients with ARS includes stabilization of the ABCs, physiologic monitoring, treatment of major injuries (burns, fractures, etc.), and blood work for CBC with total lymphocyte count and HLA prior to any transfusion. Continued treatment is based on symptoms.

Toxic Ingestion

- **Lye (sodium hydroxide)** is found in cements, clinitest tablets, drain and oven cleaners, and many household cleaners. Injury from ingestion is caused by the alkaline nature of the substance.

- **Antifreeze (ethylene glycol)** is found in antifreeze, engine coolants, and brake fluids. Ingestion is considered a medical emergency. The lethal dose is approximately 100 mL or 1.4–1.6 mL/kg, but as little as 30 mL has been known to be fatal in an adult. Inhalation of ethylene glycol is unlikely. It is only mildly irritating to the mucous membranes and skin and is not absorbed through the skin.

Clinical Manifestations

Clinical manifestations of exposure to **lye** include shortness of breath; pneumonitis; edema; burning eyes, nose, mouth, and lips; esophageal burns; bloody vomitus and diarrhea; and necrotic skin. Symptoms may progress to severe abdominal pain, cardiovascular collapse, severe metabolic acidosis, and skin necrosis within 12 hours of ingestion.

Ethylene glycol is rapidly absorbed by the gastrointestinal tract (within one to four hours of ingestion), the main route of exposure. Ingestion leads to systemic toxicity, which begins with central nervous system dysfunction. Cardiac and pulmonary failure develops within 24–72 hours. Metabolic acidosis, dehydration, and renal failure requiring hemodialysis develop within this time period also.

Collaborative Care

Initial treatment is administration of activated charcoal and gastric lavage. Vomiting is not induced as the ingested chemical will burn the GI tract a second time when the patient vomits. An initial chest x-ray is obtained; the patient is kept NPO and may undergo endoscopy or esophagoscopy. Intravenous fluid is administered to enhance renal clearance. Sodium bicarbonate is given intravenously to correct acidosis with a pH of < 7.2. With ethylene glycol ingestion, intramuscular pyridoxine and thiamine are given to control symptoms of bleeding. Fomepizole (Antizol) is given intravenously with an initial loading dose, followed by twice daily doses. Intubation, mechanical ventilation, cardiovascular support, and fluid resuscitation are necessary with large ingestions. Early hemodialysis may be instituted to augment treatment of acidosis and prevent renal insufficiency. Diagnosis and treatment must be prompt to achieve the best outcome.

Toxic Inhalation

- **Carbon monoxide**, also known as the silent killer, has a slower onset of the signs and symptoms of toxicity. Risk for exposure to carbon monoxide is high in the following: industrial workers, persons unable to escape a fire in an enclosed space, personnel at fire scenes, persons using gas-powered generators during power outages, and persons in running vehicles that are poorly ventilated.

Clinical Manifestations

Assessment of oxygen saturation is not reliable in patients with carbon monoxide poisoning because carbon monoxide binds to hemoglobin at a higher affinity than oxygen, which causes the patient's O_2 saturation to be erroneously elevated. Signs and symptoms of carbon monoxide poisoning include headache, dizziness, nausea, flulike symptoms, fatigue, shortness of breath on exertion, impaired judgment, chest pain, confusion, depression, hallucinations, agitation, vomiting, abdominal pain, drowsiness, visual changes, fainting, seizures, impaired memory, and cherry red skin (seen in 2–3 percent of severely poisoned patients). Chronic smokers normally have carboxyhemoglobin levels as high as 10 percent. Patients with carboxyhemoglobin levels of 10–20 percent begin to show signs of toxicity, and those with levels of > 25 percent show signs of severe exposure.

Collaborative Care

The priority of care for patients exposed to carbon monoxide is to administer 100 percent oxygen. Hyperbaric oxygen therapy may be indicated and will provide an immediate reduction in the carbon monoxide level and associated symptoms. This therapy may not be readily available in some locations or may require the patient to be transferred to a tertiary center that does have this service. The half-life of carbon monoxide is reduced from approximately five hours to an hour with this treatment. Collaborative care of patients with high levels of exposure to inhaled agents may include the patient being intubated, mechanically ventilated, and admitted to an intensive care unit. The patient's condition may warrant use of hemodynamic monitoring and support of circulation with the use of vasoactive and/or inotropic agents.

Asphyxia

Asphyxia, a clinical condition resulting in a severe hypoxia to the organs and tissues, can be caused by a variety of situations. If the offending cause is not resolved, long-term brain damage or death may develop within a matter of minutes.

Oxygen-deficient environment: When a person encounters atmospheric conditions where there is a very low ambient level of oxygen, asphyxia can result. Examples are carbon monoxide poisoning during a fire, intentional or accidental inhalation of helium, or being trapped in an enclosed airtight space. The available oxygen is consumed during each respiratory cycle and is replaced by carbon dioxide. The interval time from entering the oxygen-deficient environment to a completely anoxic environment depends on the level of oxygen present at the onset.

Smothering: Mechanical obstruction of the mouth and/or nostrils that prevents airflow is a form of asphyxia. This prevents inhalation and exhalation and limits the exchange of oxygen and carbon dioxide across the alveolar membranes in the lungs. The person will lose consciousness in a matter of minutes and will experience cardiac arrest and death shortly thereafter due to anoxia. Examples of smothering include objects placed over the face such as pillows, hands, and plastic bags.

Compression: Compression asphyxia results from the severe or complete restriction of the chest cavity due to outside force, which prevents inhalation and exhalation. Hypoxia results because there is no inspired air to allow for exchange of oxygen across the alveolar membranes in the lungs. Also called "crush" or "traumatic" asphyxia, examples of causes include being crushed under a large object such as a vehicle or being forced into a prone position under heavy weight, such as when an aggressive suspect is being detained. Predatory animals such as pythons and anacondas kill their prey by compressive asphyxiation.

Review Questions

1. A patient is admitted to the ICU after experiencing a severe allergic reaction to a bee sting. The patient is intubated and mechanically ventilated and has received antihistamines and steroids, as well as large quantities of IV fluids. Despite these treatments, he remains hypotensive. Based on the above information, which shock state is present?

   A. hypovolemic

   B. cardiogenic

   C. distributive

   D. obstructive

2. A patient is admitted to the ICU from the operating room after sustaining a gunshot wound to the chest during an assault. The bedside nurse receives report from the ER nurse that the patient experienced cardiopulmonary arrest in the emergency department and was rushed to surgery before a head-to-toe exam was completed. The ICU nurse prepares to assist in performing which of these exams when the patient arrives at the ICU?

   A. primary survey

   B. systems exam

   C. neurologic assessment

   D. secondary survey

3. An elderly patient is admitted to the ICU with severe pneumonia that results in septic shock. She requires intubation and mechanical ventilation followed by IV fluids, antibiotics, and vasopressors for continued treatment. Approximately 48 hours after admission, her laboratory studies reveal the following: Creatinine has doubled since admission, platelet count has fallen to 25,000, AST/ALT are increased, and cardiac enzymes are elevated. The patient is experiencing which of these conditions?

   A. severe sepsis

   B. multiple organ dysfunction syndrome (MODS)

   C. systemic inflammatory response syndrome (SIRS)

   D. normal response to severe pneumonia in elderly patients

4. A 60-year-old male is in the ICU following a bowel resection for colon cancer. He has been successfully weaned from mechanical ventilation and is receiving TPN via a central venous catheter placed during surgery. On postoperative day #7, he becomes febrile, confused, tachycardic, and hypotensive. Laboratory studies reveal a new leukocytosis and elevated lactate level. Blood cultures are obtained, which show the growth of gram positive organisms. Which of these is the most likely cause of the patient's condition?

   A. SIRS due to ventilator-associated pneumonia

   B. endocarditis resulting in embolic stroke

   C. septic shock due to infected central venous catheter

   D. urosepsis from poor perineal and Foley catheter care

5. The ICU staff is informed by the emergency department supervisor to prepare to receive multiple patients who have been exposed to a toxic agent. The agent has not yet been identified but seems to be causing respiratory failure. Which of these should be the priority of each ICU nurse?

   A. Ensure that other patients in the ICU are not exposed to the toxic agent.

   B. Ensure that visitors are restricted until the agent is identified.

   C. Isolate patients who are suspected to have been exposed to the agent.

   D. Avoid exposure to the agent by using protective clothing and equipment.

6. The ICU nurse receives report from the emergency department regarding a college student who ingested ethylene glycol (antifreeze) while intoxicated at a party. He is intubated and mechanically ventilated and has received large quantities of IV fluid as well as IV sodium bicarbonate. Despite these measures, he continues to have severe metabolic acidosis and is oliguric. The ICU nurse should anticipate which of these therapies specific to this toxic exposure?

   A. hemodialysis

   B. antibiotics and vasopressors

   C. insertion of a pulmonary artery catheter

   D. continued fluid resuscitation and sodium bicarbonate

7. A patient is admitted to the ICU after sustaining thermal burns to 50 percent of his body in a house fire. He is intubated and mechanically ventilated and currently has stable vital signs other than tachycardia. Which of these fluids would be most appropriate for the continued resuscitation of this patient?

   A. a colloid such as dextran or hetastarch

   B. 3% saline

   C. D5W

   D. lactated Ringer's

8. A patient is admitted to the ICU following a construction accident, where a large object fell on top of him and pinned him to the ground. He was not breathing after the accident, and rescuers were not able to provide artificial ventilation until the object was removed. In the ICU, the patient is showing signs of anoxic brain injury. Which of these is the most appropriate term for the patient's mechanism of injury?

   A. traumatic asphyxia

   B. penetrating trauma

   C. multisystem trauma

   D. obstructive shock

9. A critical care nurse working on the hospital rapid response team is called to evaluate a patient on the general medical/surgical nursing floor. The patient's bedside nurse states she became concerned due to a change in the patient's vital signs, which are as follows: temperature 39.1 °C, heart rate 110, respiratory rate 26, and leukocytosis present on CBC analysis. The critical care nurse recognizes which of these conditions and collaborates with the patient care team to prevent further deterioration?

   A. sepsis

   B. multiple organ dysfunction syndrome (MODS)

   C. systemic inflammatory response syndrome (SIRS)

   D. toxic exposure

10. Which of these physiologic measurements is **not** reliable in patients who have been exposed to carbon monoxide gas?

    A. carboxyhemoglobin level

    B. blood pressure

    C. coagulation studies

    D. pulse oximetry readings

Review Answers and Explanations

1. C

The patient is not experiencing hypovolemic shock (A), as there is no mention of blood loss and he has received adequate fluid resuscitation. There is no mention of a primary cardiac insult that would result in cardiogenic shock (B). There is no mention of any signs/symptoms of tension pneumothorax, pericardial tamponade, or massive pulmonary embolus to suggest obstructive shock (D). The patient is experiencing an anaphylactic reaction, which is a form of distributive shock.

2. D

The primary survey (A) would have been completed in the ER and OR, as major life threats were identified and corrected. A systems exam (B) is not applicable in this situation. A neurologic assessment (C) would be completed at some point, but this alone is not sufficient for this patient. The patient will require a secondary survey to assess for non-life-threatening injuries that may have been missed due to the emergent injuries.

3. B

Although severe sepsis (A) is the likely culprit, there are no objective criteria for severe sepsis in the scenario. Similarly, there are no objective criteria for SIRS (C). Nothing in the scenario points to normal responses to severe pneumonia to (D). The patient is experiencing dysfunction of multiple organ systems including the lungs, kidneys, liver, hematologic system, and heart. Therefore she is experiencing MODS.

4. C

Answer (C) is correct because the patient is displaying signs/symptoms of septic shock based on objective criteria, has a central venous catheter that is over a week old, and has positive blood cultures with organisms frequently associated with central line infections. Answer (A) is incorrect because the patient has been successfully weaned from mechanical ventilation and there is no mention of associated respiratory symptoms and/or positive sputum cultures. Answer (B) is possible but highly unlikely given this patient's history. Answer (D) is incorrect because there is no mention of a Foley catheter and/or positive urine culture results.

5. D

The first priority for health care workers dealing with toxic exposures is to prevent becoming exposed to the agent themselves; therefore answer (D) is correct. Answers (A), (B), and (C) may be implemented in this situation, but only after the health care workers (in this case, ICU nurses) have protected themselves.

6. A

This patient requires hemodialysis to maintain acid-base balance and provide protection for the kidneys. There is no indication that the patient is hypotensive or has an infection, so answer (B) is incorrect. There is no indication for the insertion of a pulmonary artery catheter, so answer (C) is incorrect. The patient continues to have severe acidosis despite IV fluids and sodium bicarbonate, so answer (D) is possible but does not constitute definitive treatment.

7. D

LR is a crystalloid resuscitation fluid with electrolyte levels similar to those found in human blood. Colloids (A) have not been found to be superior to crystalloids for fluid resuscitation, and they carry risks such as anaphylactic reaction and coagulopathies. Hypertonic saline (B) is not indicated in burn patients, as this solution pulls fluids from the interstitial space into the vasculature. Answer (C) is incorrect because dextrose solutions are not appropriate for resuscitation in volume-depleted patients.

8. A

Answer (A) is the most appropriate based on the patient's mechanism of injury and resulting signs/symptoms. Answer (B) is incorrect because there is no mention of penetrating injury. While answer (C) is possible, the term *multisystem trauma* is broad and does not represent this patient's specific injury pattern. Answer (D) also is possible, but there is no mention of a shock state present.

9. C

The patient meets all of the objective criteria for SIRS; therefore answer (C) is correct. While the patient has some of the signs/symptoms associated with sepsis (A), there is no mention of a source of infection. There is no mention of failure of one or more organ systems (B). Also, there is no mention of toxic exposure (D).

10. D

Answer (D) is correct because carbon monoxide has a higher affinity for hemoglobin than oxygen molecules; therefore, the pulse oximetry readings are falsely elevated. The carboxyhemoglobin level measures the degree of carbon monoxide in the bloodstream, so answer (A) is incorrect. Answer (B) is incorrect because the measurement of blood pressure is not affected by carbon monoxide. Coagulation studies (C) are not related to carbon monoxide exposure.

Professional Caring and Ethical Practice Using the Synergy Model

13

HISTORY

The American Association of Critical-Care Nurses (AACN) established the Certification Corporation in 1975 with a mandate to develop the critical care registered nurse (CCRN) certification examination program. The purpose of this program was to have a method for developing, maintaining, and promoting high standards for critical care nursing practice. The goal of the certification process is the best possible care of critically ill patients and their families in a respectful, healing, and humane health care environment. Initially, requirements for certification included hours worked in a critical care setting, the number and type of tasks performed, and an examination based on body systems.

Starting in the late 1980s, the U.S. health care system implemented multiple system changes. They included the following:

- Diagnostic related groups (DRGs) for payment of hospital care

- Legally mandated nurse-to-patient ratios

- Shorter lengths of hospitalization

- Increased use of unlicensed assistive personnel

These changes impacted the bedside nurse's ability to advocate for and provide optimal patient care. Much discussion in the media sought to identify problem areas such as critical care nurse burnout, erosion of the bedside nurse's autonomy, and how to measure quality of care.

In 1992, AACN developed a vision of health care systems driven by the needs of patients and families, where critical care nurses were able to maximize their contribution to patient care. At the same time, the Certification Corporation commissioned a think tank to develop a conceptual model of certified nursing practice. Over the next several years, the group developed the Synergy Model for Patient Care. In 1995, the Synergy Model was adopted for use in certifying critical care nursing practice. The first testing for certification with the new model was in 1999. Approximately 20 percent of the CCRN exam is comprised of questions related to professional caring and ethical practice using the Synergy Model.

SYNERGY MODEL FOR PATIENT CARE

The basic premise of the model is based on the writings of Virginia Henderson (1960). She described the nurse-patient-family relationship as nurses "doing what patients and their families need for them to do." All patients have similar needs and, therefore, experience these needs across a wide range, from health to illness. However, a severely compromised patient will have more complex needs. Nursing practice is driven by the needs of patients and their family, and it requires nurses to be proficient in multiple dimensions of care. When nurse competencies relate to patient needs and the characteristics of the nurse and patient synergize, optimal patient outcomes can result.

There are four components of the Synergy Model for Patient Care: **core concepts**, **patient and family characteristics**, **nurse competencies (characteristics)**, and **outcomes**. The core concepts include the following ideas:

- The needs and characteristics of patients and families influence and drive the competencies of the nurse.

- Synergy occurs when individuals work together in ways that move them toward a common goal.

- Active partnership between the patient and nurse will result in optimal outcomes.

Patient and family characteristics include resiliency, vulnerability, stability, complexity, resource availability, participation in care, participation in decision making, and predictability. **Nurse competencies** (characteristics) include clinical judgment, advocacy/moral agency, caring practices, collaboration, systems thinking, response to diversity, clinical inquiry, and facilitation of learning. **Outcomes** can be patient derived, nurse derived, or system derived.

PATIENT CHARACTERISTICS

Resiliency is the capacity to return to a restorative level of functioning using compensatory and/or coping mechanisms. The ability to bounce back from an insult is influenced by multiple factors such as age, comorbidities, and intact compensatory mechanisms. The levels of resiliency are as follows:

Minimal	Moderate	High
Unable to respond	Moderate response	Respond and maintain
Coping failure	Begin coping	Intact coping response
Minimal reserves	Moderate reserves	Strong reserves
Brittle		High endurance

Vulnerability is the susceptibility to actual or potential stressors that can adversely affect patient outcomes. It can be impacted by the patient's health behaviors or physiological makeup. The levels of vulnerability are as follows:

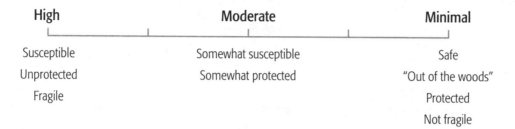

High	Moderate	Minimal
Susceptible	Somewhat susceptible	Safe
Unprotected	Somewhat protected	"Out of the woods"
Fragile		Protected
		Not fragile

Stability is the ability to maintain a steady state of equilibrium. The patient and family response to therapies and nursing interventions can have an impact on the patient's stability. The levels of stability are as follows:

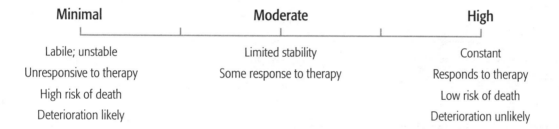

Minimal	Moderate	High
Labile; unstable	Limited stability	Constant
Unresponsive to therapy	Some response to therapy	Responds to therapy
High risk of death		Low risk of death
Deterioration likely		Deterioration unlikely

Complexity is the intricate entanglement of two or more systems. *Systems* refers to emotional or physiological states of the body, family dynamics, therapies, or the environmental interactions with the patient. When multiple systems are involved, the patient displays more complex patterns. The levels of complexity are as follows:

High	Moderate	Minimal
Intricate	Moderate dynamics	Straightforward
Complex dynamics		Routine dynamics
Ambiguous/vague		Simple/clear cut
Atypical presentation		Typical presentation

Resource availability is the level of resources (technical, fiscal, personal, psychological, social) that the patient/family/community brings to the situation. When a patient or the family brings more resources to the health care situation, there is greater potential for a positive outcome. The levels of resource availability are as follows:

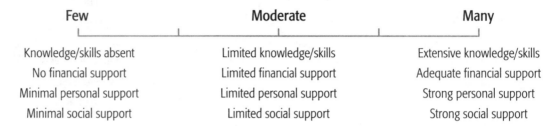

Few	Moderate	Many
Knowledge/skills absent	Limited knowledge/skills	Extensive knowledge/skills
No financial support	Limited financial support	Adequate financial support
Minimal personal support	Limited personal support	Strong personal support
Minimal social support	Limited social support	Strong social support

Participation in care is the extent to which the patient/family engages in all aspects of care. Patient and family participation can be influenced by cultural background, educational background, and resource availability. The levels of participation are as follows:

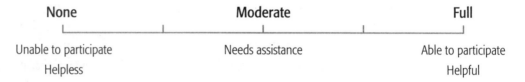

None	Moderate	Full
Unable to participate	Needs assistance	Able to participate
Helpless		Helpful

Participation in decision making refers to the extent to which patient/family engages in decision making. Patient and family involvement in clinical decision making can be influenced by their knowledge level, capacity to make decisions, cultural background, and the level of inner strength during a crisis. The levels of participation are as follows:

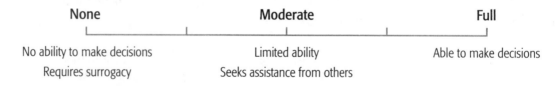

None	Moderate	Full
No ability to make decisions	Limited ability	Able to make decisions
Requires surrogacy	Seeks assistance from others	

Predictability is a characteristic that allows one to expect a certain course of events or course of illness. The levels of predictability are as follows:

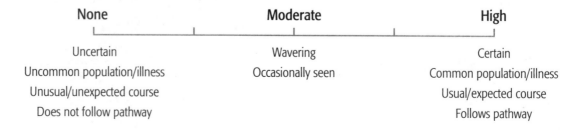

None	Moderate	High
Uncertain	Wavering	Certain
Uncommon population/illness	Occasionally seen	Common population/illness
Unusual/unexpected course		Usual/expected course
Does not follow pathway		Follows pathway

NURSE CHARACTERISTICS

Critical care nursing is an integration of knowledge, skills, experience, and individual attitudes. The nurse characteristics are bedside competencies, essential for the provision of care to critically ill patients and their families. The development of clinical knowledge was first described by Patricia Benner (1984) in her landmark book *From Novice to Expert.*

Clinical judgment includes clinical reasoning, decision making, critical thinking, and a global grasp of the situation. This is coupled with nursing skills acquired through a process of integrating formal and informal experiential knowledge and evidence-based guidelines. This integration of knowledge assists the critical care nurse to make the appropriate clinical decisions during the course of care given to the patient and her family. The levels of clinical judgment are as follows:

Novice	Competent	Expert
Collects basic level data	Collects/interprets complex data	Synthesizes multiple data
Follows written directions	Makes routine decisions	Sees the "big picture"
Questions own decisions	Seeks help appropriately	Collaborates as needed
Delegates decisions	Recognizes patterns/trends	Responds dynamically
Includes extraneous data	Focuses on key elements	Recognizes limits

Advocacy/moral agency is working on another's behalf and representing the concerns of the patient/family and nursing staff. This includes serving as a moral agent in identifying and helping to resolve ethical and clinical concerns within and outside the clinical setting. Since nurses have a unique relationship with patients and their families, they are often the voice for those who cannot speak for themselves. The levels of advocacy and moral agency are as follows:

Novice	Competent	Expert
Advocates for patient/self	Advocates for patient/family	Works for patient/family
Self assesses own values	Incorporates patient values	Advocates for patient/family
Aware of ethical conflicts	Supports ethical decisions	Uses all resources
Functions in own values	Moral decisions inconsistent	Patient rights drive decisions
Aware of patient rights	Acknowledges patient/family rights	Empowers patient/family
Accepts death as outcome	Assists with dying process	Achieves professional relationships

Caring practices are nursing interventions that create a compassionate, supportive, and therapeutic environment for patients and staff with the aim of promoting comfort, healing, and prevention of unnecessary suffering. These activities include vigilance, engagement, and responsiveness of caregivers, including family and health care personnel. These caring practices create a safe environment for sick patients. An overwhelming fear of many patients and their families is that they will experience unrelenting pain or suffering. Pain assessment and management are fundamental caring practices. The levels of caring practices are as follows:

Novice	Competent	Expert
Focuses on basic needs	Responds to subtle changes	Anticipates changes/needs
Uses standards/protocols	Provides individualized care	Engages patient/family
Maintains safe environment	Uses caring practices	Needs determine care
May overlook certain needs	Optimizes environment	Promotes safety/comfort
		Facilitates safe passage

Collaboration is working with patients, families, and health care providers in a way that promotes and encourages each person's contribution toward achieving optimal and realistic patient and family goals. This involves multidisciplinary work with colleagues and community. The bedside nurse knows the care environment best and is able to assemble a team and focus on the best interest of the patient and family. The levels of collaboration are as follows:

Novice	Competent	Expert
Willing to be taught	Willing to teach/mentor others	Serves as role model/teacher/mentor
Attends team meetings	Preceptors and teachers	Facilitates team meetings
Open to assistance	Involved in multidisciplinary care	Involved in patient outcomes
		Professional and community leader

Systems thinking includes the body of knowledge and tools that allow the nurse to manage whatever environmental and system resources exist for the patient, family, and staff within or across all systems. Integral to systems thinking is the ability to understand how one decision can impact the whole system. Nurses, using a global perspective in clinical decision making, have the ability to negotiate the needs of the patient and family through the health care system. The levels of systems thinking are as follows:

Novice	Competent	Expert
Uses standard strategies	Care based on patient need	Care driven by patient/family needs
Poor problem resolution	Finds system solutions	Global view of system problem
Patient/family isolated environment	Negotiates care decisions	Navigates problems for patient/family
Uses self as key resource	Reacts to patient/family needs	Optimizes patient/family outcomes

Response to diversity is the sensitivity to recognize, appreciate, and incorporate differences into the provision of care. Differences may include cultural beliefs, spiritual beliefs, gender, race, ethnicity, lifestyle, socioeconomic status, age, values, and the use of alternative and complementary therapies. Nurses need to recognize the individuality of each patient while observing for patterns that respond to nursing interventions. The competent nurse asks about differences and considers their impact on patient care, but the expert nurse tailors the care environment to meet the diversity needs of the patient and family. The levels of response to diversity are as follows:

Novice	Competent	Expert
Assesses; uses standards	Asks; considers impact on care	Anticipates patient/family needs
Care is based on own beliefs	Accommodates differences	Incorporates differences
Recognizes barriers to care	Assists incorporation of system culture	Adapts culture to needs
	Seeks to meet patient/family needs	Reduces/eliminates barriers; uses EBP for outcomes

Clinical inquiry is the ongoing process of questioning and evaluating practice and providing informed practice. Creating practice changes through research utilization and experiential learning. Clinical inquiry evolves as the nurse moves from novice to expert. At the expert level, the nurse individualizes standards and guidelines to meet the patient needs. Clinical inquiry requires observing, asking questions, finding the evidence, and making practice changes. The levels of clinical inquiry are as follows:

Novice	Competent	Expert
Does not question practice	Adapts standards to patient needs	Improves based on research
Uses EBP when directed	Applies EBP (if no conflict)	Questions practice
Needs more learning	Accepts direction for change	Seek answers to EBP questions
Seeks assistance	Seeks alternative care practices	Lifelong learner
Data collector	Research team member	Evaluates EBP and implements

Facilitation of learning means that the nurse is able to facilitate learning for patients and families, nursing staff, other members of the health care team, and the community using both formal and informal learning. Education is based on the individual strengths and weaknesses of the patient and family. Creative methods need to be used to ensure patient and family comprehension.

Novice	Competent	Expert
Uses standard educational materials	Adapts educational material to needs	Modifies/develops content
Keeps teaching separate from care	Educates as part of patient care	Patient/family involved in teaching
Provides information	Teaches based on needs	Individualizes teaching
Basic knowledge of needs	Uses various teach methods	Collaborates teaching needs
Patient/family are passive learners	Patient/family have input in teaching	Negotiates teaching needs

OUTCOMES

Optimal outcomes happen when the patient characteristics and nursing characteristics are matched. Since the Synergy Model views the patient and family as active participants, the outcomes measured must be patient and family driven. The *three levels of outcomes* discussed are **patient driven**, **nursing driven**, and **system driven**.

Patient-driven outcomes include functional changes, behavioral changes, comfort, trust, quality of life, and satisfaction. *Nurse-driven outcomes* include physiological changes, the presence or absence of complications, and the extent treatment objectives were obtained. *System-driven outcomes* include readmission rates, length of stay, and resource utilization for each case. One or more types of outcomes may overlap due to goals and expectations.

Patient-Driven Outcomes

Patients and their families require competence, caring, and trust from nurses when they are vulnerable and powerless. Trust is the result of the patient and family developing a caring relationship with the nurse. The nurse demonstrates competence to the patient and family by being attentive to their concerns, empowering them, and teaching them. Without trust among the nurse, patient, and family, relevant information can be lost or ignored. To patients and their family, nursing care that comforts them is the most basic service that caregivers can provide. Caring practices that create a therapeutic and compassionate environment are a large component of the patient's quality of care outcomes. Patient satisfaction measures related to nursing care usually include technical and professional factors, trusting relationships, and educational experiences.

Nurse-Driven Outcomes

The critical care nurse monitors and manages therapies, based on trends and physiological changes, in a timely and competent manner. By knowing the trajectory of specific illnesses, the nurse can respond with the appropriate changes needed to assist the patient to a positive outcome. Using vigilance and clinical judgment, the nurse creates a healing environment that provides safe passage for the vulnerable patient. Safe passage mandates the absence of complications (iatrogenic injury, infection, and hazards of immobility). The extent to which treatment objectives are attained within a predictable timeframe is a nursing-derived outcome variable. A high degree of collaboration and positive communication between critical care nurses and other health care professionals is associated with lower mortality rates, lower rates of nosocomial infections, shorter lengths of stay, and high patient satisfaction rates regarding care.

System-Driven Outcomes

The overriding goal of health care systems is to give high-quality care at reasonable cost for the greatest number of patients. Elevated readmission rates add to the personal and financial burden of providing health care. Third-party payers (insurance companies, Medicare, Medicaid) are no longer paying for multiple admissions to the same hospital for the same diagnosis or complications from that diagnosis. The critical care nursing competencies are instrumental in decreasing complications, length of stay, and readmissions. Nurses play a critical role in coordination of the patient's care, which maximizes resource utilization and minimizes cost to the health care system.

Creating a Safe Environment/Evaluating Adverse Events Using the Fair and Just Culture

The potential for adverse events or errors in critical care units is high, considering the frequency and complexity of interventions, as well as the high level of communication that must occur among the various health care professionals. In addition, CMS has determined that it is not appropriate to reimburse for care provided for or associated with what it terms "never events," or events defined as serious and costly errors in the provision of health care services that should never occur. Examples of never events in the critical care unit are a central line catheter infection and pressure ulcers. Creating a safe working environment, including the ability for the critical care nurses to initiate important conversations with other health care professionals, will help reduce these events. Developing competencies and critical thinking skills in the practice of critical care nursing will also help prevent errors. The Synergy Model and the description of nurse characteristics support this safe working environment.

If an adverse event or error occurs, it is important to evaluate both the processes and the individual actions using a fair and just culture to determine the primary cause of the event. One of the questions asked during this investigation is called the substitution test and asks,

"Would three other individuals with similar experience and in a similar situation and environment act in the same manner as the person being evaluated?" If the answer is no, then the act of the individual has to be evaluated as being due to lack of competency or knowledge deficit or negligence on their part. If the answer is yes, then the processes of the organization must be evaluated to determine the cause of the event.

ETHICAL ISSUES

Ethics is defined as the system or code of morals of a particular person, religion, group, or profession. The American Nurses Association (ANA) is the major source of ethical guidance for the nursing profession. The ANA code of ethics is based on the underlying assumption that nursing is concerned with the protection, promotion, and restoration of health; prevention of illness; and the alleviation of patient suffering. The critical care nurse encounters ethical issues on a daily basis. Some of these ethical issues include do not resuscitate (DNR) orders, withdrawal of support, new technologies, and new protocols. Since the critical care nurse may have developed a therapeutic relationship with the patient and family, it is important that the nurse be involved with any discussion of an ethical dilemma.

The American Association of Critical-Care Nurses (AACN) has included the ethics of care and ethical principles within its mission, vision, and values statements. An ethic of care is a moral orientation. Essential to an ethic of care are trust, compassion, collaboration, and accountability. Traditional nursing ethical principles provide a basis for assessment and decision making. These principles include autonomy, beneficence, nonmaleficence, futility, justice, veracity, fidelity, and confidentiality.

ANA Code of Ethics for Nurses 2015

Provision 1

The nurse practices with compassion and respect for the inherent dignity, worth, and unique attributes of every person.

Provision 2

The nurse's primary commitment is to the patient, whether an individual, family, group, community, or population.

Provision 3

The nurse promotes, advocates for, and protects the rights, health, and safety of the patient.

Provision 4

The nurse has authority, accountability, and responsibility for nursing practice; makes decisions; and takes action consistent with the obligation to promote health and to provide optimal care.

Provision 5

The nurse owes the same duties to self as to others, including the responsibility to promote health and safety, preserve wholeness of character and integrity, maintain competence, and continue personal and professional growth.

Provision 6

The nurse, through individual and collective effort, establishes, maintains, and improves the ethical environment of the work setting and conditions of employment that are conducive to safe, quality healthcare.

Provision 7

The nurse, in all roles and settings, advances the profession through research and scholarly inquiry, professional standards development, and the generation of both nursing and health policy.

Provision 8

The nurse collaborates with other health professionals and the public to protect human rights, promote health diplomacy, and reduce health disparities.

Provision 9

The profession of nursing, collectively through its professional organizations, must articulate nursing values, maintain integrity of the profession, and integrate principles of social justice into nursing and health policy.

From the American Nurses Association. (2016). Code of ethics for nurses with interpretive statements. Washington, DC: American Nurses Association.

Autonomy

The principle of autonomy recognizes the rights of individuals to self-determination. This is rooted in society's respect for individuals' ability to make informed decisions about personal matters. Autonomy has become more important as social values have shifted to define medical quality in terms of outcomes that are important to the patient rather than to medical professionals. The increasing importance of autonomy can be seen as a social reaction to a "paternalistic" tradition within health care. Respect for autonomy is the basis for informed consent and advance directives. Autonomy can often come into conflict with beneficence when patients disagree with recommendations that health care professionals believe are in the patient's best interest. Individuals' capacity for informed decision making may come into question during resolution of conflicts between autonomy and beneficence. The role of surrogate medical decision makers is an extension of the principle of autonomy. *Paternalism* is the term used when health care providers make decisions for the patient based on the rationale that it is in the patient's best interest. This practice denies the patient the autonomy to make his own decisions and should be identified and discouraged when possible.

Beneficence

Beneficence is the concept of doing good and preventing harm to humanity in general. This requires that one promote the well-being of patients and implies that harms and benefits are balanced, leading to positive or beneficial outcomes.

Nonmaleficence

The concept of nonmaleficence is embodied by the expression, "First, do no harm." The critical care nurse has a duty to remove the patient from or prevent harmful situations.

Beneficence and nonmaleficence are on opposite ends of a continuum and are incorporated differently into ethical situations.

Futility

This principle states that care should not be given if it is futile in terms of improving patient comfort or the medical outcome. In recent years, there has been increased use of advance directives, including living wills and durable powers of attorney for health care. In many cases, the "expressed wishes" of the patient are documented in these directives, and this provides a framework to guide family members and health care professionals in decision making when the patient is incapacitated. Undocumented expressed wishes can also help guide decision making in the absence of advance directives. "Substituted judgment" is the concept that a family member can give consent for treatment if the patient is unable (or unwilling) to give consent herself. The key question for the decision-making surrogate is not "What would you like to do," but instead "What do you think the patient would want in this situation?" Courts have supported families' arbitrary definitions of futility to include simple biological survival.

Justice

The principle of justice requires that health care resources be distributed fairly and equitably among groups of people. This is especially important to critical care since a majority of health care resources are allocated to this practice setting.

Veracity

The principle of veracity requires that persons are obligated to tell the truth when communicating with others. Some cultures do not place a great emphasis on informing the patient of the diagnosis, especially when cancer is the diagnosis. Even American culture did not emphasize truth telling in a cancer case up until the 1970s. In American medicine, the principle of informed consent takes precedence over other ethical values, and patients are usually at least asked whether they want to know the diagnosis. Critical care nurses should maintain truthfulness in all aspects of practice, including medication administration.

Fidelity

Fidelity involves the notions of loyalty, faithfulness, and honoring commitments. Patients and families must be able to trust the nurse and have faith in the therapeutic relationship if growth is to occur. Therefore, the nurse must take care not to threaten the therapeutic relationship or to leave obligations unfulfilled.

Confidentiality

Confidentiality is commonly applied to conversations between health care professionals and patients. Legal protections prevent health care professionals from revealing their discussions with patients, even under oath in court. Confidentiality is mandated by HIPAA laws, specifically the Privacy Rule, and various state laws, some more rigorous than HIPAA. Confidentiality is challenged in cases such as the diagnosis of a sexually transmitted disease in a patient who refuses to reveal the diagnosis to a spouse or in the termination of a pregnancy in an underage patient without the knowledge of the patient's parents. Confidentiality also applies to written medical documents such as dictated reports and flowsheets.

Ethical Decision Making

Ethical cases are not always straightforward or "black and white" and often involve circumstances with multiple side issues and distractions. The most common ethical issues seen in critical care units are allocation of scarce critical care resources, informed consent, organ donation, confidentiality, and foregoing treatment. It is often difficult to know that a true ethical dilemma exists. Rushton & Scanlon (1998) listed warning signs that can assist the critical care nurse with recognizing ethical dilemmas.

- Is the situation emotionally charged?
- Has the patient's condition changed significantly?
- Is there confusion or conflict about the facts?
- Is there increased hesitancy about the right course of action?
- Is the proposed action a deviation from customary practice?
- Is there a perceived need for secrecy around the proposed action?

When these warning signs occur, the critical care nurse needs to reassess the situation and then determine if an ethical dilemma exists. Finding a morally justifiable resolution to ethical dilemmas can be difficult for patients, families, and health care professionals. Using a systematic, structured process is a helpful way to approach ethical decision making (see table 13.1).

TABLE 13.1 *Ethical Decision-Making Models*

M.O.R.A.L. Model (Crisham, 1992)	Ethical Decision-Making Process (Aiken, 1994)	ERC Plus Model (Ethics Resource Center, 2008)
1. Massage the dilemma.	1. Collect, analyze, interpret the data or information.	1. Define the problem.
2. Outline the options/possibilities.	2. State the dilemma clearly.	2. Identify available alternative solutions to the problem.
3. Review criteria and resolve.	3. Consider choices of action based on ethical principles.	3. Evaluate the identified alternatives.
4. Affirm the position.	4. Analyze the advantages and disadvantages of each action.	4. Make the decision.
5. Look back.	5. Make a decision that resolves the dilemma.	5. Implement the decision.
		6. Evaluate the decision.

Ethical Decision-Making Process

1. **Identify the dilemma.** Gather as much information as you can that will illuminate the situation. In doing so, it is important to be as specific and objective as possible. Writing ideas on paper may help you gain clarity. Outline the facts, separating out innuendos, assumptions, hypotheses, or suspicions.

2. **Determine the nature and dimensions of the dilemma.** There are several avenues to follow in order to ensure that you have examined the problem in all its various dimensions. Consider the ethical principles of autonomy, nonmaleficence, beneficence, justice, and fidelity. Decide which principles apply to the specific situation and determine which principle takes priority for you in this case. In theory, each principle is of equal value, which means that it is your challenge to determine the priorities when two or more of them are in conflict. Review the relevant professional literature to ensure that you are using the most current professional thinking in reaching a decision. Consult with experienced professional colleagues and/or supervisors. Many organizations have *ethics committees* with highly skilled professionals including clinicians, social workers, lawyers, and theology representatives who may serve as consultants in these cases. As they review with you the information you have gathered, they may see other issues that are relevant or provide a perspective you have not considered. They may also be able to identify aspects of the dilemma that you are not viewing objectively. Consult your state or national professional associations to see if they can provide help with the dilemma.

3. **Generate potential courses of action.** Brainstorm as many possible courses of action as possible. Be creative and consider all options. If possible, enlist the assistance of at least one colleague to help you generate options.

4. **Consider the potential consequences of all options and determine a course of action.** Considering the information you have gathered and the priorities you set, evaluate each option and assess the potential consequences for all the parties involved. Ponder the implications of each course of action for the client, for others who will be affected, and for yourself as a counselor. Eliminate the options that clearly do not give the desired results or cause even more problematic consequences. Review the remaining options to determine which option or combination of options best fits the situation and addresses the priorities you have identified.

5. **Evaluate the selected course of action.** Review the selected course of action to see if it presents any new ethical considerations. Apply three simple tests to the selected course of action to ensure that it is appropriate. The three tests are justice, publicity, and universality. In applying the *test of justice*, assess your own sense of fairness by determining whether you would treat others the same in this situation. For the

test of publicity, ask yourself whether you would want your behavior reported in the press. The *test of universality* asks you to assess whether you could recommend the same course of action to another nurse in the same situation. If the course of action you have selected seems to present new ethical issues, then you'll need to go back to the beginning and reevaluate each step of the process. Perhaps you have chosen the wrong option or identified the problem incorrectly. If you can answer in the affirmative to each of the questions, thus passing the tests of justice, publicity, and universality, and you are satisfied that you have selected an appropriate course of action, then you are ready to move on to implementation.

6. **Implement the course of action.** Taking the appropriate action in an ethical dilemma is often difficult. Once a decision has been reached, it often comes after much thought and consideration, and rarely is there complete agreement among all of the interested parties.

7. After implementing your course of action, it is good practice to **follow up on the situation to assess whether your actions had the anticipated effect and consequences.** The evaluation of the outcome can be used as a basis for future decision-making. If the outcome is not as planned, it may be possible to modify the plan or to use an alternative that was not originally chosen.

Legal Accountability

Each state has a Nurse Practice Act that defines the scope of practice and provides guidance for acceptable nursing roles. Standards of care are any established measures of extent, quality, quantity, or value. There are many established standards, including usual and customary practice, institutional guidelines, association guidelines, and legal precedent. The ANA and AACN have established standards of practice. Many hospitals have developed standards for practice within the institution. Critical care units have standards of care, policies, and protocols for specific groups/types of patients or specific procedures (e.g., ACLS, intensive insulin therapy, blood transfusion policies). Critical care nurses are often obligated to meet one or more of these standards simultaneously.

Professional Liability

Professional liability includes *professional negligence, malpractice, and delegation.* **Negligence** is the failure to do what any reasonable, prudent nurse would do under similar circumstances or an act or failure to act that leads to injury of another person. There are six specific elements that must be established to determine negligence.

1. **Duty:** To protect the patient from an unreasonable risk of harm

2. **Breach of duty:** Failure to do what a reasonable, prudent nurse would do under the same or similar circumstances

3. **Proximate cause:** Proof that the harm to the patient was preventable

4. **Injury:** Proof of harm done to the patient

5. **Direct cause of injury:** Proof that the nurse's conduct was the cause or contributed to the patient's injury

6. **Damages:** Proof of actual loss, damage, pain, or suffering caused by the nurse's behavior

Malpractice

Malpractice is a specific type of negligence that takes into account the status of the caregiver and the standard of care. There are two types of malpractice: professional misconduct and malpractice. **Professional misconduct** is the improper discharge of professional duties or the failure to meet the standard of care, resulting in harm to the patient. **Malpractice** is the failure to utilize the prevailing professional standard or failure to anticipate consequences of the nurse's actions. The majority of malpractice and negligence that occurs in the critical care environment includes failure to prevent falls, medication errors, failure to assess changes in clinical status, and failure to notify the primary health care professional of changes in patient status.

Delegation and Supervision

Principles of Delegation

All decisions related to delegation and assignment are based on the fundamental principles of protection of the health, safety, and welfare of the public. A Joint Statement on Delegation issued by the American Nurses Association (ANA) and the National Council of State Boards of Nursing (NCSBN) stipulates the following principles:

- The RN takes responsibility and accountability for the provision of nursing practice.

- The RN directs care and determines the appropriate utilization of any assistant involved in providing direct patient care.

- The RN may delegate components of care but does not delegate the nursing process itself. The practice of pervasive functions of assessment, planning, evaluation, and nursing judgment cannot be delegated.

- The decision of whether or not to delegate or assign is based upon the RN's judgment concerning the condition of the patient, the competence of all members of the nursing team, and the degree of supervision that will be required of the RN if a task is delegated.

- The RN delegates only those tasks for which she or he believes the other healthcare worker has the knowledge and skill to perform, taking into consideration training, cultural competence, experience, and facility/agency policies and procedures.

- The RN individualizes communication regarding the delegation to the nursing assistive personnel, and client situation and the communication should be clear, concise, correct, and complete. The RN verifies comprehension with the nursing assistive personnel and that the assistant accepts the delegation and the responsibility that accompanies it.

- Communication must be a 2-way process. Nursing assistive personnel should have the opportunity to ask questions and/or for clarification of expectations.

- Chief Nursing Officers are accountable for establishing systems to assess, monitor, verify, and communicate ongoing competence requirements in areas related to delegation.

- There is both individual accountability and organizational accountability for delegation. Organizational accountability for delegation relates to providing sufficient resources, including:

  - Sufficient staffing with an appropriate staff mix

  - Documenting competencies for all staff providing direct patient care and for ensuring that the RN has access to competence information for the staff to whom the RN is delegating care

  - Organizational policies on delegation that are developed with the active participation of all nurses and acknowledgment that delegation is a professional right and responsibility

The act of delegation must ensure that the critical care nurse coordinates safe and effective patient care. Delegation allows the nurse to perform functions that only a registered nurse can perform, and it utilizes the full potential of the health care team to maximize positive patient outcomes. The Five Rights of Delegation provide an additional resource to facilitate decisions about delegation.

1. **Right Task**
   One that is delegable for a specific patient

2. **Right Circumstances**
   Appropriate patient setting, available resources, and other relevant factors considered

3. **Right Person**
   Right person is delegating the right task to the right person to be performed on the right person

4. **Right Direction/Communication**
   Clear, concise description of the task, including its objective, limits, and expectations

5. **Right Supervision**
   Appropriate monitoring, evaluation, intervention as needed, and feedback

If one or more of the Five Rights of Delegation are not met, then delegation should not proceed until all criteria are established.

Review Questions

1. The Center for Medicare and Medicaid Services (CMS) has identified various errors made in the course of providing health care services, with certain unacceptable occurrences resulting in nonreimbursement. The term used for these errors is

   A. serious errors.

   B. never events.

   C. nonpaying errors.

   D. central line infection.

2. Which of these is **not** a main component of the Synergy Model for Patient Care?

   A. core concepts

   B. nurse competencies (characteristics)

   C. complexity

   D. outcomes

3. The charge nurse in a busy surgical intensive care unit has just been notified of an admission from the operating room. The patient has sustained multiple traumatic injuries and is requiring constant transfusion of blood products, vasopressors, and IV fluids, yet the patient continues to have labile vital signs. Which of these nurses should you assign to care for this patient?

   A. the new graduate nurse with six months' experience, as it will be a good learning experience

   B. yourself, as you already know about these procedures

   C. the most senior nurse working in the unit that shift

   D. the nurse whose characteristics best meet the anticipated needs of the patient

4. Which of these should **never** be delegated to another health care worker, such as an unlicensed assistive caregiver?

   A. basic patient care activities such as bathing

   B. any task that requires judgment, clinical or otherwise

   C. documentation

   D. answering telephones in the ICU

5. Critical care nurses are accountable to ensure they are practicing according to many rules, policies, and guidelines. Which of these is **not** an example of a directive that a critical care nurse must follow?

   A. State Nurse Practice Act

   B. ANA Standards of Practice

   C. institutional policies

   D. instructions given by a nursing professor

6. Which of these ethical concepts describes the notion that telling the truth is important when communicating with others, especially with regard to medical diagnoses or treatments?

   A. veracity

   B. confidentiality

   C. justice

   D. beneficence

7. A patient with advanced metastatic cancer is admitted to the ICU with sepsis and respiratory failure. His condition declines despite all available treatments, and he has required resuscitation for two cardiopulmonary arrests in the past 12 hours. The health care team meets with the patient's family and informs them that there are no more treatments available and the outcome will not change. Which of these ethical principles is guiding this discussion?

   A. justice

   B. futility

   C. fidelity

   D. nonmaleficence

8. A patient with a terminal illness has written a living will, specifying that no aggressive or heroic measures be implemented to sustain life or prolong suffering should she be unable to voice her wishes. This is an example of preserving the patient's right to

   A. stability.

   B. resiliency.

   C. autonomy.

   D. confidentiality.

9. A critical care nurse is busy with two critically ill patients in the ICU. Unlicensed assistive personnel has offered to assist the nurse by providing care to one of the patients. The task is within the scope of the care partner, who has been appropriately trained, and the situation is appropriate. However, the nurse is not able to supervise, as she is busy caring for the other patient. Is this an appropriate use of delegation?

   A. Yes, all conditions for appropriate delegation have been met.

   B. Yes, the nurse is too busy to provide all the care herself.

   C. No, unlicensed assistive personnel should never provide care in the ICU.

   D. No, the nurse is not able to supervise the delegated task; therefore, delegation is not appropriate.

10. A critical care nurse focuses her education on a patient with congestive heart failure (CHF) to prevent future deterioration and promote symptom relief that will help the patient have a better quality of life. Using the Synergy Model, which of these outcomes encompasses preventing future hospital admissions for CHF?

    A. patient driven

    B. nurse driven

    C. system driven

    D. professional accountability

Review Answers and Explanations

1. B

Answer (B) is correct, as this is the term used by CMS to identify "serious and costly errors" that should not occur in the course of medical treatment. This term is important for critical care nurses to know, as it reinforces care practices geared toward avoiding these errors. Answers (A) and (C) are incorrect because these are descriptive terms and have not been used as specific labels by CMS. Answer (D) is incorrect because this is a specific error, which may or may not fall under criteria for CMS nonreimbursement.

2. C

Answers (A), (B), and (D) are three of the four components of the Synergy Model. Answer (C) is a specific patient characteristic but is not in itself a main component. It is important for the critical care nurse to know the main components of the Synergy Model, as this will facilitate further understanding of the interaction among the components. It is not necessarily important for the critical care nurse to memorize all the potential characteristics (patient, family, nurse) but rather to understand that many characteristics often interact at a given time when caring for critically ill patients.

3. D

Using the Synergy Model, answer (D) is correct, as this will match patient and nurse characteristics to support the best outcomes. Answer (A) is incorrect because a novice nurse does not yet possess the skills and competencies to care for an unstable, complex, nonresilient patient. However, it may be appropriate to facilitate learning experiences for a novice nurse to care for less complex, more stable, resilient patients. Answer (B) is incorrect because

the charge nurse may not meet the patient's needs better than another nurse working at the time. Generally, a charge nurse should not take primary responsibility for such a patient, as this will interfere with other duties. Answer (C) is incorrect because the nurse with the most seniority may not possess the appropriate characteristics needed for this patient.

4. B

Answer (B) is correct because any task that requires judgment can never be delegated; this does not fit into the decision-making process for delegation. Answer (A) is incorrect because basic patient care activities, such as bathing, are frequently delegated when safe to do so. Answer (C) is incorrect because documentation may be delegated provided that the information being documented is appropriate (such as documentation of basic vital signs). Answer (D) is incorrect because answering telephones is a basic duty that requires no special skill or education.

5. D

Answers (A), (B), and (C) are incorrect because they are all examples of directives regarding nursing practice. Instructions given by a nursing professor do not hold nurses legally accountable and do not direct nursing practice.

6. A

Answers (B), (C), and (D) are terms used for other ethical principles. It is important for the critical care nurse to know the terms and definitions of various ethical concepts, as this will support the decision-making process when an ethical dilemma presents itself.

7. B

Justice (A) is the principle that health care resources are fairly distributed, which does not directly relate to the case presented. Fidelity (C) involves loyalty, which is not the theme of the case presented. Nonmaleficence (D) is the concept of "First, do no harm," which is not related to the case presented. Futility (B) is the ethical principle related to care that will not improve patient outcome or patient comfort. Aggressive measures to sustain life in a patient such as the one described above are often considered futile.

8. C

Stability (A) and resiliency (B) are associated with patient characteristics in the Synergy Model and do not relate to ethical principles. Confidentiality (D) is an ethical principle related to keeping health care–related discussions private from the public, which is not the primary issue in this case. Autonomy (C) is the ethical principle related to preserving self-direction. An advance directive, such as a living will, is an example of a way a patient can maintain autonomy over decision making even when incapacitated.

9. D

Answer (D) is correct because a task should never be delegated unless the nurse is available to supervise and intervene if needed. Answer (A) is incorrect because all the criteria for appropriate delegation have not been met. Answer (B) is incorrect because tasks should never be delegated based on the nurse's workload alone. Answer (C) is incorrect because unlicensed assistive personnel are frequently employed to provide various aspects of care in ICUs under the direct supervision of the critical care nurse.

10. C

Patient-driven outcomes (A) relate to caring practices that create a therapeutic relationship among the patient, nurse, and family. Nurse-driven outcomes (B) relate to using vigilance, creating a healing environment, and protecting vulnerable patients. Professional accountability (D) is related to legal negligence, delegation, and malpractice. Therefore answer (C) is correct, as system-driven outcomes relate to the broader health care system by preventing unnecessary hospital admissions for the same illness.

Caring for Patients with Behavioral and Psychosocial Conditions

Knowledge of common behavioral, psychosocial, and psychiatric disorders is important for the critical care nurse. Early identification of risk factors, characteristics, and symptoms of these problems can be crucial in treating a critically ill patient.

ABUSE AND NEGLECT

Abuse is a complex psychosocial problem that affects large numbers of adults throughout the world. Abuse refers to the harmful or injurious treatment of another human being. Types of abuse include physical, sexual, verbal, financial, psychological, and emotional. Abuse often coexists with neglect, which is defined as a failure to meet a dependent person's basic physical and medical needs. Active neglect occurs when a caregiver intentionally fails to meet the responsibilities of caring for another individual, while passive neglect occurs when the failure to provide care is a result of unintentional disregard.

Physical abuse refers to intentionally causing physical harm or injury to a vulnerable party.

Emotional abuse refers to the intentional infliction of mental harm and/or psychological stress. This abuse includes insults, isolation, and threats of physical harm.

During their careers, registered nurses (RNs) will likely care for patients who have experienced all types of abuse and neglect. Patients suffering from physical and emotional abuse, however, are the most commonly encountered.

Risk Factors

In the adult population, elderly individuals are at greatest risk for abuse and neglect. Individuals 80 years of age or older are two to three times more likely to suffer from abuse than younger populations. Women are also more likely to be abused and neglected than men. Patients who are suffering from dementia are more likely to be abused and neglected than those without dementia. Abuse and neglect more commonly occur in the home, which makes the role of a vigilant RN even more important when the patient presents to an inpatient setting.

Symptoms, Diagnosis, and Treatment

The abused and/or neglected patient often presents with distinct overt symptoms and may also have abnormal laboratory values. Pressure sores, extreme weight loss, poor hygiene, and lab values indicating malnutrition are indicative of a neglected patient. (Diagnostic values found in malnutrition may be found later in this chapter.) Physical assessment findings in the abused patient include bruises, burns, and fractures of peripheral extremities, normally accompanied by inconsistent explanations from the patient and caregiver regarding the etiology. Psychological assessment findings include withdrawn behavior, guarded behavior during physical assessment, and depression.

The diagnosis of abuse and neglect can be made based upon the history, physical exam, and data collected. Once a clear diagnosis is made, the first priority is treatment of any life-threatening issues or medical problems. Next, the abuse and/or neglect situation should be addressed prior to discharge. Psychological diagnoses, once identified, should be referred to the appropriate health professional. Suspected cases of abuse should be immediately reported to an adult protective services agency or to the appropriate chain of care in the workplace. Most states mandate reporting abuse of the elderly, as well as other age populations.

ANTISOCIAL BEHAVIORS, AGGRESSION, AND VIOLENCE

Antisocial behaviors are disruptive acts characterized by covert and overt hostility and intentional aggression toward others. Antisocial behaviors exist along a severity continuum and include repeated violations of social rules, defiance of authority and of the rights of others, deceitfulness, theft, and reckless disregard for self and others. Antisocial individuals lack empathy, are excessively emotional, have a great need for admiration, and are markedly impulsive. Antisocial patients often present problems in the medical setting, including a high level of anger and attempts at caregiver manipulation.

Antisocial behavior, aggression, and violence are highly related. Aggressive behavior is based on impulsion and hostility. Violence is the worst-case result of aggression. Understanding these terms and having the ability to identify the patient with such behaviors results in a safer and more productive patient care environment.

Risk Factors

Risk factors for development and persistence of antisocial behaviors include genetic, neurobiological, and environmental stressors. The patient with antisocial behavior is at risk for becoming aggressive and violent. Other risk factors for aggression, and ultimately violence, include a history of violence, substance abuse, depression, schizophrenia, manic behavior, dementia, and delirium. Patients in long-term isolated situations are more likely to become aggressive without warning signs. Unstable hospital situations place the elderly patient at greater risk for becoming inadvertently aggressive.

Interventions

Prevention of aggressive or violent behavior is the best intervention. The RN must recognize a patient displaying antisocial or aggressive behavior in order to prevent a violent situation, which may result in staff or patient injury. To prevent a situation of possible violence, the patient with antisocial behavior is best managed with careful investigation of his or her concerns or motives, clear and concise communication in a nonpunitive manner, and the setting of clear limits. Findings, assessments, and limits must be clearly communicated to the patient. Referral to appropriate health care providers is also imperative to establish a plan of care and appropriate interventions before any escalation occurs.

Any patient at greater risk for aggression and violence should be approached cautiously with vigilant assessment skills. An assessment of orientation and memory must be done to rule out dementia, delirium, and substance withdrawal. Proper orientation to person, place, time, and situation is necessary if deemed appropriate. This simple, verbal intervention is an effective method of violence prevention. If previously mentioned conditions are uncovered, consider treatment with the appropriate medication (discussed later in this chapter).

In some situations, the use of physical restraints to prevent the patient from injuring herself or others is necessary. The "Restraints" section found later in the chapter discusses this intervention as an optional means of patient safety and protection.

DELIRIUM AND DEMENTIA

Delirium is an acute disorder of attention, memory, and perception. Delirium accounts for up to 15 percent of acute care hospital admissions, although it is often not the primary diagnosis but a result of an underlying condition. The risk factors for delirium include advanced age, preexisting brain disease, medications, and substance abuse. The most common causes of delirium are underlying dementia, electrolyte disorders, acute renal failure, cerebrovascular accident (CVA), pain, acute infection, medication overdose, substance intoxication, substance withdrawal, and unfamiliar environment.

The diagnosis of delirium is made based on clinical observation, established screening tools, and judgment. The essential features of delirium include an acute onset within hours or days, fluctuation of delirious symptoms, ease of inattention, ease of distraction, disorganized thought process, and altered level of consciousness.

Delirium is treatable in the patient care setting. Treatment is managed both pharmacologically and nonpharmacologically. The goal of treatment for the delirious patient is reorientation and prevention of aggressive and possible violent behavior. Nonpharmacologic nursing interventions should include optimizing surroundings, providing a quiet environment, providing attentive care, and including family members, if available, in the plan of care. Reorientation is best provided through verbal reminders of person, place, time, and situation. Use of pharmacological interventions, such as antipsychotics and benzodiazepines, should be implemented cautiously as they may further exacerbate delirium. It is important to address the entire clinical picture of the patient rather than simply manage behavior. Adequate pain relief must be addressed among patients in pain. Monitoring patient response to these medications is a direct nursing responsibility.

All treatment of the delirious patient should be considered emergent. When the patient poses a physical threat to himself or the staff, appropriate interventions include one-to-one direct patient observation, physical restraint use as a last resort, and sedative medication use.

In order to make a diagnosis of dementia, delirium must first be ruled out. Dementia is a progressive decline in memory and at least one other cognitive function in a previously alert person. These cognitive areas include attention, orientation, judgment, abstract thinking, and personality.

The incidence of dementia is directly related to advancing age. In patients over 80 years of age, 30 percent are at great risk for dementia. Risk factors for dementia other than age include history of head injury, lower socioeconomic status, female gender, family history, and history of developmental delay such as Down syndrome.

Dementia is a result of brain damage. Causes include Alzheimer's disease, CVA, AIDS, alcoholism, Parkinson's disease, and other neurodegenerations. The pathophysiology of these conditions is too great to discuss in this review, as the RN's focus should be on presentation of symptoms, diagnosis, and treatment. Recognizing dementia is essential in prevention of delirium, promotion of patient safety, and treatment of a possible underlying condition. A diagnosis of dementia is based on short- and long-term memory loss, plus one or more of the following: aphasia (language problems), apraxia (organizational problems), agnosia (inability to recognize objects and their purpose), and disturbed function of personality and/or inhibition. Obtainment of personal history through the patient and family members, a focused neurological physical, focused laboratory results (refer to "Diagnostics of Behavioral and Psychosocial Disorders" section), and a mini mental status exam (MMSE) are vital for dementia diagnosis.

Nonpharmacologic nursing treatment of dementia is similar to that of delirium. The nurse's perspective on dementia should be to understand pharmacologic treatment and be able to implement nonpharmacologic treatment. Adequate nutrition and hydration levels should be closely monitored to prevent decline. Also important are maintaining a schedule with the patient as much as possible and providing the appropriate stimulation for time of day. For example, lights should be off at night and on during the daytime. This will help the patient with dementia during hospital admission. These interventions are especially effective in prevention of sundowning, or the acute nighttime psychosis common in elderly, hospitalized patients.

DEVELOPMENTAL DELAYS

A developmental delay, or disability, is described as a severe chronic mental or physical disability that manifests before the age of 22 years, is likely to continue indefinitely, and results in substantial functional limitations in three or more areas of cognitive and emotional function. These areas include self-care, receptive and expressive language, learning, mobility, self-direction, capacity for independent living, and economic self-sufficiency. Developmental delays affect 1 percent to 3 percent of the population. These patients also normally present with a high prevalence of comorbid physical and mental conditions. Generalized care of the developmentally delayed adult should concentrate on increased risks of suffering from psychological stress, isolation, and abuse.

Down Syndrome

Down syndrome, or trisomy 21, is the result of an error in chromosomal division. Life expectancy for individuals with Down syndrome is now 55 years of age. These patients will present with physical symptoms of broad hands, bradycardia, lax ligaments, flat nose bridge, open mouth, and short stature in addition to other physical traits. Mental retardation is common in these patients. Important nursing considerations in caring for the patient with Down syndrome include monitoring for symptoms of sleep apnea, Alzheimer's disease, increased seizure risk, and elevated risk for diabetes mellitus type II. Behavioral issues are also common in patients with Down syndrome. The RN should always be direct, clear, and concise with this type of patient before performing any type of assessment or intervention. Employ the patient's family in as many care aspects as possible.

Fragile X Syndrome

Fragile X syndrome is the leading genetic cause of mental retardation. This syndrome is caused by a change in the FMR1 gene. A small section of the gene code (three letters only: CGG) is repeated on a fragile area of the X chromosome. Fragile X syndrome affects males more commonly than females. Patients will present with hyperactive behavior, large body size, large forehead with a prominent jaw, mental retardation, and the tendency to avoid eye contact. Focusing on decreasing negative, possibly aggressive behavior in the Fragile X patient is the goal of nursing care in an acute setting.

Cerebral Palsy

Cerebral palsy (CP) is a generalized term used to categorize a group of nonprogressive, noncontagious conditions that cause physical disability in human development. CP is caused by damage to the motor control centers of the developing brain and can occur during pregnancy, during childbirth, or after birth up to about age three. Motor disturbances in CP are often accompanied by disturbances of sensation, perception, cognition, communication, and behavior. Musculoskeletal disabilities in CP range from the minor to the extreme.

Typical symptoms include involuntary movements (such as spasms or facial gestures), unsteady gait and problems with balance, decreased muscle mass, and scissor walking or toe walking. In the most common cases of CP, the treatment is symptomatic and focuses on helping the person develop as many motor skills as possible.

Autism Spectrum Disorder

Autism spectrum disorder (ASD) describes a complex developmental delay that typically appears during the first three years of life and affects an individual's ability to communicate and interact. Adult autistic patients will present with a lack or delay in language use, repetitive behaviors, avoidance of eye contact, and fixation on certain objects. Nursing interventions for autistic patients include preventing aggressive behavior through brief, focused assessments and providing structured and organized care.

Other Developmental Delays

Other developmentally delayed patients may have the diagnosis of Williams syndrome or Prader-Willi syndrome. These are rare genetic disorders not commonly seen in the general population. The patient with Williams syndrome is at great risk for renal impairment and heart disease, both increased by the lack of production of elastin. Prader-Willi patients normally exhibit an insatiable appetite, placing them at risk for obesity, sleep apnea, and diabetes mellitus type II. Individuals with Williams syndrome or Prader-Willi syndrome most likely will have developmental delays and/or learning disabilities.

FAILURE TO THRIVE

Failure to thrive describes a state of decline that is multifactorial and may be caused by chronic concurrent diseases and functional impairments. Its prevalence increases with age, and it is most commonly seen in elderly individuals due to loss of physical and/or mental functions and/or age-related changes. Patients diagnosed with failure to thrive present with four syndromes: impaired physical function, malnutrition, depression, and cognitive impairment.

Risk Factors

The most common psychiatric condition found in elderly patients with failure to thrive is depression. Depression is often a cause of failure to thrive, and it can also be a consequence. Depression will be further discussed in the "Mood Disorders and Depression" section of this chapter. Failure to thrive is also more evident in patients with chronic obstructive pulmonary disease (COPD), chronic renal failure, end-stage diabetes, congestive heart failure (CHF), and cerebrovascular accident (CVA).

Symptoms, Diagnosis, and Treatment

Failure to thrive manifests as weight loss of greater than 5 percent below baseline, decreased appetite, poor nutrition, and inactivity. These are often accompanied by dehydration, depressive symptoms, and impaired immune function. On assessment, the failure-to-thrive patient is frail, withdrawn, and depressed. Close attention should be paid to complaints of pain and discomfort in the elderly, as these may mask an underlying depression as a cause or result of failure to thrive. The MMSE should be used to evaluate cognitive function to screen for any underlying dementia as a result of malnutrition. Malnutrition is common in failure-to-thrive patients due to poor dietary intake. Confirmation of malnutrition can be made using several diagnostic lab tests. Close monitoring of calorie intake should be instituted in patients deemed malnourished.

The ultimate goal of caring for a failure-to-thrive patient is the improvement of functional status. Nursing interventions should be directed toward correcting easily treatable causes of the patient's status. Correction of abnormal lab values should be addressed appropriately and immediately if deemed urgent. Nutritional intake should be supplemented as ordered, and psychiatric treatment should be initiated when needed.

MOOD DISORDERS AND DEPRESSION

In a given year, nearly 21 million U.S. adults are diagnosed with a mood disorder. Mood disorders include major depressive disorder, bipolar disorder, dysthymic disorder, and generalized anxiety disorder. The depressed patient is more likely to require inpatient care. The RN must have a heightened sensitivity to the possibility that these patients may have problems with substance abuse, as it is a common comorbidity with mood disorders.

Bipolar Disorder

Bipolar disorder is distinguished by periods of mania, in which a person experiences extreme "highs," followed by periods of depression, or equally extreme "lows." A person is typically diagnosed with bipolar disorder when the cyclic episodes persist for most of the day every day for at least two weeks. A diagnosis of bipolar disorder can be made in the absence of depressive symptoms if mania is present. However, some patients are misdiagnosed with bipolar disorder due to lack of investigation on the part of the provider. Depression can appear similar to bipolar disorder, and thorough investigation should be conducted prior to diagnosis.

Patients with bipolar disorder present with complaints of insomnia, irritability, low energy, difficulty with focusing, and relationship problems. Most patients present for care during a depressive state, when their functional level is decreased. If bipolar disorder is suspected, asking questions about manic symptoms should be initiated. Severe manic symptoms include grandiosity, decreased need for sleep, erratic speech, increased energy, racing thoughts, distractibility, irritable mood, and excessive sexuality. As previously mentioned, a concurrent substance abuse problem is likely to be evident in this patient.

The most extreme form of the disorder often results in hospitalization for manic episodes. Undiagnosed bipolar disorder places the patient at greater risk for significant functional disability, poor quality of life, and suicide. The goal of treatment in these patients should be mood stabilization with the control of any psychotic, manic behavior through medication.

Generalized Anxiety Disorder

Generalized anxiety disorder (GAD) is a pattern of frequent or constant worry and anxiety over many different activities and events. GAD patients often complain of restlessness, fatigue, irritability, muscle tension, decreased concentration, difficulty with controlling worry, anxiety that is out of proportion to the situation, and sleep disturbance. Sleep disturbance refers to difficulty with falling asleep or staying asleep or overall unsatisfying sleep. Somatic symptoms presenting with GAD include excessive diaphoresis, palpitations, shortness of breath, abdominal pain, diarrhea, and constipation.

Depression and substance abuse may occur with an anxiety disorder. Anxiety is also common in substance withdrawal. Common nonpharmacologic treatment methods for GAD include cognitive-behavioral therapy and relaxation techniques. Both may be performed by the RN at bedside as needed to prevent the patient from experiencing increased physical symptoms. Pharmacologic treatment options include anxiolytics or sedatives for acute anxiety symptoms and the use of antidepressants, including SSRIs and SNRIs, for consistent therapy. It is important to note that if a patient presents with both anxiety and depression, treatment of the depressive disorder is the first priority.

Depression and Dysthymic Disorder

Depression is defined as an abnormal emotional state characterized by exaggerated feelings of sadness, melancholy, dejection, worthlessness, emptiness, and hopelessness that are inappropriate and out of proportion to reality. Approximately 15 percent of persons have been diagnosed with or suffered from depression at one point in their life.

Dysthymic disorder is a chronic type of depression in which a person's moods are regularly low. The main symptom of dysthymia is a state of lowered, darkened, saddened mood nearly every day for at least two years. The symptoms are less severe than in patients with major depression. Diagnosis and treatment of dysthymic disorder is consistent with that used in depression. For this reason, the remaining discussion within this section will focus on depression: its risk factors, symptoms, diagnosis, and treatment. The large difference in treatment response is the anticipated time frame. Due to the more chronic nature of dysthymic disorder, these patients may respond more slowly to appropriate treatment options.

Patients suffering from long-term illness are more likely to suffer from depression as a result of their condition. These illnesses include AIDS, rheumatoid arthritis, CVA, dementia, diabetes mellitus, hypothyroidism, myocardial infarction, and CHF. The *Diagnostic and Statistical Manual of Mental Disorders*, or *DSM-5*, requires that a person must have depressed mood (or loss of interest) and at least four other symptoms, most of the time, most days, for at least two weeks continuously. A common mnemonic used in the diagnosis of depression that includes these symptoms is SIGECAPS.

S - sleep disturbance (insomnia, hypersomnia)
I - interest reduced, anhedonia (reduced pleasure or enjoyment)
G - guilt and self-blame
E - energy loss and fatigue
C - concentration problems
A - appetite changes (low appetite/weight loss or increased appetite/weight gain)
P - psychomotor changes (retardation, agitation)
S - suicidal thoughts

Once depression is diagnosed, the goal of antidepressant treatment is correction of suicidal thoughts (if present), mood, interest, and activity level. The RN must be aware that one of seven depressed patients will attempt to commit suicide, and up to 15 percent of patients with depression admitted to an inpatient setting commit suicide. The "Suicidal Behavior" section later in the chapter discusses the need for vigilance in these patients. Awareness of any substance abuse disorders is vital to the recovery of a depressed patient as well. As previously noted, substance dependence is a common comorbidity of depression. This topic will be further discussed in the following section, "Substance Dependence." Monitoring for symptoms for failure to thrive is also recommended in the depressed patient, as previously discussed in the "Failure to Thrive" section of this chapter.

The combination of cognitive behavioral therapy and pharmacologic therapy proves most effective in the treatment of depression. Prior to a patient beginning an antidepressant, one must make sure the patient is not experiencing mania, as such medication may worsen an episode. Common and more recent medication classifications used for treatment of depression include SSRIs, SNRIs, tricyclic antidepressants, and MAO inhibitors (rarely used).

SUBSTANCE DEPENDENCE

Twelve percent of the general population presently abuses drugs. According to the Behavioral Risk Factor Surveillance System (BRFSS) survey, in 2013 more than half of the U.S. adult population drank alcohol in the past 30 days. Approximately 17 percent of the adult population reported binge drinking, and 6 percent of the adult population reported heavy drinking. From 2006 to 2010, excessive alcohol use was responsible for an annual average of 88,000 deaths, including 1 in 10 deaths among working-age adults aged 20–64 years and

2.5 million years of potential life lost. More than half of these deaths and three-quarters of the years of potential life lost were due to binge drinking. Commonly abused substances include alcohol, tobacco, cannabis, sedatives, opioids, amphetamines, cocaine, hallucinogens, and inhalants. Substance abuse and dependence increase the risk for depression and suicide in an individual, while many patients with depression and generalized anxiety will use a substance, most commonly alcohol, to self-treat their underlying mood disorder.

Having knowledge of and identifying the "red-flag" broad signs/symptoms of substance abuse is the role of the RN. These red-flag warnings of substance abuse and dependence include frequent work or school absences, history of frequent trauma, depression or anxiety, labile hypertension, diarrhea, weight changes, and sleep disorders. On assessment, the dependent patient may present with mild tremor, nasal irritation (suggestive of cocaine inhalation), odor of marijuana on clothes, and signs of nutritional wasting. Suspected malnutrition most commonly associated with alcohol dependence may be confirmed with lab values, as well as several other tests that point to alcohol dependence (further discussed in the "Diagnostics" section).

The CAGE questionnaire is the most practical screening tool used in situations of suspected substance dependence. CAGE is a mnemonic for a questionnaire that asks about attempts to **c**ut down on substance use, **a**nnoyance with criticisms, **g**uilt about substance use, and using the preferred substance as an **e**ye opener. Although originally derived for suspicion of alcohol abuse, any substance may be referred to within the questions, making it a simple, concise, and effective screening tool. The CAGE questionnaire is thought to be 60 percent to 90 percent effective when two or more questions are positive.

Drug-Seeking Behavior

The term *drug-seeking* is frequently used but poorly and rarely defined. This term may be described as a set of behaviors in which an individual makes a directed and concerted effort to obtain a medication. The role of the RN is to be aware of these types of behavior. Inpatient drug-seeking behaviors include frequent and early pain medication administration requests, around-the-clock-as-needed medication requests while lacking the symptoms that indicate a need for medication administration (also known as "clock watching"), and the purposeful falsification of symptoms of anxiety and/or pain. Outpatient drug-seeking behavior typically includes inconsistent stories about pain or medical history, repeated requests for early refills, and purposeful visits to emergency departments with specific complaints of anxiety and/or pain.

Acute Substance Withdrawal

The best method to anticipate substance withdrawal is the acquisition of a thorough history and physical to place those at risk on higher alert. The most common substance a patient is likely to withdraw from under supervised medical care is alcohol. Alcohol withdrawal and withdrawal from benzodiazepines are both considered life threatening and share many symptoms. Early recognition of the signs and symptoms of withdrawal results in the best patient outcome. The following outlines the *Diagnostic and Statistical Manual of Mental Disorders* (DSM-5) diagnostic criteria for alcohol withdrawal:

DSM-5 Criteria for Alcohol Withdrawal

If an individual experiences the following four criteria in the time frames outlined, he is likely withdrawing from alcohol dependence.

A. Cessation of (or reduction in) heavy and prolonged alcohol use

B. Two (or more) of the following symptoms developing within a few days following criterion A:

- Autonomic hyperactivity
- Increased hand tremor
- Insomnia
- Nausea or vomiting
- Transient visual, tactile, or auditory hallucinations or illusions
- Psychomotor agitation
- Anxiety
- Seizures (grand mal)

C. Experienced symptoms, outlined in criterion B, cause clinically significant distress and/or impairment in social, occupational, or other areas.

D. The symptoms are not caused by another condition or mental disorder.

Adapted from: American Psychiatric Association (2013): Diagnostic and Statistical Manual of Mental Disorders, Fifth Edition (DSM-5). Washington, D.C.: American Psychiatric Association.

Benzodiazepine withdrawal presents with very similar symptoms as alcohol withdrawal. Again, anticipation of a possible withdrawal is the best practice when dealing with at-risk patients. A preliminary urinary drug screen (UDS) can be performed to aid this process.

During acute substance withdrawal, maintenance of stable hemodynamics, respiratory, and nutritional status are considered first priority. Patient safety must also be considered during this time, and often the use of physical and chemical restraints is indicated. Further discussion regarding the use of restraints is discussed in the "Restraints" section of this chapter.

SUICIDAL BEHAVIOR

Suicide ranks as the 10th leading cause of death in the United States. One of seven depressed patients will attempt to commit suicide, and 2 to 9 percent of patients with depression admitted to an inpatient setting commit suicide.

Risk Factors

The RN should be adept at recognizing risk factors and specific behavior indicating a suicidal attempt may be imminent. Risk factors for suicide include sex, age, ethnicity, environment, situation, medications, and underlying psychiatric diagnosis. Men are almost twice as likely to commit suicide as women; however, women attempt suicide two to three more times than men. With increasing age, the risk for suicide increases. The risk is also higher for Caucasians than for those belonging to a minority ethnic group. Patients involved in a stressful situation at home, including abuse, or perceiving a hospital admission as restrictive and hopeless are also at greater suicide risk. As previously mentioned, depressed patients are more likely to commit suicide, as are patients with a history of substance abuse.

Suicidal behavior that may indicate an **imminent attempt** includes exhibiting a sense of isolation and withdrawal, a lack of friends and family, an expressed preoccupation with death, a flat affect, an outward expression of hopelessness, and anhedonia.

Intervention

Individuals with past suicide attempts and displaying any of the above characteristics should automatically be placed on a higher watch for a repeated attempt. The potentially suicidal patient should be considered an emergent situation. Direct questions regarding any thoughts of suicidal ideation, plan, and motive should be asked. Any patient with a thought-out plan indicates greater danger for suicide. A person who is indeed suicidal should be placed on one-to-one monitoring; any objects that may be used to inflict self-harm, including medications and knives, should be removed from the environment, and the patient should be referred to direct psychiatric care. Providing a well-lit environment for a patient at risk for suicide can reduce the likelihood of an attempt, as a dark environment correlates with increased suicidal attempts.

RESTRAINTS

The Centers for Medicare and Medicaid Services (CMS) defines physical restraints as any manual method or physical or mechanical device, material, or equipment attached or adjacent to the resident's body that the individual cannot remove easily, which restricts freedom of movement or normal access to the body.

Falls do not constitute self-injurious behavior or a medical symptom that warrants the use of a physical restraint. Although restraints have been traditionally used as a falls prevention approach, they have major, serious drawbacks and can contribute to serious injuries. There is no evidence that the use of physical restraints, including but not limited to side rails, will prevent or reduce falls. Additionally, falls that occur while a person is physically restrained often result in more severe injuries.

Physical versus Chemical Restraints

Physical restraints are designed to restrict voluntary movement or behavior by the use of a device, commonly soft wrist and/or ankle wraps, for behavioral alteration purposes. Physical restraint is the most common type of restraint used by RNs in practice. Chemical restraint is the use of a medication to control an individual's behavior. This medication is used with the intention of sedation for the safety of the patient and caregivers/staff as indicated. Medications used for chemical restraint most commonly include antipsychotics and benzodiazepines or sedatives.

Physical restraints as an intervention do not treat the underlying causes of medical symptoms. Therefore, as with other interventions, physical restraints should not be used without also seeking to identify and address the physical or psychological condition causing the medical symptom. Restraints may be used, if warranted, as a temporary symptomatic intervention while the actual cause of the medical symptom is being evaluated and managed. Additionally, physical restraints may be used as a symptomatic intervention when they are immediately necessary to prevent a resident from injuring himself/herself or others and/or to prevent the resident from interfering with life-sustaining treatment, when no other less restrictive or less risky interventions exist.

Necessitation of Restraints

Arguments can be made for the use of restraints in specific patient care situations. These situations include if and when the patient poses an imminent threat to

- self (e.g., suicidal behavior, emergency situations);
- a caregiver (e.g., during substance withdrawal);
- medical equipment or surroundings that play a part in the patient's medical care (e.g., mechanical ventilation or invasive cardiac monitoring).

Managing the Restrained Patient

The restrained patient requires additional monitoring. The RN is required to review the continual need for restraints through evaluation of the patient's behavior on an hourly basis. For example, if the need for restraints was justified for a patient showing aggressive behavior during an acute alcohol withdrawal, the patient must be observed for completion or stabilization of the acute episode before the restraints are removed. In reference to observation, the restrained patient must be under observation at all times. One-to-one patient assignment, or use of another qualified, nonnursing staff member to provide constant surveillance, is a common type of close observation used in this situation. This is to not only observe changes in behavior but to also prevent patient injury. Assessment of the restrained individual should also include compliance with plan of care and evaluation of effectiveness of the restraint method. Ultimately, restraints should be removed when the patient's condition improves.

DIAGNOSTICS OF BEHAVIORAL AND PSYCHOSOCIAL DISORDERS

This section will present the most common laboratory procedures used in the assistance of diagnosing common behavioral/psychosocial disorders.

Urine Drug Screen (UDS)

Positive substance results using a UDS can help with placing a patient who is at risk for withdrawal, identifying the cause of delirium, and assessing risk for suicidal behavior (see table 14.1).

TABLE 14.1 *Urine Screening Test Time Frames*

Substance	Length of time for detection in urine
Alcohol	12 hrs
Amphetamine (methamphetamine)	48 hrs
Benzodiazepine (lorazepam, diazepam, alprazolam)	3 days
Cocaine metabolites	2–4 days
Marijuana	3 days
Opioids	
Codeine	48 hrs
Heroin	48 hrs
Morphine	2–3 days
Oxycodone	2–4 days

Urinalysis

Use of the urinalysis may aid in the diagnosis of a urinary tract infection (UTI) in the delirious, aggressive elderly patient. A UTI will present with positive leukocytes, positive nitrites, and possibly trace to positive blood when a urinalysis is performed.

Serum Lab Values

TSH—Elevated (hypothyroid) and low (hyperthyroid) may both cause dementia.

GGT—Elevated suggests alcohol abuse.

ALT/AST—Elevated suggests liver dysfunction, possible alcohol abuse, possible liver cirrhosis and or/failure, which may cause delirium and/or dementia.

Creatinine—Elevated indicates renal insufficiency, which may cause dementia.

BUN—Elevated indicates dehydration; suspect failure to thrive.

Potassium—Elevated indicates renal dysfunction; suspect failure to thrive or dementia.

Sodium—Elevated can cause dementia; low can cause delirium and/or dementia.

Glucose—Decreased (hypoglycemia) can cause delirium/dementia.

Folic acid—Deficiency indicates alcohol abuse, often with B12 deficiency.

Cobalamin (B12)—Deficiency indicates malnutrition; can cause dementia.

Thiamine (B1)—Deficiency indicates alcohol abuse.

Riboflavin (B2)—Deficiency indicates alcohol abuse, possible failure to thrive.

Niacin (B5)—Deficiency indicates alcohol abuse, possible failure to thrive.

Pyridoxine (B6)—Deficiency indicates alcohol abuse.

Vitamin D 25 hydroxy—Deficiency raises concern for failure to thrive.

Oxygen Saturation

Reduced oxyhemoglobin saturation indicates respiratory deficiency. This can cause long-term dementia symptoms, often a result of chronic obstructive pulmonary disease (COPD).

MEDICATIONS

Common psychiatric medications used in treatment of the psychosocial/behavioral patient are listed below. In a depressed patient, always monitor for increased signs of suicide risk after beginning medications.

Antidepressant and Antianxiety Therapy

Selective serotonin reuptake inhibitors (SSRIs) are the most commonly prescribed antidepressant therapy, including these brand names: Prozac, Paxil, Zoloft, Lexapro, and Celexa. SSRIs inhibit reuptake of serotonin, leaving more available to the central nervous system. **Selective serotonin and norepinephrine reuptake inhibitors (SSNRIs)**, including Effexor, Effexor XR, Cymbalta, and Pristique, inhibit reuptake of serotonin and norepinephrine, leaving more available to the CNS. SSRIs and SSNRIs may take up to four to six weeks for maximum response. Common side effects for both include tremors and nausea.

Not as commonly prescribed, **tricyclic antidepressants**, including Elavil and Sinequan, inhibit norepinephrine and serotonin reuptake with anticholinergic effect. Generally, response is seen within three to four weeks. Tricyclic antidepressants may cause drowsiness, urinary retention, and dry mouth. **Caution should be taken if administering to an elderly individual.**

Monoamine oxidase inhibitors (MAOIs), including Nardil and Parnate, are rarely prescribed due to their high interaction with other medications. These medications nonselectively inhibit monoamine oxidase. Response to MAOIs is usually seen within three to four weeks, but there are many side effects, so MAOIs should be used only as a last choice. **Caution should be taken if administering to an elderly individual.**

Bupropion, including Wellbutrin, Wellbutrin SR, and Wellbutrin XL, inhibits serotonin, dopamine, and norepinephrine uptake, leaving more available to the CNS. Response to bupropion is generally seen within three weeks. Side effects may include increased seizure activity, nausea, and tremors.

Bipolar Disorder Therapy

With any bipolar medication, the patient should be monitored closely for stabilization of manic state and prevention of increased suicide risk during depressive state.

Lithium alters neuronal sodium transport, ultimately stabilizing the individual's mood. It generally takes three to five days to reach maximum efficacy. The patient should be monitored for tremors, diarrhea, and arrhythmias.

Also used for mood stabilization, **atypical antipsychotics**, including olanzapine, risperidone, quetiapine, and aripiprazole, work by antagonizing dopamine D2 receptors, serotonin 5-HT2 receptors, and other unidentified receptors. Atypical antipsychotics typically take up to one to three weeks for response. Side effects include somnolence, dizziness, tremors, and nausea.

Benzodiazepines

Benzodiazepines are commonly used to control the acutely aggressive, violent, anxious, delirious, or restless patient. They are also commonly used to help control alcohol withdrawal symptoms. Monitoring for risk of dependence and overdose potential is important in a patient receiving these medications. These medications are not recommended for long-term use. Common brands include Xanax, Valium, Ativan, and Klonopin. These medications bind to benzodiazepine receptors and cause sedation. If administered orally, effects will be seen within 45 minutes. If administered intravenously, effects will be seen within 10 minutes. Individuals taking benzodiazepines should be monitored for dependence and increased sedation.

First-Generation Antipsychotics

Commonly prescribed to control the acutely psychotic, delirious, aggressive, violent, or confused patient, **first-generation antipsychotics** are almost always given via an intramuscular route. Common brands include Compazine, Haldol, Moban, and Loxitane. First-generation antipsychotics are potent agonists of muscarinic, alpha adrenergic, and histamine receptors and cause sedation and decreased aggression. Intramuscular administration response is usually seen within 15 to 30 minutes of administration. Individuals should be monitored for oversedation resulting in respiratory depression and/or administration site irritation.

Review Questions

1. An 83-year-old patient with dementia presents to the unit. The nurse knows that this patient is at greatest risk for which of these psychosocial disorders?

   A. developing substance dependence

   B. being abused in the home at or the hospital

   C. developing Down syndrome

   D. developing antisocial behavior

2. You suspect that a 76-year-old patient who suffers from dementia has been abused by his caregiver while at home. What signs and symptoms would you most likely base your suspicions on?

   A. hair loss, poor dental hygiene, and memory loss

   B. confused behavior, diminished heart sounds, and lower-extremity edema

   C. sacral pressure sores, guarded behavior during physical assessment, and diffuse bruising without explanation

   D. urinary incontinence, aggression, and loss of hearing

3. What is the most effective diagnostic test to assess for risk of suffering from substance withdrawal while in the hospital?

   A. a urine drug screen

   B. a mini mental status exam

   C. a urinalysis

   D. a GGT level

4. When analyzing the lab values of an underweight, inactive, and depressed patient, what results would lead the nurse to suspect failure to thrive?

   A. elevated GGT, increased glucose, and decreased B6

   B. increased B12, decreased folic acid, and normal AST/ALT

   C. elevated creatinine, decreased vitamin D 25H, decreased B12

   D. elevated TSH, decreased B1, elevated GGT

5. A patient has required physical wrist restraints due to delirium. At the end of the nurse's shift, the patient begins to follow verbal commands, speak pleasantly, and ask for water. What is the best method available to the nurse to assess the patient's cognitive function?

   A. consultation with another nurse

   B. perform a physical assessment

   C. ask the patient's family if they believe the patient is at her functional baseline level

   D. mini mental status exam

6. A patient was recently admitted to the hospital who has a known history of schizophrenia, depression, and substance abuse. The patient is presently displaying elements of antisocial behavior, including impulsiveness and aggression. What is the best nursing approach to take to prevent the behavior from becoming violent?

   A. The nurse should approach the patient cautiously with clear communication, using rigid assessment skills and setting clear patient-nurse boundaries.

   B. The nurse should quietly approach the patient and limit communication as much as possible.

   C. The nurse should be equally aggressive with the patient, as allowing the patient's behavior to alter the nurse's actions will only make the potential violent behavior more likely.

   D. The nurse should approach the patient in a punitive manner, use short phrases for communication, and use the threat of restraints to persuade the patient to retreat from potential violence.

7. A patient who is being treated for an episode of uncontrolled hyperglycemia has a history of mental retardation, sleep apnea, and diabetes mellitus type II. Physical symptoms also include broad hands, flat nose, and short stature. What is the likely developmental delay diagnosis?

   A. fragile X syndrome

   B. Down syndrome

   C. Prader-Willi syndrome

   D. autism spectrum disorder

8. The most likely class of medication to be used in treatment of a patient diagnosed with depression is a selective serotonin reuptake inhibitor (SSRI). How long would the nurse expect it to take for this patient to see relief from this medication?

   A. two weeks

   B. seven weeks

   C. three to four days

   D. five weeks

9. The nurse is caring for a patient who is considered an increased suicide risk. What symptoms might lead the nurse to believe that the patient is imminently contemplating suicide?

   A. elevated heart rate, complaints of pain

   B. outgoing behavior, aggressive behavior

   C. expressing acceptance of death, flat affect

   D. complaints of chest pain, manic behavior

10. In which of these situations would the temporary use of physical restraints be most appropriate?

   A. bipolar patient in a manic state

   B. aggressive patient trying to pull out his indwelling Foley catheter

   C. patient with a history of substance abuse resting quietly

   D. elderly patient with a history of dementia exhibiting possible sundowning behavior

Review Answers and Explanations

1. B

The most likely profile of an abused patient is elderly, female, and with dementia. Such patients are at greatest risk for abuse and neglect in the home and in the hospital due to their dependence on others for care.

2. C

Guarded behavior during assessment indicates anxiety on the part of the patient due to a history of physical abuse, while unexplained bruising is a physical sign of abuse. Sacral pressure sores often indicate a patient has been neglected with regard to proper skin care.

3. A

The urine drug screen is the quickest, most comprehensive screening that can be performed quite easily to assess for a patient's recent history of substance use. If positive, the nurse should be on high alert for substance withdrawal after the patient has been sober for 48 to 72 hours. A GGT level (D), although indicative of consistent alcohol use when elevated, does not provide a comprehensive substance use profile.

4. C

An elevated creatinine is indicative of renal insufficiency or failure, which can cause elevated potassium along with failure to thrive. Decreased vitamin D 25 hydroxy often indicates a lack of activity and malnutrition, which is associated with failure to thrive. Decreased B12 is often indicative of malnutrition due to lack of proper diet, also associated with failure to thrive.

5. D

The mini mental status exam is vital for the diagnosis of dementia, and within this exam, the nurse is able to assess for orientation, proper language use, memory, and attention. This is the best method available out of the aforementioned choices to assess for improvement of delirium.

6. A

A patient who has the increased potential to become aggressive and violent should be communicated with clearly in order to allow the nurse to assess any worsening behavior. Setting limits in a nonpunitive way helps prevent the patient's aggression level from increasing. Rigid assessment skills and the setting of boundaries allow the nurse to be in control of a possibly escalating situation.

7. B

Down syndrome patients present with broad hands, flat nose, bradycardia, open mouth, and short stature. Comorbidities commonly associated with Down syndrome include sleep apnea, diabetes mellitus, Alzheimer's disease, and mental retardation.

8. D

The selective serotonin reuptake inhibitors are the most commonly prescribed class of antidepressants. This class of medication does not provide immediate relief from depressive symptoms. Most patients will experience relief from or improvement in their depressive symptoms between four and six weeks into therapy.

9. C

Patients who are at risk for imminent suicide present with acceptance of and preoccupation with death. This preoccupation should be considered a red flag while assessing a patient at high risk for suicide. A flat affect is commonly seen in these patients, as well as an outward expression of hopelessness and anhedonia.

10. B

The patient that poses a physical threat to himself meets restraint-use criteria. This patient also meets the criteria through posing an imminent threat to medical equipment, in this case an indwelling Foley catheter, that plays a part in his medical care. Although the sundowning patient may become agitated and dangerous, this example does not specify the patient as presently suffering from delirium.

PART IV

Practice Test

Adult CCRN Practice Test

Directions: Each question or incomplete statement below is followed by 4 suggested answers or completions. In each case, **highlight** the statement that best answers the question or completes the statement. Allot 3 hours to answer the 150 questions in this test.

1. A patient with heart failure should be taught which factor is most useful in monitoring this condition clinically?

   A. ejection fraction

   B. cholesterol panel

   C. cardiac output

   D. coronary atherosclerosis

2. A 73-year-old male is admitted to the ICU. He appears to be in respiratory distress with worsening tachypnea (rate of 41) and use of accessory muscles. He is also anxious. Oxygenation with supplemental oxygen has been unsuccessful due to noncompliance. What is the most appropriate next step?

   A. prompt initiation of BiPAP with FiO_2 of 100%

   B. prompt initiation of CPAP with FiO_2 of 100%

   C. prompt administration of sedation to increase compliance

   D. prompt intubation and initiation of mechanical ventilation

3. One complication associated with endovascular procedures is compartment syndrome due to multiple vascular puncture sites. A nurse can determine if compartment syndrome is present by

   A. performing a neurological assessment.

   B. measuring capillary perfusion pressure (CPP).

   C. measuring interstitial fluid pressure.

   D. performing a neurovascular and extremity girth assessment.

4. A critical care nurse working on the hospital's rapid response team is called to the medical floor for a patient who is acutely agitated. The patient's bedside nurse reports that the patient was admitted with pneumonia and upon the last assessment was found to be very agitated and nearly combative with the staff. The critical care nurse should immediately assess for which of these common causes of agitation in hospitalized patients?

   A. medication-induced psychosis

   B. hypoxia

   C. seizures

   D. acute cerebral vascular attack (stroke)

5. The nurse is caring for a patient admitted after being found acting erratically outside the hospital. The patient continues to rant in an unrecognizable language, makes sexual advances toward staff, and refuses to lie down in bed. Based on this patient's symptoms, what is his likely underlying diagnosis?

A. depression

B. bipolar disorder

C. alcohol withdrawal

D. antisocial behavior

6. A ruptured plaque occluding a cerebral artery is a common cause of

A. transient ischemic attack (TIA).

B. hemorrhagic stroke.

C. myocardial infarction.

D. ischemic stroke.

7. The use of sequential compression devices (SCDs), Ted hose, and/or low molecular weight heparin (LMWH) are important measures to directly prevent which of these conditions?

A. myocardial infarction

B. pulmonary embolus

C. deep vein thrombosis (DVT)

D. COPD exacerbation

8. A patient is admitted for chest pain. The symptoms are presently considered stable, and any acute cardiovascular issues have been previously ruled out. The nurse has observed that the patient is asking for her as-needed pain medication on a continual basis without showing any physical signs or symptoms of pain. If the nurse suspects a history of opioid substance abuse in this patient, which of these is the best method for assessment?

A. using the CAGE questionnaire

B. monitoring for early signs of substance withdrawal, including tachycardia and confused behavior

C. asking for lab orders to include B12 level, folic acid level, and GGT

D. checking the dental hygiene status of the patient

9. A patient is recovering in the ICU after suffering from severe community-acquired pneumonia. After extubation, the patient is having difficulty clearing copious, thick, and "tacky" secretions from his respiratory tract. The critical care nurse collaborates with the health care provider and respiratory therapy to add which of these treatments to the patient's plan of care?

A. inhaled bronchodilators

B. antifungal agents

C. humidified oxygen

D. reintubation

10. Which of these nursing interventions will help the patient feel safe in the critical care setting?

    A. not allowing family members to remain at the bedside

    B. asking for the charge nurse's help before making any decisions

    C. conversing with him by telling him your plans for after work

    D. responding quickly to his call bell or need for assistance

11. The nurse is caring for a patient with a known history of alcohol abuse who has been hospitalized for two days. What symptoms would make the nurse highly suspicious of early alcohol withdrawal in this patient?

    A. drowsiness and bradycardia

    B. visual hallucinations and vomiting

    C. delirium and violent behavior

    D. hand tremors and nausea

12. A patient is admitted to the ICU after being found unresponsive at home. The patient is suspected to have carbon monoxide poisoning from using a portable heater in an enclosed space. Which of these lab values will **not** be accurate in a patient with carbon monoxide poisoning?

    A. carboxyhemoglobin

    B. lactic acid

    C. leukocytes

    D. pulse oximetry

13. Leukopenia in a patient with viral infection, overwhelming bacterial infection, or bone marrow disorder may demonstrate that

    A. the patient has used all the available leukocytes to fight the infection and is unable to reproduce them at the necessary rate to post a successful immune response.

    B. the patient has no need for the body to stimulate an immune response with these types of infections, and therefore there is no need to produce additional leukocytes.

    C. the bone marrow is selective in the production of cells for the body and may inhibit production in these situations.

    D. the CBC is unable to count WBC accurately when antibiotics are being used.

14. Which of these statements is a warning sign that can alert the critical care nurse that an ethical dilemma may exist?

    A. There is no need for secrecy about a proposed intervention.

    B. Family members are confused about what is happening to the patient.

    C. The proposed course of action follows customary practices.

    D. The situation is emotionally stable.

15. A nurse should recognize that a patient who is taking Lopressor (metoprolol) is at most risk for developing which of these clinical manifestations?

    A. hypertension

    B. hypersensitivity

    C. bradycardia

    D. tachycardia

16. Which of these factors is the primary consideration when applying a model for ethical decision making?

    A. court's wishes

    B. family's wishes

    C. patient's wishes

    D. staff's wishes

17. What percentage of the resting cardiac output do the kidneys receive?

    A. 40 percent

    B. 20–25 percent

    C. 10–15 percent

    D. 5 percent

18. Bilirubin is the result of a breakdown of

    A. hemoglobin.

    B. white blood cells.

    C. amylase.

    D. bile.

19. A patient with 4 hours of chest pain has acute ST elevation in leads V_1–V_2. You understand that the location of the infarction is to be

    A. lateral.

    B. septal.

    C. inferior.

    D. anterior.

20. The lateral aspect of the skull beneath the temporal bone just above the ear is the most common site of injury for

    A. epidural hematoma.

    B. intracerebral hemorrhage.

    C. subarachnoid hemorrhage.

    D. subdural hematoma.

21. A patient presents with tachypnea, tachycardia, and hypotension. A pulmonary embolus is suspected. Which of these is the quickest/easiest imaging to order to make the diagnosis, assuming normal renal function and no known allergies?

    A. pulmonary angiography

    B. CT chest with IV contrast

    C. CT chest without IV contrast

    D. V/Q perfusion scan

22. The capacity to return to a restorative level of functioning using compensatory or coping mechanisms is referred to as

    A. vulnerability.

    B. resiliency.

    C. complexity.

    D. stability.

23. The anterior pituitary receives stimulation from the hypothalamus through the

    A. vascular system.

    B. sympathetic nervous system.

    C. parasympathetic system.

    D. central nervous system.

24. A 52-year-old patient is alert, intubated, and on a ventilator following cardiac bypass surgery. Which of these assessment tools would be the most appropriate to determine the patient's pain level?

    A. FACES scale

    B. pain intensity scale

    C. PQRST method

    D. Jacox scale

25. Which of these terms refers to nursing competencies or characteristics in the Synergy Model?

    A. resiliency

    B. response to diversity

    C. complexity

    D. stability

26. A patient diagnoses with acute pericarditis, as evidenced by global ST elevation. How many of the 12 leads will show reciprocal ST segment depression?

    A. one

    B. two

    C. three

    D. none of the leads

27. There are three levels of resiliency pertaining to patient characteristics. Which of these are the noted levels?

    A. low, medium, high

    B. minimal, moderate, high

    C. anger, denial, acceptance

    D. confusion, fear, depression

28. A 67-year-old patient with hypertensive emergency is being monitored for response to a new antihypertensive medication. The husband asks if he can sit next to the patient and hold her hand. Which of these responses would be best for you to say?

    A. "No, further stimulation may make her blood pressure worse."

    B. "No, your presence may make her anxious."

    C. "No, it interferes with my taking her blood pressure."

    D. "Yes, and I will continue to monitor her."

29. Patient characteristics that include susceptibility to actual or potential stressors that can adversely affect outcomes are known as

    A. stability.

    B. resiliency.

    C. complexity.

    D. vulnerability.

30. Cerebral perfusion pressure is calculated by

    A. adding the ICP to the MAP.

    B. multiplying the MAP by the ICP.

    C. subtracting the ICP from the MAP.

    D. subtracting the MAP from the ICP.

31. A patient with advanced Parkinson's disease was admitted to the ICU with hypoxia 8 hours ago. A tracheal aspirate showed the presence of multiple organisms. The CCRN may expect antibiotic coverage for

    A. aspiration pneumonia.

    B. community-acquired pneumonia.

    C. nosocomial pneumonia.

    D. COPD exacerbation.

32. Electrocardiographic changes that result from hyperkalemia are

    A. widened QRS, elevated ST segment, lengthening PR interval.

    B. prolonged QT segment, bradycardia.

    C. U waves, ST depression, ventricular irritability (i.e., PVCs).

    D. tachycardia, ventricular irritability.

33. An ethical dilemma is a situation requiring a choice between which of these?

    A. morally acceptable but opposing alternatives

    B. morally unreasonable but legal alternatives

    C. legal but immoral alternatives

    D. illegal but morally acceptable alternatives

34. A common clinical finding of SIADH (syndrome of inappropriate antidiuretic hormone) may include which symptoms?

    A. mental status changes

    B. tachycardia

    C. polyuria

    D. polydipsia

35. A healthy 40-year-old patient is admitted to the ICU postoperatively from an elective surgical procedure requiring a general anesthetic. The patient is somnolent. The provider requests an ABG, which returns as pH of 7.2, $PaCO_2$ 62, PaO_2 75, and HCO_3^- 25. This patient has a

    A. respiratory alkalosis.

    B. metabolic acidosis.

    C. metabolic alkalosis.

    D. respiratory acidosis.

36. The medication fenoldopam (trade name: Corlopam) is ordered for a patient with hypertensive crisis. The nurse will need to monitor for which of these side effects?

    A. hypokalemia, headache, and reflex tachycardia

    B. hypokalemia, headache, and bradycardia

    C. hyperkalemia, headache, and reflex tachycardia

    D. hyperkalemia, headache, and bradycardia

37. A patient is transferred to the ICU following an outpatient endoscopy procedure. Shortly after receiving topical benzocaine spray to the oropharynx, the patient became hypoxic, which did not resolve with oxygen therapy. While the critical care nurse is obtaining a sample for an arterial blood gas, she notices that the blood is a dark "chocolate" brown color. She recognizes this condition as

    A. carbon monoxide poisoning.

    B. methemoglobinemia.

    C. pulmonary embolus.

    D. normal reaction to benzocaine administration.

38. Which of these manifestations should a nurse recognize as most significant when assessing a patient with intestinal obstruction?

    A. vomiting

    B. fever

    C. constipation

    D. sweating

39. Which of these is an **unacceptable** way to administer a central painful stimulus?

    A. pinching and twisting the trapezius muscle

    B. pressing on the superior orbital rim

    C. pushing up and inward at the angle of the jaw

    D. twisting a nipple

40. A 68-year-old female, recovering in the ICU from complications following an emergency colostomy, expresses concern about who will take care of her at home. The nurse learns that she and her 75-year-old husband live on the second floor of an apartment building that has no elevator. In addition, the husband is having difficulty understanding how to care for the patient's wounds. Which of these nursing interventions would be most appropriate?

    A. Ask the patient's grown daughter to move in for a short time to provide care.

    B. Consult with the patient's insurance carrier for nursing home placement.

    C. Contact case management or social work for a home nursing consult.

    D. Reinforce information about wound care and provide reassurance to the spouse.

41. Approximately 90 percent of erythropoietin is manufactured in the

    A. bone marrow.

    B. kidneys.

    C. liver.

    D. lungs.

42. The nurse is caring for a patient diagnosed with systemic inflammatory response syndrome (SIRS). Which statement accurately describes the difference between SIRS and sepsis?

    A. Blood cultures are positive with SIRS but are negative with sepsis.

    B. Blood cultures are negative with SIRS but are positive with sepsis.

    C. Temperature elevation is found only in SIRS.

    D. Tachycardia is found only in sepsis.

43. As an ICU nurse caring for a patient with oat cell carcinoma of the lung, which patient characteristic would the nurse expect in this patient?

    A. predictability

    B. resource availability

    C. vulnerability

    D. stability

44. A patient is brought into the ICU after being involved in a motor vehicle crash. He is in respiratory distress. On physical exam, the nurse noticed that the left side of the chest is moving inward as the patient inhales and the remaining chest wall expands. Based on this observation, the nurse suspects that the patient is suffering from

    A. pneumothorax.

    B. pulmonary hemorrhage.

    C. flail chest.

    D. atrial fibrillation.

45. Which of these modalities would **not** be used to treat SIADH?

    A. fluid restriction

    B. diuretic administration

    C. administration of 3% saline

    D. kayexalate enemas

46. A Native American patient who is DNR is near death. The family, after consultation with tribal leaders, has requested that a tribal drummer be allowed to drum and sing at the bedside as the patient expires. A staff member has expressed concern about the noise and disruption this will cause. Which of these would be the most appropriate response to the coworker?

    A. "We will have the ceremony outside in the garden."

    B. "The physician has approved the ceremony in the room."

    C. "Don't you understand what this ceremony means to them?"

    D. "What concerns do you have about the ceremony?"

47. Using the Parkland Formula, calculate the first eight-hour fluid resuscitation needs of a 40 kg patient with a 65 percent total body surface area (TBSA) burn.

    A. 502 mL

    B. 10,400 mL

    C. 5200 mL

    D. 1040 mL

48. A goal of therapy for a patient with congestive heart failure is to

    A. decrease preload, increase afterload, and increase cardiac output.

    B. increase preload, increase afterload, and increase cardiac output.

    C. increase preload, decrease afterload, and increase cardiac output.

    D. decrease preload, decrease afterload, and increase cardiac output.

49. Ischemic injury to the kidney will usually commence when

    A. mean arterial pressure is < 60 mm Hg for > than 40 hours.

    B. mean arterial pressure is > 60 mm Hg; however, urine output is < 30 mL/hr.

    C. mean arterial pressure is intermittently < 60 mm Hg over a 60-hour period.

    D. systolic BP < 100 mm Hg.

Questions 50–51 refer to the following scenario:

The nurse is caring for a 75-year-old patient currently restrained by soft wrist wraps due to acute delirium and erratic behavior. This patient has a standing order from the provider for intramuscular Haldol as needed.

50. What type of behavior would best warrant the as-needed administration of intramuscular Haldol to this patient?

    A. decline in cognitive level

    B. acceptance with plan of care

    C. increased aggression and attempts at violence directed toward the staff

    D. sexual advances toward the nurse

51. After the intramuscular administration of Haldol to the patient, how long should the nurse anticipate until the medication elicits a sedative response?

    A. 2 hours

    B. 45 minutes

    C. 20 minutes

    D. 1 hour

52. The nurse is reviewing the medication records of a 35-year-old patient admitted to the ICU. Which one of these would suggest an increased risk of deep vein thrombosis?

    A. use of oral contraceptive pills

    B. use of daily ASA

    C. use of a daily multivitamin

    D. use of a proton pump inhibitor for acid reflux

53. Meningeal irritation is indicated by

    A. nuchal rigidity.

    B. Homan's sign.

    C. Babinski's reflex.

    D. flaccid paralysis.

54. Four days after a patient sustains a partial thickness or second-degree burn of the hand, what would be the highest priority of care for this patient?

    A. pain management

    B. body image

    C. airway maintenance

    D. fluid volume management

55. An elderly patient is admitted to the ICU for COPD exacerbation. The medical history also includes hypertension and coronary artery disease. The treatment regimen includes oxygen, antibiotics, steroids, and inhaled beta-2 agonist bronchodilators. The critical care nurse should monitor the patient for which of these medication side effects that may compromise his preexisting cardiac conditions?

    A. leukocytosis related to steroids

    B. tachycardia related to beta-2 agonists

    C. allergic reaction to antibiotics

    D. depressed respiratory drive due to oxygen therapy

56. Which assessment maneuver should be done to determine if a patient has hepatojugular reflux?

    A. Place patient's head-of-bed at 45 degrees, compress the upper right abdomen for 30 to 45 seconds, assess for pronounced jugular vein distension.

    B. Place patient's head-of-bed at 45 degrees, compress the upper left abdomen for 30 to 45 seconds, assess for pronounced jugular vein distension.

    C. Place patient in Trendelenburg, compress the lower left abdomen for 30 to 45 seconds, assess for pronounced jugular vein distension.

    D. Place patient in Trendelenburg, compress the upper left abdomen for 30 to 45 seconds, assess for pronounced jugular vein distension.

57. The critical care nurse should recognize that major complications of diabetes insipidus (DI) could include

    A. dehydration.

    B. hyponatremia.

    C. hyperkalemia.

    D. bradycardia and hypertension.

58. A 65-year-old patient with a history of COPD, diagnosed by pulmonary function tests, is admitted to the ICU in respiratory distress after his wife called 911 because he was gasping for air. He is hypoxic with oxygen saturation of 83 percent and has a mildly elevated WBC count. What are the appropriate measures to treat this patient?

    A. beta agonist and steroids

    B. beta agonist, steroids only, and chest x-ray

    C. beta agonist, steroids, and broad spectrum antibiotics

    D. beta agonist, steroids, broad spectrum antibiotics, chest x-ray, blood/urine cultures

59. The critical care nurse is precepting a novice-level nurse. At the novice level, the clinical judgment that can be expected would **not** include which of these?

    A. collecting basic-level data

    B. including extraneous data

    C. questioning own decisions

    D. recognizing patterns and trends

60. A 28-year-old patient is in the ICU recovering from a motorcycle crash, during which he experienced bilateral femur fractures. The patient suddenly complains of dyspnea, and then experiences decreasing pulse oximetry readings. The bedside monitor displays what appears to be new-onset atrial fibrillation. The critical care nurse synthesizes this information and suspects that the patient is experiencing

    A. acute pulmonary embolus due to fat embolus.

    B. acute pulmonary embolus due to mobilization of a lower-extremity DVT.

    C. acute myocardial infarction.

    D. normal response to immobility due to femur fractures.

61. Which of these behaviors is an example of families trying to obtain some control over the situation?

    A. going to work and visiting once a day

    B. sleeping at the patient's bedside

    C. refusing to help feed the patient

    D. closing their eyes when entering the room

62. Which of these changes is consistent with pericarditis?

    A. widened QRS complex

    B. inverted T waves

    C. no P waves

    D. diffuse pattern of ST elevation

63. Which cerebral component is responsible for reabsorbing cerebrospinal fluid?

    A. lateral ventricle

    B. dura mater

    C. arachnoid villi

    D. subarachnoid cisterns

64. You have been working with a nurse who has been on the unit for more than 10 years. You notice that the nurse synthesizes multiple data points, looks at the "big picture," collaborates well with others, and recognizes limitations. At what level of clinical judgment would you consider the nurse to be at this time?

    A. novice
    B. competent
    C. expert
    D. certified

65. The categories of clinical conditions that may result in acute renal failure would **not** include

    A. prerenal.
    B. intrarenal.
    C. postrenal.
    D. uremic.

66. While suctioning an intubated and ventilated patient, the nurse notes that the ventilator alarm is malfunctioning. Which of these would be the most appropriate action for the nurse to take?

    A. Reset the ventilator alarm and monitor it closely for the next few hours.
    B. Notify the physician of the problem.
    C. Report the occurrence to the FDA.
    D. Contact the monitoring respiratory therapist to ensure the patient is safe and prepare to replace the ventilator, and report the occurrence to the appropriate department.

67. Which of these illustrate collaborative management for the critically ill patient with septic shock?

    A. Ambulate three times a day, withhold nutrition, and consult speech therapy.
    B. Consult physical therapy, reposition patient as tolerated, withhold nutrition.
    C. Administer enoxaparin sodium (Lovenox) for deep vein thrombosis prophylaxis, reposition patient as tolerated, administer nasoenteral feedings.
    D. Monitor vital signs once a shift, move out of bed to the chair, give regular diet.

68. The nurse is assigned to care for 4 patients. The nurse would **first** examine the patient with?

    A. cirrhosis without ascites.
    B. pancreatitis with ascites.
    C. a palpable right kidney.
    D. hepatitis and peripheral edema.

69. A 42-year-old patient is admitted to the ICU for the initiation and titration of Flolan (epoprostenol) for the treatment of pulmonary hypertension. A pulmonary artery catheter is placed, and the medication is initiated at the lowest dose possible. The best way to assess for response to this medication is to

    A. frequently assess pulmonary artery pressures.
    B. obtain daily transesophageal echocardiograms to assess for left ventricular function.
    C. obtain frequent arterial blood gas samples to assess for improvement in hypoxia.
    D. assess hourly urine output.

70. A patient on the unit has suffered frontal head injuries from an auto accident. Which type of impairment may result from injury to the frontal lobe?

    A. loss of sensation

    B. loss of vision

    C. alterations in hearing

    D. alterations in personality

71. A client with a recent bowel obstruction is prescribed all of these medications. Which medication should the nurse question?

    A. Celebrex

    B. Lortab

    C. Lipitor

    D. Caduet

72. When assessing a patient who has undergone coronary artery bypass grafting, which of these findings would indicate hypovolemic shock secondary to postoperative hemorrhage?

    A. low CO, low CVP, low BP, and increased heart rate

    B. low CO, normal CVP, low BP, and normal heart rate

    C. high CO, normal CVP, low BP, and increased heart rate

    D. high CO, low CVP, low BP, and normal heart rate

73. A 49-year-old female is admitted to the ICU with a diagnosis of massive pulmonary embolus. She is intubated, mechanically ventilated, and requiring vasopressors to support her blood pressure. The critical care nurse recognizes that one of the last treatment possibilities for this patient would include

    A. pressure control ventilation.

    B. addition of a second vasopressor.

    C. insertion of an intraaortic balloon pump.

    D. administration of fibrinolytics such as tPA.

74. A patient is diagnosed with a hypercoagulopathy disorder and is to begin therapy with warfarin (Coumadin) to prevent future blood clots; however, the patient is receiving IV heparin as well. The critical care nurse knows that the heparin infusion must be continued until

    A. the patient is discharged from the hospital.

    B. the patient is transferred out of the ICU.

    C. the patient has reached a therapeutic INR with warfarin.

    D. it is ordered to be discontinued.

75. Priority nursing care for a patient with an acute dissecting descending aortic aneurysm includes

    A. maintaining above-normal blood pressure.

    B. monitoring BUN and creatinine laboratory values.

    C. pain relief and blood pressure control.

    D. maintaining below-normal blood pressure.

76. A patient was in respiratory distress and found to have a pneumothorax. The patient fully recovered after a needle thoracostomy and chest tube placement. Repeat routine chest radiograph shows air in the mediastinum. Chest tube is functioning properly. Which of these is the correct course of action?

    A. Do nothing and simply observe.

    B. Remove the chest tube.

    C. Insert the chest tube further.

    D. Prepare to place the patient on BiPAP.

77. A patient with an inter-aortic balloon-pump is admitted to the cardiovascular intensive care unit. The charge nurse utilizes the Synergy Model by assigning which of these to care for him?

    A. the nurse with the most seniority on the unit

    B. the nurse with the most experience with inter-aortic balloon-pumps

    C. the new graduate, who will gain experience from this assignment

    D. the nurse who has the room next to this patient

78. A 23-year-old patient has a significant contusion to the right retroperitoneal region. Upon evaluation, the patient's vital signs are stable; however, he has severe tenderness in the right retroperitoneal region. The most likely initial radiology procedure the provider would order is

    A. abdominal CT scan.

    B. intravenous pyelogram (IVP).

    C. renal arteriogram.

    D. chest x-ray.

79. The patient's lactic acid level has risen from 2 mmol/L to 6 mmol/L 8 hours after admission. This finding likely indicates

    A. appropriate fluid resuscitation.

    B. the need to start total parenteral nutrition (TPN) immediately.

    C. inadequate tissue perfusion.

    D. the need to transfuse 20 units of cryoprecipitate immediately.

80. The nurse is asked to meet with a multidisciplinary team to update them about recent nursing assessments. The nursing characteristic expected of the nurse based on the Synergy Model is

    A. advocacy/morals.

    B. system thinking.

    C. caring practice.

    D. collaboration.

81. A patient is admitted to the ICU and is mechanically ventilated on volume control. The family is at the bedside and is curious as to what this means. Which of these statements correctly explains the nature of volume control ventilation?

    A. "The ventilator prevents the patient from taking in too much volume."

    B. "The ventilator controls the amount of tidal volume delivered to the patient in each breath."

    C. "The ventilator has a set volume to deliver in a day and will stop after this volume has been administered to allow the patient to breath on his own."

    D. "The patient controls the amount of tidal volume in each breath, but the ventilator controls the IPAP and EPAP."

82. The primary purpose of the cerebrospinal fluid (CSF) is to

    A. transport oxygen to the brain.

    B. manufacture neurotransmitters.

    C. cushion the brain and spinal cord.

    D. maintain cerebral perfusion pressures.

83. A 65-year-old patient has been in the ICU for nearly two weeks for pneumonia and sepsis. History includes CHF, hypertension, diabetes, and chronic renal failure for which she is dependent on dialysis. Suddenly the patient becomes tachypneic, hypoxic, and tachycardic. A pulmonary embolus is suspected. The critical care nurse expects the patient to undergo which of these diagnostic tests given the patient's history?

    A. spiral CT scan with contrast

    B. D-dimer

    C. chest x-ray

    D. ventilation/perfusion scan

84. A 79-year-old patient is admitted to the ICU with a diagnosis of congestive heart failure (CHF). During routine care, the critical care nurse notices a swollen and reddened right calf. Ultrasound confirms the presence of a large DVT in that area. Which of these treatments would prevent this DVT from traveling to the lungs and causing a pulmonary embolus?

    A. IV heparin infusion

    B. massaging the area of the DVT

    C. placement of an IVC filter (Greenfield filter)

    D. initiation of warfarin (Coumadin) therapy

85. Which statement best describes an arterial occlusive problem?

A. Affected limb is pink, warm, painful, and it has a pulse.

B. Affected limb is white, cold, painful, and pulseless.

C. Affected limb is cyanotic, cool, edema, and pulseless.

D. Affected limb is white, cool, edema, and it has a pulse.

86. A narrow pulse pressure and pulsus alternans are commonly associated with which type of cardiomyopathy?

A. hypertrophic

B. dilated

C. restrictive

D. idiopathic

87. The patient asks the nurse what a Billroth II procedure involves. The best answer by the nurse is that there will be

A. a partial removal of part of the large intestine.

B. a complete excision of the stomach.

C. an anastomosis of the gastric remnant to the jejunum.

D. the creation of a rectangular stomach flap.

88. The parietal lobe is responsible for which function?

A. hearing

B. sensory integration

C. motor function

D. vision

89. In a patient who has a pituitary tumor, the nurse would **not** expect to see stimulation or inhibition of the secretion of which of these?

A. growth hormone

B. corticotropin

C. aldosterone

D. prolactin

90. A 72-year-old female is admitted to the ICU with a diagnosis of congestive heart failure (CHF) exacerbation. She is hypoxic and hypertensive and has increased work of breathing. Her chest x-ray reveals severe pulmonary edema. The critical care nurse should question which of these treatment orders?

A. IV diuretics

B. IV nitroglycerin

C. 1000 mL bolus of IV normal saline

D. IV morphine

91. For a patient who has an intraaortic balloon pump, which of these findings requires immediate nursing intervention?

A. 150 mm Hg pressurized heparin (1,000 U/500 mL NS) bag connected to arterial pressure line

B. low helium alarm warning

C. similar aortic and arterial blood pressure readings

D. loss of left arm distal pulses, chest discomfort, or low urine output

92. When the initial insult is a result of damaged tissues or trauma, which coagulation pathway is stimulated or initiated?

    A. intrinsic pathway

    B. extrinsic pathway

    C. hypercoagulability

    D. erythropoietin mechanism

93. In the polyuric stage of acute tubular necrosis (ATN), what are the most important nursing considerations?

    A. restricting fluid intake, monitoring electrolyte levels

    B. monitoring for fluid depletion and electrolyte levels

    C. administering hypertonic solution

    D. administering diuretic therapy

94. Which of these findings is more indicative of hypoglycemia than of hyperglycemia?

    A. altered mental status

    B. rapid breathing

    C. warm skin

    D. tachycardia

95. A 62-year-old male who has recently had valve replacement and been discharged on Coumadin presents to the emergency department with hematuria. His INR is 2.1, Hgb is 9.5, and Hct 29%. What would be the initial course of treatment?

    A. FFP infusion

    B. cryoprecipitate infusion

    C. platelet infusion

    D. administration of vitamin K

96. System thinking includes a body of knowledge and the tools that help nurses manage environmental and system resources that exist for which of these?

    A. staff

    B. patients

    C. families

    D. all the above

97. A patient with pancreatitis calls the nurse to report trouble breathing, and his pulse oximetry shows a saturation of 89 percent. What action should receive priority?

    A. Assess blood pressure.

    B. Check oxygen saturation levels.

    C. Administer oxygen.

    D. Give the prescribed medication for pain.

98. The nurse cares for a client with acute respiratory distress syndrome (ARDS) who has a PaO_2/FiO_2 of less than 95 mm Hg. Which statement best describes the client's ARDS?

    A. mild ARDS

    B. moderate ARDS

    C. severe ARDS

    D. end-stage ARDS

99. The most common cause today of chronic renal failure is

    A. poorly controlled diabetes.

    B. sepsis.

    C. glomerulonephritis.

    D. renal vein thrombosis.

100. A stroke in which area of the brain would cause aphasia?

A. left hemisphere

B. right hemisphere

C. pons

D. cerebellum

101. A 36-year-old female is seen to the Emergency Department. The patient and her family do not speak English and are unable to communicate with the health care team. Which of these methods would be most effective when coordinating care with the family of this patient?

A. Use a translation service.

B. Have a bilingual family member translate.

C. Use ancillary staff for explanations.

D. Use a communication board.

102. Which of these should the nurse expect to find in a patient with decorticate posture?

A. flexion of both upper and lower extremities

B. flexion of elbows, extension of the knees, and plantar flexion of the feet

C. extension of upper extremities and flexion of lower extremities

D. extension of elbows and knees, plantar flexion of feet, and flexion of the wrists

103. Which of these manifestations, if identified in a patient who has suffered a myocardial infarction, should a nurse associate with the development of a papillary muscle rupture?

A. abrupt onset of shortness of breath and no neck vein distension

B. abrupt onset of chest pain and holosystolic murmur

C. abrupt onset of shortness of breath and acute neck vein distention

D. abrupt onset of chest pain and no murmur or neck vein distension

104. Which of these findings is indicative of diabetes insipidus (DI)?

A. serum sodium of 160 mEq/L

B. serum osmolality of 284 mOsm/L

C. central venous pressure (CVP) of 10 mm Hg

D. urine specific gravity of 1.032

105. When caring for a patient with acute respiratory distress syndrome (ARDS), the critical care nurse recognizes the importance of which of these ventilator parameters?

A. pressure support

B. FiO_2

C. PEEP (positive end expiratory pressure)

D. pressure control

106. The renin-angiotensin-aldosterone cascade is initiated by

A. hyponatremia.

B. fall in mean arterial pressure/renal artery hypotension.

C. fluid retention/overload.

D. elevated BUN/creatinine.

107. An elderly patient is admitted to the ICU from the emergency department with a diagnosis of severe community-acquired pneumonia. The critical care nurse knows that community-acquired pneumonia in the elderly often results from exposure to

    A. *Legionella* species.

    B. *Streptococcus* species.

    C. any one of a number of organisms.

    D. none of the above.

108. A 63-year-old patient is recovering from a Whipple procedure and the abdominal wound is healing by secondary intention. Wound care is complex, and the son is having difficulty successfully demonstrating the skill. Which intervention would be the most appropriate next step for the nurse?

    A. Provide written step-by-step instructions for the son.

    B. Eliminate dressing changes from the skills the son must perform.

    C. Provide coaching and the opportunities to repeat the skill.

    D. Consult the wound care specialist.

109. A 55-year-old patient in the ICU has been admitted for potential organ rejection after a recent kidney transplant. What is the most likely manifestation the patient would demonstrate?

    A. increased urine output

    B. decreased BUN/creatinine

    C. elevated creatinine

    D. elevated platelet count

110. The patient presents the following signs and symptoms—temperature 102.6 °F, heart rate 136, blood pressure 90/50, urine output of 40 mL over the last hour, white blood cell count 10,000, and negative urine, sputum, and blood cultures. You suspect the patient has

    A. cardiogenic shock.

    B. septic shock.

    C. multiple organ dysfunction syndrome (MODS).

    D. systemic inflammatory response syndrome (SIRS).

111. A patient who has narrow QRS supraventricular tachycardia with heart rate of 188 and hypotension may require

    A. cardioversion.

    B. defibrillation.

    C. pacing.

    D. automatic implantable cardioverter defibrillator (AICD).

112. A patient with acute metabolic acidosis would present with which of these arterial blood gases results?

    A. pH 7.55, pCO_2 32, pO_2 75, HCO_3^- 24

    B. pH 7.50, pCO_2 45, pO_2 73, HCO_3^- 30

    C. pH 7.30, pCO_2 55, pO_2 67, HCO_3^- 28

    D. pH 7.31, pCO_2 40, pO_2 75, HCO_3^- 14

113. Which of these groups of patient data support the diagnosis of multiple organ dysfunction syndrome (MODS)?

    A. urine output of 30 mL/hr, blood urea nitrogen (BUN) of 18 mg/dL, and white blood cell count (WBC) or 5,120 white blood cells/mcL

    B. upper GI bleeding, a Glasgow coma score (GCS) of 15, and a hematocrit (Hct) of 25%

    C. a total bilirubin of 15 mg/dL, a serum creatinine of 8 mg/dL, and a platelet count of 2,300 mm^3

    D. a respiratory rate of 45/minute, a $PaCO_2$ of 60 mm Hg, and a chest x-ray with diffuse bilateral infiltrates

114. A 25-year-old male is admitted to the ICU after sustaining multiple severe injuries in a motorcycle crash. He underwent 12 hours of surgery and arrives at the ICU intubated and mechanically ventilated, with multiple blood products transfusing. The critical care nurse should be aware of what "deadly cascade" of early complications related to the critically injured trauma patient?

    A. alkalosis, hypertension, decreased GI motility

    B. acidosis, hypothermia, coagulopathy

    C. hypotension, dysrhythmias, pulmonary edema

    D. hemorrhage, infection, altered skin integrity

115. Which of these is a serious conduction defect that occurs when the left bundle branch is blocked, causing a widening of the QRS complex on a 12-lead ECG?

    A. PVC

    B. hemiblock

    C. Wolfe-Parkinson-White

    D. endocarditis

116. Optimal outcomes for patients are achieved when which of these occurs?

    A. Patients and nurses are in active partnerships.

    B. Nurses are in complete control of the patient needs.

    C. Nurses and physicians work together to complete patient care.

    D. Patient and families control their own plan of care.

117. When caring for a patient with receptive dysphasia, which of these interventions is most appropriate?

    A. talking in a loud voice so that the patient can hear you

    B. correcting the client for every miscommunicated word

    C. avoiding conversation since the patient does not understand

    D. using gestures while talking to the patient

118. A patient with a BP of 96/66 mm Hg took a sublingual 0.04 mg nitroglycerin tablet five minutes ago and continues to experience chest pain. Which of these actions should a nurse take next?

    A. Take the patient's blood pressure.

    B. Give another dose of nitroglycerin.

    C. Check the patient's ECG rhythm.

    D. Advise the patient to lie down with legs elevated.

119. A patient's family expresses concern regarding the meaning of numbers on the patient's monitor and asks the nurse for clarification. Which of these is the most appropriate response for the nurse to give?

    A. "The numbers tell us when the patient is having problems."

    B. "Which numbers on the monitor concern you?"

    C. "The numbers help us determine the best treatment."

    D. "What don't you understand about the monitor?"

120. Which is the primary responsibility of the nurse when preparing a patient for bowel resection and placement of an ostomy?

    A. Maintain the patient NPO the day prior to surgery.

    B. Administer oral medication on the morning of surgery.

    C. Give antibiotics prior to surgery.

    D. Insert a nasogastric tube.

121. A patient is admitted to the ICU after experiencing a seizure while visiting a family member in another part of the hospital. The patient was initially treated with Ativan (lorazepam) and is now to receive "1 gram of Dilantin (phenytoin) IV push." The critical care nurse questions this order because she knows that giving this medication rapidly causes which of these reactions?

    A. hypotension and bradycardia

    B. phlebitis and tachycardia

    C. diarrhea and unequal pupillary reactions

    D. hives and bronchoconstriction

122. The critical care nurse is caring for a patient who is admitted to the ICU with a diagnosis of severe alcohol intoxication. The patient is very lethargic and has vomited multiple times. The critical care nurse identifies this patient is at highest risk for

    A. community-acquired pneumonia.

    B. hospital-acquired pneumonia.

    C. aspiration pneumonia.

    D. alcohol withdrawal symptoms.

123. Before administering nesiritide (brand name: Natrecor) to a patient who has congestive heart failure, which of these should the nurse check?

    A. blood pressure

    B. cardiac output

    C. heart rate

    D. electrocardiogram

124. A patient is admitted to the ICU after experiencing a traumatic brain injury. In order to prevent complications from "secondary injury" in the early critical care phase, the nurse should focus the care to prevent

    A. infection, hypertension, and skin breakdown.

    B. diuresis, electrolyte imbalances, and acidosis.

    C. hypotension, hypoxia, and increased intracranial pressure.

    D. coagulopathy, malnutrition, and agitation.

125. A cardiac surgeon has complained that most of the nurses in the ICU do not know how to care for a temporary pacemaker and wants to designate certain nurses to care for the patients. Several of the nurses in the unit have formed a task force to evaluate the problem and develop a workable solution. Which of these is the best first step for the nurses to take to resolve this problem?

    A. Refer the surgeon to the administrative manager to resolve the issue.

    B. Set up mandatory pacemaker in-services for all of the unit nurses.

    C. Include pacemaker care as part of the annual competency review.

    D. Meet with the surgeon to discuss his specific concerns.

126. A patient with gallbladder disease may experience increased pain after a meal of

    A. noodles and broth.

    B. baked chicken and rice.

    C. pizza.

    D. lean beef and vegetables.

127. A patient with a two-week history of progressive lower-extremity weakness is admitted to the ICU for possible Guillain-Barré syndrome. The critical care nurse should monitor the patient closely for which of these potential complications?

    A. skin breakdown

    B. suicidal ideation

    C. urinary tract infection

    D. respiratory depression

128. The appropriate blood component that should be administered for thrombocytopenia is

    A. whole blood.

    B. fresh frozen plasma.

    C. platelets.

    D. RBCs.

129. The patient has a Glasgow Coma Score (GCS) of 5 two weeks after sustaining a head injury. The patient is currently not being sedated. You interpret the GCS score as

    A. not an appropriate measure of neurologic function in a head-injured patient.

    B. a devastating traumatic brain injury.

    C. an injury that will not leave the patient with any limitations.

    D. brain death.

130. The nurse is planning diabetic teaching with a patient who is visually impaired. Which of these strategies would be most useful for this patient?

A. Eliminate use of the food models during the meal planning session.

B. Provide a simplified description of the complete diabetes teaching program.

C. Provide verbal descriptions of diabetes care to the patient.

D. Show an educational videotape to the patient's family.

131. An elderly female is admitted to the surgical floor for recovery from a total hip replacement. On postoperative day four, she develops fever and dyspnea. Chest x-ray reveals bilateral lower lobe infiltrates. The patient is transferred to the ICU, and the critical care nurse expects treatment to be initiated for which of these conditions?

A. hospital-acquired pneumonia

B. aspiration pneumonia

C. pulmonary embolus

D. congestive heart failure

132. Examples of prerenal conditions that may lead to renal failure would **not** include

A. dehydration.

B. hypovolemia.

C. hemorrhage/blood loss.

D. ureter obstruction.

133. The experienced critical care nurse is precepting a novice ICU nurse in caring for a patient with a COPD exacerbation. When discussing causes of COPD and risk factors, the experienced nurse explains that

A. COPD is caused by one condition and has only one treatment.

B. COPD exacerbations are frequently fatal.

C. COPD has many causes and many different treatments.

D. COPD is treated in the same way as pneumonia and congestive heart failure.

134. A patient who has congestive heart failure is receiving nesiritide (brand name: Natrecor). Which of these responses should a nurse expect the patient to have if the medication is achieving the desired therapeutic effect?

A. increased SVR

B. decreased BNP level

C. increased contractility

D. decreased SVR

135. Your elderly ICU patient is at risk for developing shock. You know that cyanosis of which of these indicates decreased perfusion in an elderly patient?

A. sclera of the eyes

B. oral mucous membranes

C. skin of the forehead

D. nail beds of the fingers and toes

136. Which technique is recommended for eliciting a response to peripheral pain?

A. sternal rub

B. trapezius muscle squeeze

C. nail bed pressure

D. mandibular pressure

137. A 53-year-old male patient is admitted to the ED after three days of nausea and vomiting. Initial blood tests reveal the following: BUN 28.0, creatinine 1.0, K+ 5.9, and Hct 58.0. The patient is alert and oriented and has been only able to drink small quantities of fluids over the last two days. The findings indicate that the patient is showing evidence of

    A. acute renal failure.

    B. chronic renal failure.

    C. dehydration.

    D. acute tubular necrosis.

138. Which of these lab results should be most concerning to the nurse caring for a patient with liver disease receiving possible hepatotoxic drugs?

    A. AST 28 units/L

    B. ALT 32 units/L

    C. ALT 50 units/L

    D. AST 10 units/L

139. The American Association of Critical-Care Nurses (AACN) developed the certification program for which of these reasons?

    A. to increase the likelihood that critical care nurses would receive pay raises

    B. to educate and test on issues involving critical care patients

    C. to develop, maintain, and promote high standards for critical care nursing practice

    D. to maintain records on critical nurses across the nation for database information

140. The primary precursor for all blood cells is the

    A. megakaryocyte.

    B. reticulocyte.

    C. pluripotential stem cell.

    D. granulocyte.

141. The adult daughter of a mechanically ventilated patient has agreed to learn how to suction her mother. What is the first task that the nurse must do when developing a teaching plan?

    A. Obtain written information about the procedure.

    B. Determine a schedule for demonstrating the procedure.

    C. Assess the knowledge and skills the daughter needs to learn.

    D. Encourage the daughter to observe the procedure on other patients.

142. A patient is in the post-anesthesia care unit (PACU) after a femoral-popliteal bypass graft to the right leg. A heparin drip is currently running at 1,000 units per hour. The patient is awake and following commands and is scheduled to be transferred to the surgical unit. The nurse receives report from the laboratory that the patient's aPTT is 21 seconds. Which of these interventions is most appropriate?

    A. Adjust the heparin drip per standing orders.

    B. Contact the surgeon for heparin adjustment orders.

    C. Contact the laboratory for a STAT aPTT redraw.

    D. Assess the patient's right leg for signs of ischemia.

143. A patient has been given instructions about his automated implantable cardioverter defibrillator (AICD). Which of these statements, if made by the patient, would indicate that he needs further instruction?

    A. "I will have my device routinely checked to ensure its battery life."

    B. "I won't need to take Betapace [sotalol is the generic], since I have an AICD."

    C. "I will need to alert medical staff if I need an MRI exam."

    D. "I won't need hospitalization since I rarely receive electric shocks."

144. What model for patient care was adopted for use in the certification of critical care practice?

    A. Synergy

    B. Cyclic

    C. Nightingale

    D. Darwin

145. Based on Virginia Henderson's writings from 1960 adopted for the Synergy Model, critical care nurses are there for compromised patients and the more severe or complex the needs of the patient, the more the critical care nurse needs to do which of these?

    A. Assess more thoroughly.

    B. Obtain proficiency in multiple dimensions of care.

    C. Provide advocacy for the critical care patient.

    D. Involve family and friends in care.

146. In status epilepticus, seizure activity is best described as

    A. controlled.

    B. absent for at least one year.

    C. escalating in intensity.

    D. a rapid succession of tonic-clonic activity.

147. The four components of the Synergy Model do **not** include which of these?

    A. critical test results and values

    B. patient and family characteristics

    C. nurse competencies and characteristics

    D. patient outcomes

148. The critical care nurse receives a report on these four patients. Which patient should the nurse check first?

    A. the patient with gallbladder disease who exhibits Murphy's sign

    B. the patient with gastrointestinal reflux who has a positive Chvostek's sign

    C. the patient with hepatitis who has blood on rectal exam

    D. the patient with abdominal pain who has Grey-Turner's sign

149. A patient presents to the ICU after a penetrating trauma to the chest. The object is a tree branch and is still present. The patient appears to be relatively hemodynamically stable with BP 95/45 and heart rate 121. Which of these would be an appropriate course of action?

A. Remove the impaled object.

B. Do not remove the impaled object.

C. Attempt to trim the impaled branch so it does not appear to "sticking" out of the patient.

D. Remove the object and hold pressure for at least 45 minutes.

150. In the late stages of COPD, the right ventricle may start to fail as the pulmonary vascular resistance increases. The term for isolated right ventricular failure in the setting of COPD is

A. cor pulmonale.

B. pulmonary hypertension.

C. congestive heart failure.

D. jugular venous distension.

Practice Test Answers and Explanations

ANSWER KEY

1. A	26. D	51. C	76. A	101. A	126. C
2. D	27. B	52. A	77. B	102. B	127. D
3. D	28. D	53. A	78. A	103. C	128. C
4. B	29. D	54. A	79. C	104. A	129. B
5. B	30. C	55. B	80. D	105. C	130. C
6. D	31. A	56. A	81. B	106. B	131. A
7. C	32. A	57. A	82. C	107. C	132. D
8. A	33. A	58. D	83. D	108. C	133. C
9. C	34. A	59. D	84. C	109. C	134. D
10. D	35. D	60. A	85. B	110. D	135. B
11. D	36. A	61. B	86. B	111. A	136. C
12. D	37. B	62. D	87. C	112. D	137. C
13. A	38. B	63. C	88. B	113. C	138. C
14. B	39. D	64. C	89. C	114. B	139. C
15. C	40. C	65. D	90. C	115. B	140. C
16. C	41. B	66. D	91. D	116. A	141. C
17. B	42. B	67. C	92. B	117. D	142. A
18. A	43. A	68. B	93. B	118. B	143. B
19. B	44. C	69. A	94. A	119. B	144. A
20. A	45. D	70. D	95. D	120. C	145. B
21. B	46. D	71. B	96. D	121. A	146. D
22. B	47. C	72. A	97. C	122. C	147. A
23. A	48. D	73. D	98. C	123. A	148. D
24. A	49. A	74. C	99. A	124. C	149. B
25. B	50. C	75. C	100. A	125. D	150. A

1. A

Patient education for heart failure is now focused on the patient's ejection fraction. While cholesterol panels remain important, new research from AHA and research centers such as the Cleveland Clinic Kaufman Center for Heart Failure has shown that treating heart failure from the aspect of the patient's ejection fraction has better outcomes than previous clinical pathways. A normal ejection fraction is 50–75 percent or greater and an indirect measurement of contractility. Cardiac output is not as specific as a cardiac index. Coronary atherosclerosis is not a measure for monitoring this condition.

2. D

The patient's respiratory status is worsening, and he is not able to comply with face mask with supplemental oxygen. The patient needs to be intubated immediately. There is no time to wait to see if he passes a trial of NPPV. Answers (A) and (B) are both NPPV. These should only be used in stable clinical situations, not with patients with worsening respiratory distress and/or increasing hypoxemia. Choice (C) is clearly wrong, because sedation will suppress respiratory drive and likely mandate intubation if it is not warranted earlier.

3. D

Compartment syndrome is caused by an increased pressure within a confined compartment related to swelling or bleeding. Compartment syndrome is a potential threat following any endovascular procedure due to multiple vascular puncture sites. When pressure is elevated in a compartment, nerve damage and extremity girth is present. A neurovascular assessment will reveal compartment syndrome. A neurovascular assessment consists of monitoring for the 5 Ps: pain, pallor, pulse, paresthesia, and paralysis. Performing a neurological exam is the assessment of level of consciousness (LOC), motor, and sensory function. The pathophysiology of compart-

ment syndrome includes a compromised capillary blood flow and elevated interstitial fluid pressure; however, a nurse has no means of determining these conditions.

4. B

One of the most common and easily corrected causes of hypoxia in hospitalized patients is pneumonia, and hypoxia should be suspected in any patient who becomes agitated. Answer (A) is possible but not a common cause of agitation. Answer (C) is possible, especially in the postictal period; however, there is no mention of a seizure disorder in the question. Answer (D) is incorrect because patients with acute CVA rarely present with agitation, as they often have focal neurologic deficits such as facial droop and hemiparesis.

5. B

Bipolar disorder is distinguished by periods of mania, in which a person experiences extreme "highs," followed by periods of depression, or equally extreme "lows." This patient is in a manic state, in which symptoms such as erratic speech, increased sexuality, grandiosity, decreased need for sleep, and increased energy are common.

6. D

Ischemic stroke results from low cerebral blood flow, usually due to occlusion of a blood vessel by clots, plaque, etc. Transient ischemic attacks (TIA) are reversible and last less than 24 hours, sometimes only minutes. Etiologies of TIA can include arteritis, thrombus emboli, arterial dissection, drugs (e.g., cocaine), stenosis due to atherosclerosis, etc. Hemorrhagic stroke is bleeding into brain tissue. Myocardial infarction is the interruption of coronary perfusion to the heart muscle.

7. C

The use of SCDs, Ted hose, and LMWH (e.g., Lovenox) can be used for the direct prevention of deep vein thromboses. It is true that a pulmonary embolus may originate from a DVT and that the use of the above measures decreases the incidence of PE, but this is secondary to its prevention of DVTs. Myocardial infarctions and COPD exacerbations have no connection with the use of the above measures.

8. A

The CAGE questionnaire is the most practical screening tool used in situations of suspected substance dependence. CAGE is a mnemonic for a questionnaire that asks about attempts to cut down on substance use, annoyance with criticisms, guilt about substance use, and using the preferred substance as an eye opener. Although originally developed for suspicion of alcohol abuse, any substance may be referred to within the questions, making it a simple, concise, and effective screening tool. The CAGE questionnaire is thought to be 60 percent to 90 percent effective when the responses to two or more questions are positive. None of the other choices directly assesses potential for substance abuse.

9. C

Adding humidification to supplemental oxygen serves to keep the respiratory tract moist and prevents secretions from becoming dry and difficult to expectorate. Answer (A) is incorrect because inhaled bronchodilators are used in reactive airway disease and are not helpful to assist with clearing of secretions related to pneumonia. Answer (B) is incorrect because antifungal agents are rarely indicated in community-acquired pneumonia and are not helpful in clearing secretions. Answer (D) is incorrect because there is no indication that reintubation is needed, and patients should not be reintubated simply to assist clearing of secretions.

10. D

Patients feel safe when nurses exhibit technical competence and meet their needs. Not allowing family to stay at the bedside, asking the charge nurse for help with decision making, and talking about your after-work plans does not demonstrate competence or create synergy with the patient or her family.

11. D

Autonomic hyperactivity, increased hand tremors, insomnia, and nausea are the earliest signs of alcohol withdrawal. Although vomiting, visual hallucinations, delirious behavior, and possible violent behavior may occur during acute alcohol withdrawal, these symptoms occur later in the progression.

12. D

Carbon monoxide poisoning causes falsely elevated pulse oximetry values, which may lead to under-utilization of oxygen therapy unless recognized. Answer (A) is incorrect because this value measures the degree of carbon monoxide poisoning. Answers (B) and (C) are incorrect because carbon monoxide poisoning does not falsely change these values.

13. A

In overwhelming infections, the body uses of all its available resources to respond to the process. In the event that it is sustained over a long period of time, the availability of leukocytes may be significantly reduced, as the body may not be able to mobilize them quickly enough. As a person ages, the ability to produce and respond to stimulus decreases as well. Answer (B) is incorrect—this scenario would absolutely need to have the immune system stimulated. The bone marrow responds to stimulus from those mechanisms to increase production and release of WBCs. In this case, there would be a need to increase release. Answer (D) is an inaccurate statement.

14. B

When family members are confused, they may not trust the nurse's decisions, or they may feel powerless to help their family member. The nurse needs to advocate for the patient by assessing the family members, empowering them to let their needs be known, and assisting them to resolve any ethical issues. Choices (A), (C), and (D) do not indicate any ethical issues.

15. C

Metoprolol blocks stimulation of beta$_1$ (myocardial) adrenergic receptors. Major side effects associated with beta-blockers are hypotension and bradycardia. Hypersensitivity reactions are not associated with metoprolol.

16. C

According to the ethical decision-making process, decisions should be made based on the patient's wishes (autonomy). Wishes of the staff or a court would interfere with the patient's autonomy. The family's wishes, while important, are not the primary factor when seeking an answer to an ethical dilemma.

17. B

The kidneys filter 180 liters of blood each day. (A) is inaccurate: No organs individually (not even heart or lungs) receive 40 percent of the cardiac output. (C) and (D) are too small. To accomplish this, approximately one-fourth of the cardiac output must go to the kidneys.

18. A

Bilirubin is a product of hemoglobin breakdown. The other choices are incorrect.

19. B

Leads V_1–V_2 view the septal region of the heart muscle. The septal wall receives its blood flow from the left anterior descending coronary artery.

ST-elevation in leads I and aVL reflects a high lateral wall infarction. ST-elevation present in leads II, III, and aVF reflects an inferior wall infarction. ST-elevation present in leads V2–V4 reflects an anterior wall infarction.

20. A

Epidural hematoma is usually caused by a blow to the head and is often associated with a skull fracture. The artery involved is the middle meningeal artery. The rough edges of the fracture or skull surface impinge on the blood vessels, causing bleeding that accumulates between the skull and the dura mater. Intracerebral hemorrhage is bleeding into the brain tissue. Subarachnoid hemorrhage is bleeding into subarachnoid space, usually from a ruptured aneurysm. Subdural hematoma is usually caused by venous bleeding of bridging veins that occurs below the dura mater.

21. B

The quickest and easiest imaging study to order in an emergent situation is a CT with IV contrast. Although pulmonary angiography is the gold standard, it will not be obtained in time to obtain a diagnosis. A V/Q perfusion scan is useful but it is not immediately available. Further more, the V/Q results are reported vaguely as high, moderate, or low probability—making the usefulness of the results marginal as a first-line study. Finally, without contrast, the pulmonary vessels will not be visualized.

22. B

Although the other answers are components of patient characteristics, resiliency is the ability of the patient to bounce back from psychological and physical stressors influenced by multiple factors.

23. A

Communication between the hypothalamus and the anterior pituitary occurs via a network of capillary vessels, referred to as portal circulation. The connection with the posterior pituitary is via nerves.

24. A

The FACES scale can be used by simply having the patient point to the appropriate face. Because of this, it is the easiest to use with children, people with language barriers, and intubated patients. The PQRST method, the pain intensity scale, and the Jacox scale all require verbalization and/or writing to communicate pain level.

25. B

Response to diversity is a nurse characteristic. (A) resiliency, (C) complexity, and (D) stability are patient characteristics.

26. D

Pericarditis is characterized by global ST elevation due to abnormal repolarization secondary to pericardial inflammation. Pericarditis is often mistaken for an inferior wall MI. However, there is no reciprocal ST depression found with pericarditis.

27. B

Resiliency is the capacity to return to a functioning state using compensatory or coping mechanisms. At the minimal level, the patient is unable to respond, has coping failure and minimal reserves, and is brittle. At the moderate level, the patient has moderate response, begins coping, and has moderate reserves. At the high level of resiliency, the patient responds with and maintains and displays intact coping responses, strong reserves, and high endurance. All the other choices are inaccurate descriptors of resiliency.

28. D

This patient is vulnerable and susceptible to potential stressors that could negatively affect her outcome. The best response is to ensure that patient and family needs are met in a caring environment. Answers (A), (B), and (C) do not consider the patient characteristics according to the Synergy Model.

29. D

The other three answers are patient characteristics, while what was defined in the question is the definition of vulnerability.

30. C

To calculate the cerebral perfusion pressure, the nurse subtracts the ICP from the MAP. Subtracting the MAP from the ICP will give a negative number. Adding or multiplying the numbers would give inappropriate results.

31. A

The patient has a neurological condition that may impair her gag reflex and ability to swallow. Hence, the patient is at risk for aspiration. Results of the tracheal aspirate are consistent with this diagnosis of aspiration pneumonia. As a result, the antibiotic coverage will likely include anaerobic organisms. The patient was just admitted to the hospital and does not meet the timeline criteria for nosocomial pneumonia. Although CAP is possible, the clinical situation highly suggests aspiration pneumonia, especially given the tracheal aspirate. COPD is not mentioned in the case, so there is no reason to suspect it.

32. A

Hyperkalemia decreases the rate of ventricular depolarization, shortens repolarization, and depresses AV conduction. Therefore, the ECG changes associated with these phenomena are those in (A). Prolonged QT segment is commonly due to drug effects such as quinidine or other electrolyte disturbances. Hypokalemia causes the ECG changes that are specified in (C). There are many causes of tachycardia (e.g., fever, stress, etc.) and ventricular irritability such as ischemia, hypokalemia, etc.

33. A

A moral dilemma is a choice between alternatives that can be justified by moral rules or principles. Answers (B), (C), and (D) are either illegal or immoral.

34. A

The most common symptoms of SIADH include personality changes, headache, decreased mentation, lethargy, nausea, vomiting, diminished DTRs, seizures, and coma. These are attributed to the electrolyte disturbances associated with SIADH. Choices (B), (C), and (D) are more likely to be seen in diabetes insipidus (DI).

35. D

Following the rules outlined in chapter 6, the pH is less than normal. This eliminates choices (A) and (C), because we know the patient is acidotic. Next, the $PaCO_2$ is greater than 45 mm Hg; hence, we know that this is a respiratory acidosis. Finally, the HCO_3^- is within the normal range, so there is no combined disorder or compensation yet. This is consistent with the short-term/acute nature of the occurrence (immediately post-op).

36. A

The major side effects associated with the medication fenoldopam are the following: headache, reflex tachycardia, and hypokalemia. The other side effects listed are not associated with fenoldopam infusion. It should be noted that nitroprusside is considered the "gold standard" medication in the treatment of hypertensive crisis. Nitroprusside itself causes cyanide toxicity (blurred vision, confusion, tinnitus, and seizures); therefore, thiosulfate is added to these infusions. Thiosulfate converts cyanide into thiocyanate, which is then excreted in the urine.

37. B

Methemoglobinemia often results from receiving topical anesthetics or nitrates, and it alters the oxgen-carrying capacity of the hemoglobin molecules. Hallmark signs of the condition include hypoxia that does not respond to oxygen therapy and a "chocolate" brown discoloration of the blood. Answer (A) is incorrect because there is no mention of exposure to carbon monoxide and the signs/symptoms do not match. Answer (C) is incorrect because pulmonary embolus does not cause a brown discoloration of the blood. Answer (D) is incorrect because this is not a normal reaction to receiving benzocaine.

38. B

Fever may indicate that the intestinal obstruction has progressed to necrotic bowel, sepsis, and/or perforation. Vomiting, constipation and sweating are expected with patients having an intestinal obstruction.

39. D

Twisting of a nipple is a peripheral pain stimulus, not a central pain stimulus. Answers (A), (B), and (C) are appropriate methods of administering a central painful stimulus.

40. C

This patient is highly complex with impaired resources and decreased ability to participate in self-care. The nurse uses system thinking and collaboration by contacting case management or social work for evaluation of the couple's situation. Answers (A) and (B) are not appropriate for meeting the patient's stated needs. Answer (D) is not an appropriate use of nursing time or skills, and case management or social work is better prepared to assist the patient.

41. B

The kidneys are the main organ for the synthesis of erythropoietin. Only about 10 percent of the erythropoietin is manufactured in the liver. Bone marrow is the site of RBC production but not erythropoietin. Lungs play no role in the production of either erythropoietin or RBCs.

42. B

SIRS is widespread inflammation with accompanying tachycardia, fever, and sometimes hypothermia. When it is accompanied by documented infection, it is called sepsis.

43. A

Predictability is a patient characteristic that allows one to expect a certain course of events or course of illness. With the high risk of morbidity/mortality involved in oat cell carcinoma, this would be the correct choice.

44. C

The patient is demonstrating paradoxical chest wall movement after trauma. It is highly likely that he has multiple rib fractures in multiple places and has compromised the connection of the chest wall with the pleura. Hence, the chest wall is "sucked" into the thorax with the air when there is negative pressure generated by the intact chest wall. With pulmonary hemorrhage you would expect hemoptysis. Pneumothorax would be diagnosed by chest radiograph and an absence of breath sounds. There was no mention of the heart rhythm being irregularly irregular; hence, atrial fibrillation is wrong.

45. D

Treatment of SIADH includes fluid restriction, administration of 3 percent saline, administration of Lasix, and potassium supplements as needed.

46. D

The nurse addresses the situation by indicating that the coworker does not understand the meaning of the request. Using caring practices, moral advocacy, responses to diversity, and clinical inquiry, the nurse works on behalf of the patient's family. She can also act as a facilitator of learning by educating the coworker regarding specific cultural issues. Answers (A), (B), and (C) are inappropriate responses to the coworker's concerns.

47. C

Using the Parkland Formula, 4 mL × %TBSA × weight in kg, one gets $4 \times 65 \times 40 = 10,400$ mL over 24 hours. Fifty percent of this infuses over the first 8 hours, and the rest is spread evenly over the next 16 hours. Half of 10,400 mL is 5,200 mL.

48. D

A patient with congestive heart failure has a high preload and afterload with a decreased cardiac output. The goal of treatment is to decrease both preload and afterload and increase cardiac output. Therefore, all other options are incorrect.

49. A

A sustained hypotensive episode greater than 40/hours will result in a decreased blood flow to the kidney and damage to the tubules. As tubules desecrate, renal damage occurs, and the ability to filter will decrease. Decreased urine output alone does not indicate injury to the kidneys. It may simply be the body's attempt to preserve water in a dehydrated state. Intermittent drops in mean blood pressure that are not sustained most likely will not cause ischemia, as the body responds with shifts in electrolytes or fluid to compensate. Systolic blood pressure alone is not a good indicator of ischemia, as the patient's normal BP may have a lower systolic BP.

50. C

The other choices do not warrant Haldol administration. Haldol is a first-generation antipsychotic. These medications are commonly prescribed to control the acutely psychotic, delirious, aggressive, violent, or confused patient. They are almost always given via the intramuscular route.

51. C

Antipsychotics elicit a sedative response within 15 to 30 minutes when administered intramuscularly.

52. A

The use of oral contraceptive medications is a known risk factor for the development of a deep vein thrombosis. The other medications listed—ASA, vitamin, and PPI—have not been found to increase the risk of a DVT.

53. A

Nuchal rigidity is a clinical manifestation of meningeal irritation in which rigidity of neck muscles limits movement of the neck, including preventing its flexion. Homan's sign is the dorsiflexion of the foot that elicits pain in posterior calf and is considered positive for DVT. Babinski's reflex indicates pyramidal tract damage, an alteration in the motor tracts of the brain. Flaccid paralysis is a clinical manifestation characterized by weakness or paralysis and reduced muscle tone without other obvious cause.

54. A

Partial thickness or second-degree burns are very painful, as the nerve endings are exposed when the dermis is burned off. Body image would not be the highest priority. Four days post-burn, airway maintenance and fluid volume management are not an issue in a patient with a burn to the hand.

55. B

Tachycardia in the setting of cardiac/coronary artery disease may induce myocardial ischemia. Answer (A) is incorrect because while leukocytosis is a side effect of steroid therapy, it will not compromise the patient's cardiac status. Answer (C) is incorrect because allergic reactions are not considered expected side effects of therapy. Answer (D) is incorrect because depressed respiratory drive due to oxygen therapy in COPD patients is more of a theoretical side effect than an actual one.

56. A

Choice (A) provides the correct steps in the determination of hepatojugular reflux. This assessment indicates right-sided heart failure.

57. A

Polyuria is the key symptom of DI, leading to dehydration or hypovolemia.

58. D

The patient is presenting with a COPD exacerbation. He should receive bronchodilator therapy via nebulizer or inhaler, steroids for airway inflammation, antibiotics, chest radiograph, and cultures prior to antibiotic administration for an infectious workup. The wrong answer choices are not complete.

59. D

Recognizing patterns and trends is consistent with the competent level of the novice to expert model. Answers (A), (B), and (C) are all novice-level clinical judgment expectations.

60. A

Patients who have experienced long bone fractures such as femur fractures are at high risk for developing a fat embolus, which can travel to the lungs and cause a pulmonary embolus. The patient's symptoms suggest a pulmonary embolus. Answer (B) is partially correct; however, it is not likely that this patient's symptoms are from a DVT. Answer (C) is incorrect because the patient is not displaying signs/symptoms of myocardial infarction. Answer (D) is incorrect because these signs/symptoms are not normal responses to immobility due to femur fractures.

61. B

Sleeping at the bedside is a coping mechanism when families feel powerless. Answers (A), (C), and (D) are methods of avoiding a situation where families feel helpless and powerless.

62. D

The "syndrome" that accompanies the signs of pericarditis include fever, chest pain, presence of pericardial friction rub, diffused ST elevation, and the potential for pericardial effusion, which may cause pericardial tamponade.

63. C

Cerebrospinal fluid is reabsorbed by the arachnoid villi and drains into the venous sinuses. The lateral ventricle is where the CSF circulates. The dura mater is the fibrous membrane that lines the interior of the skull. The subarachnoid cisterns are expanded areas of the subarachnoid space.

64. C

This nurse is exhibiting all the characteristics of the expert clinical judgment level.

65. D

Uremic syndrome is a condition that results from renal failure when the patient continues to ingest water and inappropriate food intake (e.g., high in salt), and impairment of renal failure is extensive. The three categories of acute renal failure are prerenal, intrarenal, and postrenal. Therefore, the answer is (D), which is not a category of renal failure but a stage of ATN.

66. D

The nurse is using systems thinking and collaboration by making sure that the patient is safe and by working with the appropriate department to ensure that equipment is functioning properly. In choice (A), resetting a malfunctioning alarm does not solve the problem and puts patient safety at risk. Choices (B) and (C) are incorrect, since the physician cannot repair equipment and the FDA takes reports but does not repair or replace malfunctioning equipment.

67. C

Critically ill patients need DVT prophylaxis; to prevent skin breakdown they must be repositioned as tolerated, and feeding through a nasoenteral tube is usually well tolerated. Speech therapy is needed after the patient is extubated to evaluate swallowing, nutrition is an integral part of treatment in septic patients, and vital signs need to be monitored much more frequently than each shift. Physical therapy could be consulted to provide passive range of motion exercises.

68. B

Ascites may cause dyspnea and respiratory depression. All the other choices are to be expected and not potentially life threatening.

69. A

The medication Flolan (epoprostenol) dilates pulmonary arteries and is used to reduce the pulmonary artery pressures and often requires ICU observation until a stable dose has been reached. Answer (B) is incorrect because daily transesophageal echocardiograms are not indicated for patients with pulmonary hypertension and will not allow true measurement of pulmonary artery pressures. Answer (C) is incorrect because the degree of hypoxia is not always related to the actual pulmonary artery pressures and Flolan is not titrated according to ABG results. Answer (D) is incorrect because hourly urine output is not useful for the titration of Flolan.

70. D

Functions of the frontal lobe include thought, reasoning, behavior, memory, smell, and movement. Hearing and sensation are functions of the parietal lobe. Vision is processed in the occipital lobe.

71. B

Lortab (acetaminophen and hydrocodone) is an opioid and may cause decreased gastric motility. All the other choices are permissible.

72. A

A patient in hemorrhagic shock will experience hypotension, since there is less circulating blood volume resulting from blood loss. Less circulating blood causes a low central venous pressure (CVP). A rapid loss of blood volume leads to sympathetic compensation by peripheral constriction, tachycardia, and increased myocardial contractility. A low cardiac output and blood pressure with a normal heart rate do not indicate compensation. A normal cardiac output with a low blood pressure is indicative of septic shock.

73. D

Patients with massive pulmonary embolus with hemodynamic instability are candidates for fibrinolytics unless there are contraindications. Answer (A) would not help the patient because pressure control ventilation is used primarily for ARDS and other lung tissue problems. Answer (B) is incorrect because the addition of a second vasopressor will not correct the underlying problem. Answer (C) is incorrect because an IABP will not correct the underlying problem.

74. C

At the beginning of warfarin therapy, the anticoagulant effects are not immediate. Therefore, another form of anticoagulant must be used as a "bridge." The critical care nurse should be aware of this and incorporate it in the patient's plan of care. Answer (A) is incorrect because the heparin infusion may not be needed up until discharge. Answer (B) is incorrect because the patient's plan of care must continue regardless of her location. Answer (D) is incorrect because this answer does not reflect critical care nursing knowledge and collaboration needed for the CCRN.

75. C

An aortic dissection is a tear in the wall of the aorta that causes blood flow among the layers of the arterial wall (intima, media, and tunica adventitia) and forces the layers apart. A false lumen is created. Some organs are perfused by the true lumen, and others are perfused by the false lumen. Hypertension is not only the cause of this condition, but it also contributes to further tearing. Rupture and massive blood loss can occur if the tear occurs through all layers of the aorta. For this reason, the top priority for a patient suffering from this condition is blood pressure control. Distal circulation and absence of neurologic symptoms are other real concerns. Thus, (A) and (D) are incorrect. While it is important to monitor renal laboratory values to ascertain kidney perfusion, it is not a top nursing priority of care.

76. A

Pneumomediastinum is what the patient currently has and is not an emergency. She likely developed air in this space when she suffered the pneumothorax, although you cannot be sure. Either way, she is hemodynamically stable, and the air collection in the mediastinum in this scenario is benign. Inserting the chest tube further or removing it may compromise the patient's status. Again, the patient is stable and not in respiratory distress, so she does not need BiPAP.

77. B

This patient is highly complex and vulnerable and has a decreased ability to participate in self-care. The nurse with the most experience will demonstrate to him and his family a high level of clinical competence, caring practices, and systems thinking that can win their trust. Choice (A) may not have ever taken care of a patient with a balloon-pump. Choice (C) would not have the level of skills to demonstrate clinical competence. Choice (D) is not appropriate if the only reason is that the patients would be next to each other.

78. A

The most commonly ordered study used to evaluate renal trauma patients is the CT of the abdomen, which views the retroperitoneal region as well. A chest x-ray is a simple film that will give only basic information about the lungs and bone structure. A rib fracture may cause injury to the kidney, so the chest x-ray will demonstrate the fracture but will not define the damage to the kidney. IVPs evaluate urine filtration and internal tissues. This exam may be used at a later date to evaluate or stage an injury. A renal arteriogram evaluates the arterial blood flow in the kidneys. This may be premature in the evaluation of a patient with no initial clinical evidence of bleeding.

79. C

Increasing lactic acid is most likely indicative of inadequate tissue oxygenation and perfusion. Lactic acid levels should fall with adequate resuscitation—not rise. Elevations in lactic acid may also be seen in patients with metabolic disorders such as diabetic ketoacidosis. Patients with diabetic ketoacidosis develop metabolic acidosis primarily from an accumulation of ketone bodies in the blood from free fatty acid oxidation. They can, however, have an elevated lactate level if they have poor tissue perfusion due to severe dehydration.

80. D

Although answers (A), (B), and (C) are nurse characteristics, collaboration is an important characteristic to display when working with a team because it involves communication with other care providers in order to achieve the best outcome for the patient.

81. B

In volume control, the ventilator is set to control the tidal volume of each breath received by the patient. The PEEP and respiratory rate will also be set. The current belief is that this mode of ventilation is beneficial because the physician can set a low tidal volume and prevent large volume from being drawn in by the patient. Referred to as low-volume ventilation, it is believed to minimize volutrauma in the lungs of ventilated patients.

82. C

The purpose of the CSF is to absorb shock and cushion the brain and spinal cord. Oxygen is transported in the blood vessels. Neurotransmitters are manufactured and released by the neurons. Cerebral perfusion pressure is maintained by autoregulation, chemo-metabolic factors, and intrinsic/extrinsic neurogenic factors.

83. D

Answer (D) is the best choice. This test does not require the use of IV contrast, which would be contraindicated in this patient due to her renal failure. Answer (A) is incorrect because this test requires the use of IV contrast, which is contraindicated in patients with renal failure. Answer (B) is incorrect because this test is not specific and would likely yield positive results regardless of the presence of a pulmonary embolus because of the patient's other conditions. Answer (C) is incorrect because signs of PE are rarely seen on chest x-ray.

84. C

An IVC filter is the only measure that will prevent a lower-extremity DVT from traveling to the lungs should it mobilize. Answer (A) is a common treatment for DVT but will not prevent the clot from moving to the lungs. Answer (B) is incorrect because this is contraindicated, as it may cause the DVT to mobilize. Answer (D) is incorrect because warfarin therapy will only prevent future clots, not prevent a current clot from mobilizing and traveling to the lungs.

85. B

Arterial occlusion symptoms include white, painful, and pulseless extremity. Venous occlusion symptoms include cyanotic, warm, red, painful, and edematous extremity. You can remember this by recalling the three Ps: pale, pulseless, and painful.

86. B

Dilated cardiomyopathy is the most common cardiomyopathy of the three classifications (dilated, hypertrophic, and restrictive). The clinical manifestations associated with each type of cardiomyopathy are very different. Restrictive cardiomyopathy is the least common, and physical findings associated with it are edema, ascites, right upper quadrant pain, and hepatojugular reflux (HJR). Clinical manifestations associated with hyptertrophic cardiomyopathy are displaced apical pulse and systolic thrill presence. Idiopathic cardiomyopathy is not a type of cardiomyopathy.

87. C

Billroth II procedure includes anastomosis of the gastric remnant to the jejunum. The other answer choices are incorrect. When such situations arise, there also may be a moral dilemma, as the patient may not fully understand the operation. Hence, notifying the physician in such cases is also appropriate.

88. B

Sensory input is integrated in the parietal lobe. Hearing is processed in the temporal lobe. Vision is the primary function of the occipital lobe. Voluntary motor control occurs in the frontal lobe.

89. C

Aldosterone is produced in the adrenal cortex, and it is stimulated by the renin-angiotensin system. Growth hormone, corticotropin, and prolactin are released from the pituitary in response to stimulation by the hypothalamus.

90. C

The patient is volume overloaded and has pulmonary edema. Administration of additional fluids will worsen the condition. The other answers are all common and appropriate treatments for CHF exacerbation with pulmonary edema.

91. D

The intra-aortic radiopaqued tip should be located at the two to three intercostal space on x-ray. The IABP catheter can migrate higher in the aorta and occlude the subclavian artery, causing a loss in the left arm pulses. This is the reason it is important to assess and document the left arm pulse presence besides the assessment of the pulse in the affected leg. All of the other options (A–C) are not urgent findings that require immediate intervention.

92. B

The two primary pathways in the coagulation cascade are the intrinsic and extrinsic pathways. The intrinsic pathway is initiated when there is endothelium damage and the collagen released comes in contact with factor XII. The extrinsic pathway is when tissue trauma occurs and factor III is released from the damaged tissues and comes in contact with factor VII circulating in the blood. It is called the common pathway. The erythropoietin mechanism is the cascade that precipitates the production of red blood cells when tissue oxygenation occurs. Hypercoagulability is the condition where the normal mechanisms of hemostasis are disrupted and the blood clots inappropriately.

93. B

In this stage of ATN, the patient may excrete up to four liters of fluid per day. If the fluid is not replaced as needed, the patient may become dehydrated, and electrolyte levels may increase. Restricting fluid intake would only further compound the problem. In addition, administering hypertonic solution may cause a shift from the intracellular space to the intravascular space for a temporary period of time, though as a long-term treatment it would worsen the condition. Diuretic therapy is not indicated, as the kidneys are appropriately filtering.

94. A

The effect of hypoglycemia on the central nervous system varies by individual, from bizarre behavior to coma. All the other choices are nonspecific and could result from any other causes.

95. D

Initial treatment of patient with elevated INR should be administration of vitamin K to attempt to reverse the effect of the Coumadin. The patient's lab studies do not justify administration of RBCs or FFP, since he is not supratherapeutic or actively bleeding—at least that you know of. Cryoprecipitate is not indicated in this situation. It is important that the lab values, such as hemoglobin, in these patients always be compared to those of previous admissions to determine how far off their baseline is to their current value. It is *not* uncommon for such patients to have anemia, possibly from hemolysis or chronic disease, etc.

96. D

System thinking is also the ability to understand how one decision can impact the whole system.

97. C

Correcting hypoxia is the priority. Continued assessment of blood pressure or oxygen level will not help the patient. Giving pain medication may decrease respirations more.

98. C

Based on the Berlin definition for ARDS diagnosis, severe ARDS is PaO_2/FiO_2 less than 100 mm Hg. Answer (A) is incorrect because mild ARDS is PaO_2/FiO_2 between 200 and 300 mm Hg. Answer (B) is incorrect because moderate ARDS is PaO_2/FiO_2 between 100 and 200 mm Hg. Answer (D) is incorrect because end-stage ARDS is not a standard descriptor in ARDS severity.

99. A

Quite some time ago, the most common cause of chronic renal failure was glomerulonephritis due to undetected infections, which caused renal damage. In more recent times, diabetes has overtaken this condition as the primary cause of chronic renal failure. Thrombosis is not common, but it does occur. Sepsis is often the cause of acute renal failure.

100. A

A stroke in the left hemisphere causes aphasia, intellectual impairment, right visual field defects, and slow/cautious behavior. Right hemisphere stroke symptoms include spatial-perceptual deficits, left side neglect, impulsive behavior, and left visual deficits. Stroke in the pons impairs respiratory control. Lesions of the cerebellum cause an inability to coordinate voluntary muscle movement, altered equilibrium, and trunk instability.

101. A

When patients and families are unable speak English, they are considered fragile in terms of vulnerability and can have limited resources available to them. The nurse needs to respond to diversity and systems-think to develop proactive strategies for the patient and family. The most effective method of communicating is by using a translation service. Relying on a family member, ancillary staff, or a communication board is not the most effective method of communicating. Note also that the patient's family is not English speaking in this scenario.

102. B

Decorticate posture is flexion of the elbows, extension of the knees, and plantar flexion of the feet. Decerebrate posture is extension of elbows and knees, plantar flexion of feet, and flexion of the wrists. Flexion of both upper and lower extremity position and the extension of upper extremities and flexion of lower extremity positions are used by physical therapists in rehabilitation of injuries.

103. C

Abrupt onset of shortness of breath, chest pain, murmur, and acute development of signs and symptoms of congestive heart failure (due to mitral valve insufficiency) are associated with the development of a papillary muscle rupture. Chest pain and holosystolic murmur manifestations are associated with the development of a perforated ventricular septum, which is another major complication postmyocardial infarction.

104. A

Normal serum sodium is 135–145 mEq/L. Hypernatremia, polyuria, polydipsia, hyperosmolality, hypotension, and mental status changes are the classic indicators of DI. Normal serum osmolality is 280–300 mOsm/L; answer (B) is within normal limits. Normal CVP is 2–6 mm Hg; answer (C) indicates fluid overload not depletion as seen with DI. Answer (D) indicates concentrated urine. DI patients have very dilute urine with a specific gravity of <1.005.

105. C

This parameter is considered the most important for alveolar recruitment and maintaining patency of collapsed alveoli, which promotes oxygenation and ventilation. Patients with ARDS typically require high levels of PEEP to maintain oxygenation. Answer (A) is incorrect because pressure support is a setting typically used during weaning trials. Answer (B) is partially correct, but this parameter is important for all patients requiring mechanical ventilation. Answer (D) is incorrect because pressure control is a setting used in advanced modes of ventilation, which are not within the scope of the CCRN.

106. B

The initiation of the renin-angiotensin-aldosterone cascade stimulates the sympathetic nerve activation. This must be stimulated by the reduction of arterial blood flow to the kidneys and may be the result of prerenal conditions such as hypovolemia. Electrolyte abnormalities do not stimulate this cascade. Initiation of the renin-angiotensin-aldosterone cascade actually causes the release of aldosterone, which further retains water and sodium.

107. C

Community-acquired pneumonia can be caused by many different organisms, and treatment is directed at the likely or confirmed organism. While answers (A) and (B) can cause community-acquired pneumonia, they are not necessarily the likely culprits. Answer (D) is incorrect because it excludes the correct answer.

108. C

Since the son is participating in his father's care, it is important for the nurse to act as a facilitator of learning and provide adequate opportunities to successfully demonstrate the skill. The best intervention is choice (C). Choices (A), (B), and (D) will not provide this opportunity and are not appropriate.

109. C

The patient who is evidencing organ rejection would have lab values demonstrating potential renal insufficiency. (A) or (B) would be indicative of appropriate renal function. In organ rejection scenarios, the platelet count would most likely decrease; therefore, (D) is also incorrect.

110. D

The string of data does not support cardiogenic or septic shock or MODS. SIRS is characterized by an increased temperature and heart rate with no documented signs of infection.

111. A

Cardioversion is performed in hopes of converting the abnormal supraventricular rhythm back to normal by delivering low energy joules. Defibrillation and an AICD are not necessary, since the heart is not fibrillating and has narrow QRS complexes. Pacing is not required, because the rhythm is not bradycardic.

112. D

In metabolic acidosis, the pH and bicarbonate should both be low. If it is acute, then the carbon dioxide will be about normal since there has not been any time for compensation. The other answers are wrong because

(A) pH 7.55, pCO_2 32, pO_2 75, HCO_3^- 24 signifies respiratory alkalosis.

(B) pH 7.50, pCO_2 45, pO_2 73, HCO_3^- 30 signifies metabolic alkalosis.

(C) pH 7.30, pCO_2 55, pO_2 67, HCO_3^- 28 signifies respiratory acidosis.

113. C

The values in answer (C) show that the liver, kidneys, and bone marrow are failing. The values in answer (A) are all within normal limits. Answer (B) has a normal Glasgow Coma Score, and answer (D) is related to the pulmonary system.

114. B

The critically injured, multiple-trauma patient is at high risk for these early complications because of poor perfusion, prolonged exposure to the elements (including the temperature of the surgical suite), and infusion of multiple blood products (which contributes to hypothermia and coagulopathy). The other answers are either not early complications in the critically injured multiple-trauma patient or are not commonly related to such patients (such as answer C).

115. B

A hemiblock is a blockage in the bundles that causes the widening of the QRS complex.

116. A

Based on the Synergy Model, critical care nurse and patient collaboration increases likelihood of positive outcomes.

117. D

These patients are moderately resilient and vulnerable. Resource availability is needed to assist with recovery. The nurse uses caring practices and individualizes care by using gestures while talking to the patient. Choice (A) is not appropriate; the patient is not deaf, just having difficulty understanding spoken language. Choice (B) would only frustrate the patient. Choice (C) is not helping the patient to recover.

118. B

Chest pain relief usually occurs within five minutes of taking sublingual nitroglycerin. Patients can take up to three sublingual tablets every 5 minutes over 15 minutes. Because this patient's chest discomfort is unrelieved and continues to have an acceptable blood pressure, the administration of another sublingual nitrate may resolve the chest discomfort. If the chest discomfort continues after three sublingual tablets, then the patient should go immediately to an emergency room. Although, knowing the ECG would be helpful, more important is that the patient continues to have chest pain with an acceptable blood pressure. Patients should be instructed to lie down and use this medication at first sign of chest discomfort. However, simply lying down and elevating the patient's legs is not enough.

119. B

This family is vulnerable and feeling powerless. The nurse uses compassion to assess the family's concerns and then act as a facilitator of learning by teaching them about the monitor and what the numbers of concern mean. Choices (A) and (C) are vague and do not address the family's concerns. Choice (D) is not appropriate.

120. C

Antibiotics are given preoperatively to prevent bacterial growth in the colon and postoperative infection. The patient is kept NPO after midnight or for 12 hours prior to surgery. A nasogastric tube can be inserted once the patient is in surgery.

121. A

The rapid infusion of Dilantin (phenytoin) is well known to cause hypotension and bradycardia; therefore this medication should always be given slowly. Answer (B) is partially correct, as infusion of this medication can cause phlebitis; however, it does not cause tachycardia. Answers (C) and (D) are incorrect because these are not reactions to this medication. The patient may experience an allergic reaction to this medication, but this would occur regardless of the rate of administration.

122. C

The patient is intoxicated and has a decreased mental status. Vomiting with failure to completely protect the airway increases the risk of aspiration. Answer (A) is incorrect because there is no indication that the patient was admitted with pneumonia symptoms. Answer (B) is potentially correct but not the highest risk. Answer (D) is incorrect because there is no indication that the patient has a history of alcohol abuse, and withdrawal symptoms do not occur while patients are still intoxicated.

123. A

A major side effect of Natrecor is hypotension. Oftentimes, a fluid bolus is given before starting this medication. If hypotension occurs after the start of this medication, Trendelenburg or an IV fluid bolus may be ordered. The half-life of Natrecor is 18 minutes; therefore, hypotension may last for hours.

124. C

Hypotension and increased intracranial pressure results in decreased cerebral perfusion pressure, which leads to secondary injury to the brain tissue. Hypoxia also leads to secondary injury and contributes to worsening cerebral edema. The answers in choice (A) are not related to secondary injury and are not complications in the acute phase. The answers in choices (B) and (D) are incorrect because they are not related to secondary injury in these patients.

125. D

Before setting up mandatory in-services or competency review changes, the best first step should be to meet with the surgeon and identify all of the issues. Meeting with the surgeon shows a high level of collaboration.

126. C

High-fat meals stimulate bile to be excreted from the gallbladder into the duodenum. None of the other choices exacerbate gallbladder pain.

127. D

Patients with neuromuscular disorders such as Guillain-Barré syndrome are at risk for respiratory depression due to progressive weakness, which may impair movement of the diaphragm. Answer (A) is a potential complication of any ICU admission and is not the highest priority for this type of patient. Answer (B) is not related to this diagnosis. Answer (C) is also a potential complication of any ICU admission and is not the priority for this type of patient.

128. C

Thrombocytopenia is a low platelet count. The patient should be transfused for platelet counts <50,000 when there is evidence of bleeding. Whole blood does contain platelets; however, for simple thrombocytopenia it is not recommended. The indication for FFP is a need for clotting factors. RBCs are given for anemia.

129. B

Glasgow Coma Score was developed to assess brain injury. A GCS less than 8 indicates a significant brain injury. A patient who is brain dead would have a GCS of 3.

130. C

For this patient, resource availability is a high need, and predictability is moderately wavering. To facilitate learning for this patient, the nurse must locate supportive resources that will optimize learning. By using verbal descriptions, the nurse will maximize the patient's learning. Choice (A) should not be eliminated, the patient can use touch to feel the food size and weight. Choice (B) eliminates depth to areas that may need reinforcement. Choice (D) bypasses the patient, who needs the learning.

131. A

The patient had been in the hospital for over 72 hours when the pneumonia symptoms began, which is a criterion for hospital-acquired pneumonia. Answer (B) is incorrect because there is no indication that the patient is at risk for aspiration. Answer (C) is a possibility; however, her symptoms are more consistent with pneumonia. Answer (D) is incorrect because there is no mention of a history of congestive heart failure and her symptoms do not support a diagnosis of heart failure.

132. D

Any condition that results in reduced blood flow to the kidneys may be considered prerenal. All of the responses except ureter obstruction could potentially reduce blood flow to the kidneys. That would be a postrenal condition.

133. C

COPD has many causes and many different treatments. The other answers are incorrect because COPD has many causes and many treatments, is not frequently fatal, and is not treated the same way as pneumonia or CHF.

134. D

Natrecor causes venous and arterial dilation. A false increase in BNP is normal for a patient receiving the medication Natrecor. This is an important consideration if asked to obtain a BNP level on a patient who is receiving this medication for congestive heart failure. Natrecor has no effect on contractility.

135. B

Cyanosis is most evident in the mucous membranes of older adults. The color of the sclera does not indicate decreased perfusion; skin color is difficult to assess, especially if the patient has dark skin; nail beds may have ridges, fungal infections, and yellowing in older patients—therefore they are not good choices.

136. C

Nail bed pressure elicits a peripheral response. Sternal rub, trapezius muscle squeeze, and mandibular pressure elicit a central response.

137. C

The normal BUN to creatinine ratio is less than 20:1. In this situation, the ratio is 28:1 which is strongly indicative of dehydration consistent with his history of nausea and vomiting and the normal creatinine level. The elevated potassium and hematocrit could also result from a dehydration state. It is unlikely that he developed acute renal failure as a result of dehydration over a few days, although a prerenal condition leading to ATN and acute renal failure is hypovolemia.

138. C

Normal ALT and AST should be below 40 units/L.

139. C

The basis for the certification program is to develop, maintain, and promote high standards for critical care nursing practice through certification preparation and examination. All the other choices are inaccurate.

140. C

The precursor for all blood cells is the pluripotential stem cell. The other cells listed are the final formations of either white blood cells or red blood cells.

141. C

The nurse is demonstrating facilitation of learning by assessing the daughter's overall level of knowledge and skills prior to planning for teaching sessions. Choices (A), (B), and (D) may be used after identifying the daughter's learning needs.

142. A

This patient is highly vulnerable and has minimal resiliency related to the coagulation status. The nurse uses clinical judgment based on knowing that tight control of the aPTT helps to prevent clotting of the graft and limb ischemia. By using standing orders, the nurse adjusts the heparin drip in the most efficient manner possible. The goal of heparin IV infusion is to maintain the aPTT between 60 to 80 seconds. Choice (B) may take precious time and delay the appropriate drip change. Choice (C) is not acceptable, since delaying the drip adjustment puts the patient at risk. Choice (D) is not acceptable since delay risks graft occlusion and limb ischemia.

143. B

Concurrent use of antiarrhythmic agents is necessary to decrease the frequency of events. All the other statement choices are evidence that the patient understands information that was taught pertaining to his device.

144. A

Based on the Synergy Model, the patient is the center of focus surrounded by the medical intervention. More compromised patients require advanced knowledge and skills from nurses.

145. B

The Synergy Model encompasses complete and total care of the patient, including family and the patient's community.

146. D

Status epilepticus is either continuous seizures lasting more than five minutes or two or more different seizures with incomplete recovery of consciousness between them. They are not controlled. There is no time frame in duration or occurrence of status epilepticus. There is no escalation of seizure intensity.

147. A

The four components of the Synergy Model include core concepts, patient and family characteristics, nurse competencies and characteristics, and patient outcomes. Although delivering critical test results and values in a timely manner is important to patient care, it is not one of the four components of the Synergy Model.

148. D

Grey-Turner's sign (bruising in the lower abdomen and flank) indicates retroperitoneal hemorrhage. This patient is most at risk for shock or early changes. Murphy's sign is expected in gallbladder disease. Many normal people exhibit Chvostek's sign (contraction of the facial muscles with light tapping on the facial nerve). Blood on rectal exam is not an emergent condition in a patient with hepatitis with no other indicators of a problem.

149. B

In no case should an impaled object from a penetrating trauma be removed unless the patient has received indicated diagnostic imaging and is in the operating room where emergent surgical exploration can be conducted. Hence, choices (A) and (D) are clearly wrong. Choice (C) should never be considered. Manipulating an impaled object in any way can result in increased damage to internal organs, as well as acute decomposition. Further, choice (C) is simply not reasonable or logical.

150. A

Cor pulmonale is the term for isolated right ventricular failure in the setting of COPD. Answer (B) is incorrect because pulmonary hypertension is a cause of right ventricular failure but itself is not the term. Answer (C) is incorrect because CHF refers to pulmonary congestion resulting from left ventricular failure. Answer (D) is a symptom of rather than the term for right heart failure.

Resources

Chapter 5

Alspach J. The cardiovascular system. In: *Core Curriculum for Critical Care Nursing*. 5th ed. Philadelphia: W.B. Saunders; 1998:137–338.

American Association of Critical Care Nurses. AACN practice alert: severe sepsis practice alert. *http://www.aacn.org/wd/practice/content/practicealerts.pcms?menu=practice*. Accessed July 16, 2010.

American Heart Association. Acute coronary syndrome: What is acute coronary syndrome? *http://www.americanheart.org/presenter.jhtml?identifier=3010002*. Accessed July 16, 2010.

Cleveland Clinic—Heart & Vascular Institute. Transmyocardial laser revascularization. *http://www.clevelandclinic.org/heartcenter/pub/guide/disease/cad/TMR.htm*. Accessed April 12, 2008.

Furukawa K, Motomura T, Nose Y. Right ventricular failure left ventricular assist device implantation: The need for an implantable right ventricular assist device. *Artificial Organs*. 2005;29(5):369–377.

Guyton A, Hall J. *Textbook of Medical Physiology*. 11th ed. Philadelphia: Elsevier Saunders; 1998.

Hailey L. Therapeutic hypothermia after cardiac arrest. *http://www.cardiology.utmb.edu/slides/sec-2-clinical/therapeutic%20hypothermia%20after%20cardiac%20arrest_03.pdf*. Accessed April 12, 2008.

Hamel WJ. Femoral artery closure after cardiac catheterization. *Crit Care Nurse*. 2009; 29(1):39–46.

Lewis R, Mabie W, Burlew B, Sibai BM. Biventricular assist device as a bridge to cardiac transplantation in the treatment of peripartum cardiomyopathy. *South Med J*. 1997;90(9):955–958.

Shinn JA. Implantable left ventricular assist device. *J Cardiovasc Nurs*. 2005;20(5 Suppl): S22–30.

Shoulders-Odom B. Management of patients after percutaneous coronary interventions. *Crit Care Nurse*. 2008;28(5):26–41.

Thachi, J, Toh, C H. Current concepts in the management of disseminated intravascular coagulation. *Thrombosis Research.* 2012; 129 Suppl 1:S54–9. doi: 10.1016/S0049-3848(12)70017-8.

Thelan L, Lough M, Urden L, Stacey K. Unit 3: cardiovascular alterations. In: *Critical Care Nursing: Diagnosis and Management.* 3rd ed. St. Louis: Mosby; 1998.

Walkes J, Smythe W, Reardon M. Cardiac neoplasms. In: *Cardiac Surgery in the Adult.* New York: McGraw Hill; 2005:1479–1510.

Chapter 6

American Thoracic Society; Infectious Diseases Society of America. Guidelines for the management of adults with hospital-acquired, ventilator-associated, and healthcare-associated pneumonia. *Am J Respir Crit Care Med.* 2005;171:388–416.

ARDS Definition Task Force. Acute respiratory distress syndrome: The Berlin definition. *JAMA.* 2012; 307(23):2526–2533. doi: 10.1001/jama.2012.5669.

Centers for Disease Control and Prevention. Pneumonia (ventilator-associated [VAP] and non-ventilator-associated pneumonia [PNEU]) event. https://www.cdc.gov/nhsn/pdfs/pscmanual/6pscvapcurrent.pdf. Accessed December 16, 2016.

Centers for Disease Control and Prevention. *http://www.cdc.gov.*

Mayo Clinic. Pulmonary Hypertension. *http://www.mayoclinic.org/pulmonary-hypertension/.* Accessed August 28, 2011.

National Heart and Lung and Blood Institute; National Institutes of Health. *http://www.nhlbi.nih.gov/.*

Prendergast T, Ruoss S, Seeley EJ. Pulmonary disease. In: McPhee SJ, Hammer GD, eds. *Pathophysiology of Disease: An Introduction to Clinical Medicine.* 6th ed. New York: McGraw Hill; 2009:184–221.

Talban OC, Anderson LJ, Besser R, Bridges C, Hajjeh R; CDC; Healthcare Infection Control Practices Advisory Committee. Guidelines for preventing health-care associated pneumonia, 2003: Recommendations of CDC and Healthcare Infection Control Practices Committee. *MMWR Recomm Rep.* 2004;53:1–36.

World Health Organization. *http://www.who.int/en/.*

Chapter 7

Alspach JG, ed. *AACN Core Curriculum for Critical Care Nursing.* 6th ed. Philadelphia: Saunders; 2006.

American Diabetes Association. Standards for medical care in diabetes—2007. *Diabetes Care.* 2007;30:S4–41.

Benner Z. Management of hyperglycemic emergencies. *AACN Clinical Issues*. 2006;17(1):56–65.

Chulay M, Burns S. *AACN Essentials of Critical Care Nursing*. New York: McGraw Hill; 2006.

Ganong W. *Review of Medical Physiology*. 2nd ed. New York: McGraw Hill; 2005.

Gearhart M, Parbhoo S. Hyperglycemia in the critically ill patient. *AACN Clinical Issues*. 2006;17(1):50–55.

Guller U, Turek J, Eubanks S, DeLong E, Oertli D, Feldman J. Detecting pheochromocytoma: Defining the most sensitive test. *Ann Surg*. 2006;243(1):102–107.

Johnson K, Renn C. The hypothalamic-pituitary-adrenal axis in critical illness. *AACN Clinical Issues*. 2006;17(1):39–49.

Kaplow R, Harin S. *Critical Care Nursing: Synergy for Optimal Outcomes*. Sudbury, MA: Jones and Bartlett; 2007.

Kitabchi A. E., Nyenwe E. Hyperglycemic crises in diabetes mellitus: diabetic ketoacidosis and hyperglycemic hyperosmolar state. *Endocrinol Metab Clin North Am*. 2006;35(4):725–751.

Kitabchi A E, Umpierrez G E, Miles J M, Fisher J N. Hyperglycemic crises of adult patients with diabetes. *Diabetes Care*. 2009; 32:1335–1343.

Singer P, Sevilla L. Postoperative endocrine management of pituitary tumors. *Neurosurg Clin N Am*. 2003;14(1):123–138.

Sole M, Klein D, Moseley M. *Introduction to Critical Care Nursing*. 4th ed. Philadelphia: Saunders; 2005.

Urden L, Stacy K, Lough M. *Priorities in Critical Care Nursing*. 4th ed. St. Louis: Mosby; 2003.

Utz A, Swearingen B, Biller B. Pituitary surgery and postoperative management in Cushing's disease. *Endocrinol Metab Clin North Am*. 2005;34:459–478.

Wartofsky L. Myxedema coma. *Endocrinol Metab Clin North Am*. 2006;35:687–698.

Weeks BH. Graves' disease: The importance of early diagnosis. *Nurse Pract*. 2005;30(11): 34–36, 41–42, 44–45.

Chapter 8

Alspach JG, ed. *AACN Core Curriculum for Critical Care Nursing*. 5th ed. Philadelphia: Saunders; 1998.

Guyton AC, Hall JE. Renal physiology. In: *Textbook of Medical Physiology*. 11th ed. Philadelphia: W.B. Saunders; 2006:419–467.

Chapter 9

Albano C, Commandante L, Nolan S. Innovations in the management of cerebral injury. *Crit Care Nurs Q.* 2005;28(2):135–149.

Alspach JG, ed. *AACN Core Curriculum for Critical Care Nursing.* 6th ed. Philadelphia: Saunders; 2006.

Atkinson S, Carr R, Maybee P, Haynes D. The challenges of managing and treating Guillain-Barré syndrome during the acute phase. *Dimens Crit Care Nurs.* 2006;25:256–263.

Bader M, Littlejohns L. *AANN Core Curriculum for Neuroscience Nursing.* 4th ed. Philadelphia: Saunders; 2004.

Centers for Disease Control and Prevention. Stroke Facts. *http://www.cdc.gov/stroke/facts.htm.* Last updated March 24, 2015.

Center for Head Injury Services. Brain Injury Statistics. *http://www.headinjuryctr-stl.org/statistics.html.* Accessed April 17, 2015.

Chulay M, Burns S. *AACN Essentials of Critical Care Nursing.* New York: McGraw-Hill; 2006.

Estep M. Meningococcal meningitis in critical care: An overview. *Crit Care Nurs Q.* 2005;28(2):111–121.

Fowler S, Mancini B. Predictive value of biochemical markers of stroke. *J Neurosci Nurs.* 2007;39:58–60.

Ganong W. *Review of Medical Physiology.* 22nd ed. New York: McGraw-Hill; 2005.

Haines D. *Neuroanatomy: An Atlas of Structures, Sections, and Systems.* Philadelphia: Lippincott Williams & Wilkins; 2004.

Hanel R, Demetrius K, Wehman J. Endovascular treatment of intracranial aneurysms and vasospasms after aneurysmal subarachnoid hemorrhage. *Neurosurg Clin North Am.* 2005;16:317–353.

Hickey J. *The Clinical Practice of Neurological and Neurosurgical Nursing.* 6th ed. Philadelphia: Lippincott Williams & Wilkins; 2008.

Howard J Jr. Healthcare professionals: clinical overview of MG: myasthenia gravis—a summary. Myasthenia Gravis Foundation of America. *http://www.myasthenia.org/hp_clinicaloverview.cfm.* Accessed July 22, 2010.

Kaplow R, Hardin S. *Critical Care Nursing: Synergy for Optimal Outcomes.* Sudbury, MA: Jones & Bartlett; 2007.

Kosty T. Cerebral vasospasm after subarachnoid hemorrhage. *Crit Care Nurs Q.* 2005;28(2):122–134.

Mayo Clinic. *http://www.mayoclinic.org.*

Mortimer D, Janik J. Administering hypertonic saline to patients with severe traumatic brain injury. *J Neurosci Nurs.* 2006;38:142–146.

Muscular Dystrophy Association. *http://mda.org.*

Myasthenia Gravis Foundation of America. *http://myasthenia.org/.*

National Heart and Lung and Blood Institute; National Institutes of Health. *http://www.nhlbi.nih.gov/.*

Oyama K, Criddle L. Vasospasm after aneurysmal subarachnoid hemorrhage. *Crit Care Nurse.* 2004;24(5):58–67.

Presciutti M. Nursing priorities in caring for patients with intracerebral hemorrhage. *J Neurosci Nurs.* 2006;38(Supp 4):296–299, 315.

Rossetti A, Logroscino G, Liaudet L, et al. Status epilepticus. *Neurology.* 2007;69:255–260.

Sheerin F. Spinal cord injury: Acute care management. *Emergency Nurse.* 2005;12(10):26–34.

Sole M, Klein D, Moseley M. *Introduction to Critical Care Nursing.* 4th ed. Philadelphia: Saunders; 2005.

Urden L, Stacy K, Lough M. *Priorities in Critical Care Nursing.* 4th ed. St. Louis: Mosby; 2003.

Chapter 10

Azer S. Esophageal varices: treatment and medication. Medscape Reference. *http://emedicine.medscape.com/article/175248-treatment.* Accessed July 1, 2009.

Bickely LS. *Bates Guide to Physical Examination and History Taking.* 7th ed. Philadelphia: Lippincott Williams & Wilkins; 1999.

Black JM, Hawks JH, Keene AM. *Medical-Surgical Nursing.* 6th ed. Philadelphia: Saunders; 2001.

Brozenec SA, Russell SS. *Core Curriculum for Medical-Surgical Nursing.* 2nd ed. New Jersey: Academy of Medical-Surgical Nurses.

Bucher L, Melander S. *Critical Care Nursing.* Philadelphia: W.B. Saunders; 1999.

Fischbach F, Dunning MB. *A Manual of Laboratory and Diagnostic Tests.* 7th ed. Philadelphia: Lippincott Williams & Wilkins; 2004.

Ignatavicius DD, Workman ML. *Medical-Surgical Nursing.* 4th ed. Philadelphia: W.B. Saunders; 2002.

Kidd PS, Wagner KD. *High Acuity Nursing.* 3rd ed. Upper Saddle River, NJ: Prentice Hall; 2001.

Lilley LL, Harrington S, Snyder JS. *Pharmacology and the Nursing Process*. 4th ed. St. Louis: Mosby; 2005.

London ML, Ladewig PW, Ball JW, Bindler R. *Maternal & Child Nursing Care*. 2nd ed. Upper Saddle River, NJ: Pearson/Prentice Hall; 2007.

Mims BC, Toto KH, Luecke LE. *Critical Care Skills: A Clinical Handbook*. Philadelphia: Saunders; 1996.

McNally P. *GI/Liver Secrets*. 2nd ed. Philadelphia: Hanley & Belfus/Elsevier; 2001.

Pagana K, Pagana T. *Mosby's Manual of Diagnostic and Laboratory Tests*. 3rd ed. St. Louis: Mosby; 2005.

Skidmore-Roth L. *Mosby's 2004 Nursing Drug Reference*. St. Louis: Mosby; 2004.

Smeltzer S, Bare BG. *Brunner and Suddarth's Textbook of Medical-Surgical Nursing*. 10th ed. Philadelphia: Lippincott Williams & Wilkins; 2003.

Sole ML, Hartshorn J, Lamborne ML. *Introduction to Critical Care Nursing*. 3rd ed. Philadelphia: W.B. Saunders; 2001.

Sommers MS, Johnson SA, Berry TA. *Diseases and Disorders*. 3rd ed. Philadelphia: FA Davis; 2007.

Stillwell S. *Mosby's Critical Care Nursing Reference*. 3rd ed. St. Louis: Mosby; 2002.

Tucker SM, Canobbio MM, Paquette EV, Wells MF. *Patient Care Standards*. 7th ed. St. Louis: Mosby; 2000.

Urden L, Lough ME, Stacy KL. *Thelan's Critical Care Nursing: Diagnosis and Management*. 5th ed. St. Louis: Mosby; 2005.

Chapter 11

Alspach JG, ed. *AACN Core Curriculum for Critical Care Nursing*. 5th ed. Philadelphia: Saunders; 1998.

Chmielewski C. Anatomy and overview of nephron function. *Nephrol Nurs J*. 2003; 30(2):185–190.

Dirkes S, Hodge K. Continuous renal replacement therapy in the adult critical care unit. *Crit Care Nurse*. 2007;27(2):61–80.

Edwards S. Tissue viability: understanding the mechanisms of injury and repair. *Nurs Stand*. 2005;21(13):48–56.

French S, Banerjee D. Diagnosis and care of nephritic syndrome. *General Practitioner*. 2007:30–31.

Goof C, Collin G. Management of renal trauma at a rural, level 1 trauma center. *Am Surg*. 1998;64(3):226–230.

Guyton AC, Hall JE. Renal physiology. In: *Textbook of Medical Physiology*. 11th ed. Philadelphia: W.B. Saunders; 2006:264–379.

Henke K, Eigsti J. Renal physiology: review and practical application in the critically ill patient. *Dimensions of Critical Care Nursing*. 2003;22(3):125–132.

Kellum J, Palevski P. Renal support in acute kidney injury. *Lancet*. 2006;368(9533):344–345.

Klabunder R. Cardiovascular physiology concepts: renin-angiotensin-aldosterone system. *http://www.cvphysiology.com/Blood%20Pressure/BP015.htm*. Accessed February 14, 2008.

Star R. Treatment of acute renal failure: perspectives in renal medicine. *Kidney Int*. 1998;54:1817–1829.

Thelan L, Urden L, Lough M, Stacy K. Unit IV: renal alterations. In: *Critical Care Nursing: Diagnosis and Management*. 3rd ed. St. Louis: Mosby; 1998:847–916.

Weglicki W, Quamme G, Tucker K, Haigney M, Resnick L. Potassium, magnesium, and electrolyte imbalance and complications in disease management. *Clin Exp Hypertens*. 2005;27:95–112.

Figure 11.1: This article was published in Guyton AC, Hall JE. *Textbook of Medical Physiology*. 11th ed. Philadelphia: W.B. Saunders; 2006:309, Figure 26.3. Copyright Elsevier.

Figure 11.2: This article was published in Guyton AC, Hall JE. *Textbook of Medical Physiology*. 11th ed. Philadelphia: W.B. Saunders; 2006:310, Figure 26.4. Copyright Elsevier.

Figure 11.3: This article was published in Guyton AC, Hall JE. *Textbook of Medical Physiology*. 11th ed. Philadelphia: W.B. Saunders; 2006:314, Figure 26.8. Copyright Elsevier.

Figure 11.4: This article was published in Guyton AC, Hall JE. *Textbook of Medical Physiology*. 11th ed. Philadelphia: W.B. Saunders; 2006:318, Figure 26.12. Copyright Elsevier.

Figure 11.5: This article was published in Guyton AC, Hall JE. *Textbook of Medical Physiology*. 11th ed. Philadelphia: W.B. Saunders; 2006:358, Figure 28.8. Copyright Elsevier.

Figure 11.6: This article was published in Guyton AC, Hall JE. *Textbook of Medical Physiology*. 11th ed. Philadelphia: W.B. Saunders; 2006:375, Figure 29.12. Copyright Elsevier.

Figure 11.7: This article was published in Guyton AC, Hall JE. *Textbook of Medical Physiology*. 11th ed. Philadelphia: W.B. Saunders; 2006:414, Figure 31.8. Copyright Elsevier.

Chapter 12

American College of Surgeons. *Advanced Trauma Life Support for Doctors, Student Course Manual*. 8th ed. Chicago: American College of Surgeons; 2008.

Black J, Hawks J. *Medical Surgical Nursing: Clinical Management for Positive Outcomes*. Philadelphia: Saunders; 2005.

Bullock B, Henze R. *Focus on Pathophysiology*. Philadelphia: Lippincott Williams & Wilkins; 2000.

Centers for Disease Control and Prevention. Bioterrorism agent/diseases. *http://emergency.cdc.gov/agent/agentlist-category.asp*. Accessed August 28, 2011.

Caravati EM, Erdman AR, et al. for American Association of Poison Control Centers. Practice guideline: ethylene glycol exposure: an evidence-based consensus guideline for out-of-hospital management. *Clinical Toxicology*. 2005;43(5):327–345.

Centers for Disease Control and Prevention. Smallpox. *http://emergency.cdc.gov/agent/smallpox/*. Accessed July 16, 2010.

Dellinger R P, Levy M M, Rhodes A, et al. Surviving sepsis campaign: International guidelines for management of severe sepsis and septic shock: 2012. *Critical Care Medicine*. 2013; 41:580–637.

Levy M M, Rhodes A, Phillips G S, et al. Surviving sepsis campaign: Association between performance metrics and outcomes in a 7.5-year study. *Intensive Care Medicine*. 2014; 40:1623–1633.

Medscape Reference. Drugs, diseases & procedures. *http://emedicine.medscape.com/*. Accessed July 16, 2010.

Morton P, Fontaine D, Hudak C, Gallo B. *Critical Care Nursing: A Holistic Approach*. Philadelphia: Lippincott Williams & Wilkins; 2008.

National Kidney & Urologic Diseases Information Clearinghouse; U.S. Department of Health and Human Services. Hemolytic uremic syndrome in children. *http://kidney.niddk.nih.gov/kudiseases/pubs/childkidneydiseases/hemolytic_uremic_syndrome/*. Accessed July 22, 2010.

Safe Kids USA. *http://www.safekids.org/*.

Society of Critical Care Medicine. *Fundamentals of Critical Care Support*. 4th ed. Mount Prospect, IL: Society of Critical Care Medicine; 2007.

Sole M, Klein D, Moseley M. *Introduction to Critical Care Nursing*. 5th ed. Philadelphia: Saunders; 2008.

Tomaszewski C. Carbon monoxide poisoning: early awareness and intervention can save lives. *Postgrad Med*. 1999;(105):1, 39–40.

University of Maryland Medical Center. Sodium hydroxide poisoning. *http://www.umm.edu/ency/article/002487.htm*. Updated September 29, 2009.

U.S. National Library of Medicine, National Institutes of Health. PubMed. *http://www.ncbi.nlm.nih.gov/pubmed*.

Chapter 13

Aiken TD. *Legal, Ethical, and Political Issues in Nursing*. Philadelphia: FA Davis; 1994.

Alspach JG, ed. *AACN Core Curriculum for Critical Care Nursing*. 6th ed. Philadelphia: Saunders; 2006.

American Nurses Association. *Code of Ethics for Nurses with Interpretive Statements*. Washington, DC: American Nurses Association; 2001.

Beauchamp T, Childress J. *Principles of Biomedical Ethics*. 5th ed. New York: Oxford University Press; 2001.

Benner P. *From Novice to Expert: Excellence and Power in Clinical Nursing Practice*. Menlo Park, CA: Addison Wesley; 1984.

Crisham P. Resolving ethical and moral delimmas of nursing interventions. In: Snyder M, ed. *Independent Nursing Interventions*. Albany, NY: Delmar Publishers; 1992:25–43.

Curley M. Patient-nurse synergy: optimizing patients' outcomes. *Am J Crit Care*. 1998;7:64–72.

Ethics Resource Center. Plus model. *http://www.ethics.org/resources/decision-making-process.asp*. Accessed June 3, 2008.

Hardin S, Kaplow R. *Synergy for Clinical Excellence: The AACN Synergy Model for Patient Care*. Sudbury, MA: Jones & Bartlett; 2005.

Henderson V. *Basic Principles of Nursing Care*. London: International Council of Nurses; 1960.

Kaplow R. AACN synergy model for patient care: a framework to optimize outcomes. *Crit Care Nurs*. 2003;23:S27–30.

Rushton C, Scanlon C. A road map for negotiating end-of-life care. *Med Surg Nurs*. 1998;7:57–59.

Thompson J, Thompson H. *Bioethical Decision-making for Nurses*. Norwalk, CT: Appleton Century Crofts; 1985.

Chapter 14

American Academy of Family Physicians. Case study: screening for bipolar and other mood disorders. *http://www.aafp.org/online/etc/medialib/aafp_org/documents/cme/courses/conf/assembly/2010handouts/224.Par.0001.File.tmp/224-225.pdf*. Accessed July 1, 2010.

American Foundation for Suicide Prevention. Risk factors for suicide. *http://www.afsp.org/index.cfm?page_id=05147440-E24E-E376-BDF4BF8BA6444E76*. Accessed July 1, 2010.

Barr J, Pandharipande P P. The pain, agitation, and delirium care bundle: Synergistic benefits of implementing the 2013 Pain, Agitation, and Delirium Guidelines in an integrated and interdisciplinary fashion. *Critical Care Medicine*. 2013; 41(9 Suppl 1):S99–115. doi: 10.1097/CCM.0b013e3182a16ff0.

Centers for Disease Control and Prevention. Alcohol and Public Health. https://www.cdc.gov/alcohol/data-stats.htm. Accessed December 20, 2016.

Centers for Disease Control and Prevention. Leading Causes of Death. https://www.cdc.gov/nchs/fastats/leading-causes-of-death.htm. Accessed December 20, 2016.

Centers for Medicare and Medicaid Services. Clarification of Terms Used in the Definition of Physical Restraints as Applied to the Requirements for Long Term Care Facilities. https://www.cms.gov/Medicare/Provider-Enrollment-and-Certification/SurveyCertificationGenInfo/downloads/SCLetter07-22.pdf. Accessed December 20, 2016.

Citrome L. Aggression. *http://emedicine.medscape.com/article/288689-overview*. Accessed July 2, 2010.

Collins LG. Restraining devices for patients in acute and long-term care facilities. *Am Fam Physician*. 2009;79(4):254, 256.

Daily DK. Identification of mental retardation. *Am Fam Physician*. 2000;61:1059–1067, 1070.

Edelstein BH, Martin RR, Koven LP, Duberstein PR. Development and psychometric evaluation of the reasons for living—older adults scale: a suicide risk assessment inventory. *Gerontologist*. 2009;49(6):736–745.

Encyclopedia of Mental Disorders. Abuse. *http://www.minddisorders.com/A-Br/Abuse.html*. Accessed July 2, 2010.

Encyclopedia of Mental Disorders. Neglect. *http://www.minddisorders.com/Kau-Nu/Neglect.html*. Accessed July 2, 2010.

Gerstein PS. Delirium, dementia, and amnesia. *http://emedicine.medscape.com/article/793247-overview*. Accessed July 1, 2010.

Larson M. Psychosis among substance users. *Curr Opin Pysch*. 2006;19(3):239–245.

Lessenger JE, Feinberg SD. Abuse of prescription and over-the-counter medications. *J Am Board Fam Med*. 2008;21(1):45–54.

McCaffrey MG, Pasero C, Ferrell B, Uman G. On the meaning of "drug seeking." *Pain Manag Nurs*. 2005;6(4):122–136.

Mersey DJ. Recognition of alcohol and substance abuse. *Am Fam Physician*. 2003;67(7):1529–1532.

Muscari ME. How can I detect the warning signs of extreme violence in my patients? *http://www.medscape.com/viewarticle/708159*. Accessed July 28, 2010.

National Institutes of Health. The numbers count: mental disorders in america. *http://www.apps.nimh.nih.gov/health/publications/the-numbers-count-mental-disorders-in-america.shtml*. Accessed July 28, 2010.

Prince M, Saxena S. No health without mental health: mental health is integral for the achievement of several millennium developmental goals. *Lancet.* 2007;370:859–877.

Robertson RG. Geriatric failure to thrive. *Am Fam Physician.* 2004;70(2):343–350.

Viken R. Curbside consultation, combative delirium. *Am Fam Physician.* 2008;77(2): 237–237.

Ward RK. Assessment and management of personality disorders. *Am Fam Physician.* 2004;70(8):1505–1512.

Woolf LM. *Elder Abuse and Neglect.* New York: Webster University; 2008.

Index

A

ABCDE survey of trauma, 306
abdominal trauma, 252–253
ablation therapy, 74, 83–84
absence seizures, 233
abuse, 353–354
accountability, 346
ACE inhibitors, 57, 97
acetylcholine, 194
acid-base balance by kidneys, 283–284, 288. *See also* bicarbonate buffer system
acid-control in stomach, 263
acquired immunity, 180–181
active transport in kidneys, 277–278
    ATP for, 277, 278, 281
acute abdominal trauma, 252–253
acute adrenal insufficiency, 145–146
acute anemia, 170
acute chest pain MONA, 59
acute coronary syndromes (ACS), 58–61
acute GI hemorrhage, 253–254
acute hemolytic reaction, 169
acute hepatitis panel, 251
acute hypoglycemia, 153–154
    emergency foods for, 154
acute hypoxemic respiratory failure, 107–109
acute kidney injury (AKI), 288–291
    trauma sequelae, 310
acute liver failure causes, 258
acute lymphocytic leukemia (ALL), 175
acute mitral regurgitation, 60, 79
acute myelogenous leukemia (AML), 175

acute pulmonary embolus, 105–107
acute radiation syndrome (ARS), 320–321
acute renal failure. *See* acute kidney injury
acute respiratory distress syndrome (ARDS), 107–109
    trauma sequelae, 310
acute tubular necrosis (ATN), 289, 293
    BUN levels and, 283
    renal ischemia and, 280
adaptive immunity, 180–181
Addisonian crisis, 145–146
adenoids, 178
adenosine, 88, 89
adrenal glands, 129, 133–134
adrenal insufficiency
    acute, 145–146
    adrenal cortex, 134
    pituitary gland, 132
adrenocorticotropic hormone (ACTH), 131, 132
advance directives, 340
advocacy of nurses, 333
afterload of heart, 55, 97
age-related neurologic changes, 202. *See also* elderly population
aggressive behavior, 354–355
    UTI and, 366
"air leaks," 114–115
albumin
    calcium levels and, 281
    normal lab values, 250
    transfusion, 167, 168–169
alcohol
    esophageal varices and, 253, 254

pancreatitis and, 260, 262
serum lab values and, 367
subdural hematomas and, 220, 221
substance abuse, 361–362
urine screening, 366
withdrawal, 362–363, 369
aldosterone, 133
    Addisonian crisis, 145–146
    atrial natriuretic factor and, 54
    renin-angiotensin-aldosterone system, 59, 64, 279–280, 281
    water reabsorption, 272, 279
allergic response, 181–182
    anaphylactic shock, 170, 182, 310–311
    urticaria from transfusion, 169
allogenic bone marrow transplant, 177
alpha natriuretic factor, 54
Alumnus CCRN status, 10
American Association of Critical-Care Nurses (AACN)
    application addresses, 5
    Certification Corporation, 3, 5, 6, 329
    eligibility for CCRN Exam, 4, 5–6, 20
    ethical principles, 338, 340–341
    ethics of care, 338
    experiences-recommended list, 20
    Honor Statement, 5, 6
    standards of practice, 344
American College of Cardiology (ACC), 61